Progress in Colorectal Surgery

John Beynon, BSc, MS, FRCS
Nicholas D. Carr, MD, FRCS
Department of Colorectal Surgery, Singleton Hospital, Swansea, UK
Editors

Progress in Colorectal Surgery

With 79 Illustrations

Springer

John Beynon, BSc, MS, FRCS
Nicholas D. Carr, MD, FRCS
Department of Colorectal Surgery
Singleton Hospital
Swansea, UK

British Library Cataloguing in Publication Data

Progress in Colorectal Surgery
1. Colon (Anatomy)—Surgery 2. Rectum—Surgery
3. Laparoscopic surgery 4. Proctology
I. Beynon, J. (John), 1956– II. Carr, Nicholas David, 1951–
617.5′547

ISBN 1852336773

Library of Congress Cataloging-in-Publication Data

Progress in colorectal surgery / [edited by] John Beynon, Nicholas D. Carr.
p. ; cm.
Includes bibliographical references and index.
ISBN 1-85233-677-3 (s/c : alk. paper)—ISBN 1-85233-823-7 (h/c : alk. paper)
1. Colon (Anatomy)—Surgery. 2. Rectum—Surgery. 3. Colon (Anatomy)—Cancer—Surgery. I. Beynon, J. (John) II. Carr, Nicholas David, 1951–
[DNLM: 1. Colonic Diseases—surgery. 2. Rectal Diseases—surgery. WI 520 P964 2004]

RD544.P765 2004
617.5′54—dc22 2004048206

ISBN 1-85233-823-7 (hardcover) 1-85233-677-3 (softcover)
Springer Science+Business Media
springeronline.com

Printed in the United States of America. (BS/EB)

Printed on acid-free paper SPIN 10990469 (hardcover) 10866296 (softcover)

Preface

In a previous publication, the authors attempted to cover not only topical issues but also difficult problems that might confront recently appointed trainees in the decisions they make that confront these individuals in their future practices.

Since that time, much of the thrust of coloproctology and government directives have centred around various aspects of colorectal cancer. The editors are thus of the opinion that they must not shy away from political incentive and have dedicated just over half of the present book to the diagnosis, presentation, and management of colorectal carcinoma.

By contrast, the editors have also tried to draw attention to the fact that many patients with benign disorders of the colorectum have symptoms which are incompatible with a constructive and useful quality of life. Crohn's disease is paramount in this respect and continues to provide challenges in both medical and surgical management. Moreover, coloproctologists continue to be vexed by the problems presented by the diagnosis and treatment of functional bowel disorders, and it is hoped that the chapters in this book will help to demystify the investigation and treatment of incontinence and constipation.

John Beynon, BSc, MS, FRCS
Nicholas D. Carr, MD, FRCS

Contents

Contributors

Arthur Allan, MD, FRCS, EBSQ
Department of Gastrointestinal Surgery, Good Hope Hospital, Sutton Coldfield, UK

Ponnandai J. Arumugam, MS, FRCS
Department of Colorectal Surgery, Royal Cornwall Hospital, Cornwall, UK

Wendy S. Atkin, PhD, MSc, MPH
Colorectal Cancer Unit, St Mark's Hospital, Harrow, UK

Philip E. Bearn, MS, FRCS
Department of Colorectal Surgery, St Peter's Hospital, Chertsey, UK

John Beynon, BSc, MS, FRCS
Department of Colorectal Surgery, Singleton Hospital, Swansea, UK

Finlay J.M. Curran, MD, FRCS
Department of General Surgery, Stepping Hill Hospital, Stockport, UK

Sunil Dolwani, MD, MRCP
Institute of Medical Genetics, University of Wales College of Medicine, Cardiff, UK

Brian G. Ellis, BSc, MBA, MBBSS, PhD, MRCP, FRCP
The Swan Surgery, Petersfield, UK

Michael J.G. Farthing, DSc, MD, FRCP, FmedSci
St George's Hospital Medical School, London, UK

Ian G. Finlay, BSc, FRCS
Department of Coloproctology, Lister Surgical Unit, Glasgow Royal Infirmary, Glasgow, UK

Iona C. Heath, MB BCh, MRCP, FRCGP
Caversham Group Practice, London, UK

David J. Kerr, CBE, MA, MD, DSc, FRCP, FMedSci
National Translational Cancer Research Network, Department of Clinical Pharmacology, University of Oxford, Oxford, UK

Robert D. Madoff, MD
Department of Surgery, University of Minnesota, Minneapolis, MN, USA

Najjia N. Mahmoud, MD
Department of Surgery, University of Pennsylvania, Philadelphia, PA, USA

Sara McCartney, MB BS, PhD, MRCP
Department of Gastroenterology, University College Hospitals, The Middlesex Hospital, London, UK

Alan D. McGregor, MD, FRCS
Welsh Centre for Burns and Plastic Surgery, Swansea NHS Trust, Morriston Hospital, Swansea, UK

Rachel Midgley, BSc, MRCP
CRC Institute for Cancer Studies, University of Birmingham, Birmingham, UK

Shibani Nicum, BSc, MRCP
CRC Institute for Cancer Studies, University of Birmingham, Birmingham, UK

Sarah T. O'Dwyer, BSc, MB ChB, MD, FRCS
Department of Colorectal Surgery, Christie Hospital, Manchester, UK

Susan C. Parker, MD
Department of Surgery, University of Minnesota, St Paul, MN, USA

Bharat Patel, MB BCh, FRCR
Department of Radiology, Singleton Hospital, Swansea, UK

Andrew A. Renwick, MB ChB, FRCS
Lister Surgical Unit, Glasgow Royal Infirmary, Glasgow, UK

Susan J. Ritchie, MB ChB, DRCOG
Department of Clinical Genetics, Nottingham City Hospital, Nottingham, UK

Julian R. Sampson, DM, FRCP
Institute of Medical Genetics, University of Wales College of Medicine, Cardiff, UK

John H. Scholefield, ChM, FRCS
Division of Gastrointestinal Surgery, Nottingham City Hospital, Nottingham, UK

Nigel A. Scott, MD, FRCS
Colorectal Surgery and Intestinal Failure, Hope Hospital, Manchester, UK

Edwin T. Swarbrick, MBBS, MD, FRCP
Department of Gastroenterology, New Cross Hospital, Wolverhampton, UK

Michael R. Thompson, MD, FRCS
Department of Surgery, Queen Alexandra Hospital, Portsmouth, UK

Amy Thorsen, MD
Department of Surgery, University of Minnesota, St Paul, MN, USA

L. Faulds Wood
Bowel Cancer Campaign, Twickenham, UK

1
The Effective and Efficient Management of Patients with Rectal Bleeding to Identify the Few with Cancer

Michael R. Thompson, Edwin T. Swarbrick, Brian G. Ellis, Iona C. Heath, L. Faulds Wood, and Wendy S. Atkin

There are currently insufficient resources to fully investigate all patients with rectal bleeding to exclude the small possibility of cancer, and this is the dominant factor in developing strategies for the management of rectal bleeding. However, even if there were unlimited resources it may not be desirable to investigate all patients because the small risks associated with the investigative procedure might outweigh the benefits, particularly in groups at very low risk of having cancer.

The importance of efficient as well as effective delivery of healthcare was the subject of the Rock Carling Lectures delivered by Archie Cochrane in 1972 [1], and continues to be an essential aspect of clinical medicine. In the context of the management of rectal bleeding, effectiveness is achieved if all patients with colorectal cancer are promptly diagnosed, and efficiency is achieved by limiting the number of patients without cancer investigated. In view of the high prevalence of rectal bleeding in the community and the potential demand for its investigation, the efficient management of all patients presenting with rectal bleeding will profoundly affect the prompt diagnosis of those with cancer.

The management of rectal bleeding as a symptom of bowel cancer begins with advice to the general public through disease awareness campaigns, proceeds through referral guidelines to general practitioners (GPs), and finishes with the efficient use of resources for its investigation. The varying prevalence and predictive value of rectal bleeding for cancer in different cohorts of patients is important to all stages of its management.

Rectal bleeding is also important in the diagnosis of adenomatous polyps [2–7] and colitis [7] as well as colorectal cancer [2,4–11]. Overall, 40% of all colorectal cancers and 70%–80% of rectal and sigmoid cancers present with overt rectal bleeding [9–11]. It may be a sign of an early-stage curable cancer [12–15] and of large adenomatous polyps, which, with subsequent colonoscopic surveillance, may be a valuable way of reducing the prevalence and overall mortality from colorectal cancer [16]. It is perhaps not surprising, therefore, that advice on the management of rectal bleeding stresses the importance of its detection [17,18] and prompt investigation [4,5,19].

This advice has been supported by reports that rectal bleeding has a high predictive value for cancer in primary care [4,5,19], and that it is impossible to differentiate between rectal bleeding from benign and malignant disease [4,5,19,20–24]. It is further supported by the unproven assumption that early referral of all patients with rectal bleeding will improve the survival of those with cancer [25].

These ideas have formed the basis for the current paradigm governing the approach to the management of rectal bleeding, which advises an aggressive policy of full colonic examination in all patients over the age of 40 [4,5,19]. This is partly the reason for the serious mismatch between demand and the resources for investigation—some cancer patients have long waits to be seen due to the unnecessary investigation of patients at very low risk of cancer.

We question these assumptions, and propose that it is possible to classify patients on the basis of their cancer risk for different investigation strategies.

The British government has recently introduced the "Two-Week Standard" [26], which promises that all patients suspected by their GPs of having bowel cancer will be seen within two weeks. This has focused attention on the problem, which may be partly addressed by a reconfiguration of referrals by identifying precisely which patients should qualify for urgent referral and investigation [27–30]. However, it is yet to be seen whether this will cause a greater delay in patients who do not fulfil these criteria, which in turn might exacerbate the problem with no overall benefit to all cancer patients. The introduction of referral guidelines [27–29] must not deflect the government from the long-term solution, which is for a substantial increase in hospital resources for all patients requesting and needing investigation, not just those patients at higher risk.

1. The High Prevalence of Rectal Bleeding in the Community

The high prevalence of all symptoms in the community, regardless of their nature, was first described in the Peckham experiment in 1946 [31] and subsequently by Wadsworth [32] and Hannay [33]. These studies demonstrated that most people have various symptoms most of the time, which they either self-treat or which resolve spontaneously without medical consultation. Only a small proportion of patients who eventually consult their doctors are referred to hospital for investigation [31–33]. This observation is also true for rectal bleeding [34–36].

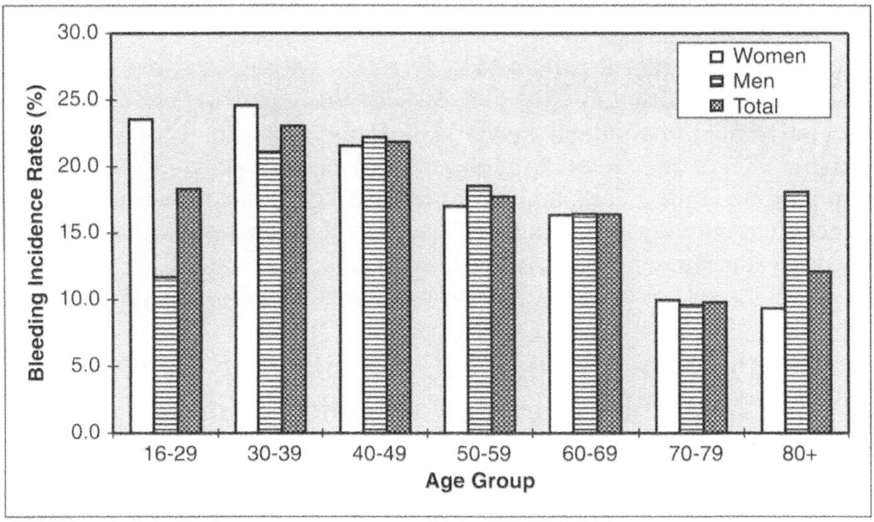

FIGURE 1.1. Incidence rates of rectal bleeding in men and women for a one year period in 1996 as a percentage of the total population.

Several studies have shown that 17%–20% of patients in the community have rectal bleeding each year [34–44]. Prevalence is inversely related to age, with young women being most affected and the elderly being least affected [34–36]. Two thirds of patients who bleed each year will have had an episode in the past [36] (Figure 1.1, Figure 1.2). It has been calculated

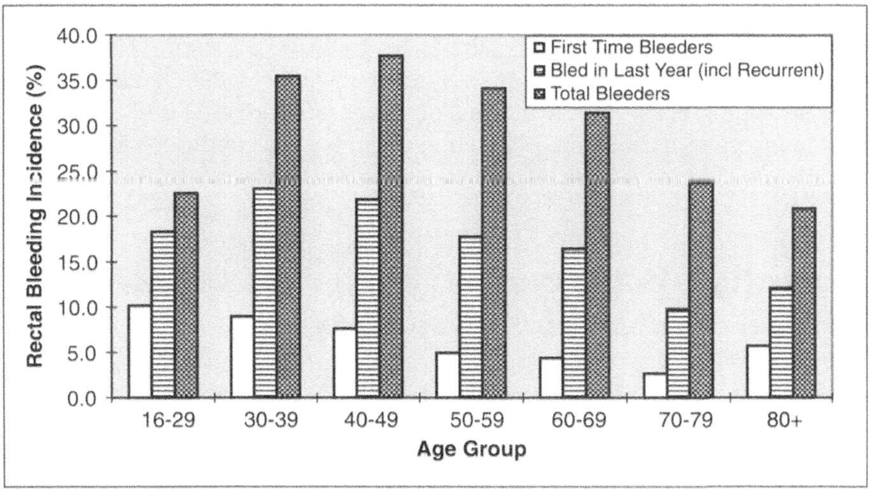

FIGURE 1.2. Incidence rates of rectal bleeding for the first time in the previous year (1996), as a percentage of the total population, and for patients having rectal bleeding at any time previously, including 1996.

that in a city with a population of 1 million people, 140000 will have rectal bleeding each year [36].

It is fortunate that less than 15% of patients with rectal bleeding seek medical help [35,36] and only 40%–50% of those patients are referred to hospital [36]. Thus, patients seen in hospital represent the "tip of the iceberg" [33] of all patients with these symptoms and we ignore this important piece of clinical epidemiology at our peril [45]. Clearly, a great deal of selection is already occurring before referral for investigation and this needs to continue.

2. The Predictive Value of Rectal Bleeding for Cancer in the Community, Primary Care, and Hospital

In view of the high prevalence of rectal bleeding and as a result of the considerable selection process, the predictive value of rectal bleeding for cancer varies from 1:705 in the community [23] to 1:17 in a surgical outpatient department [46].

Two studies on the predictive value of rectal bleeding in primary care have shown a 1:10 prevalence of cancer [3,5], which is considerably higher than that in the hospital study [46] and two others in primary care that showed a 1:29 and 1:30 prevalence [6,36]. It is likely that the two studies showing a higher prevalence [3,5] was the result of not all patients identified with rectal bleeding in primary care being referred for investigation. About one half of all patients with rectal bleeding in the community have an associated change in bowel habit. In two thirds of cases the change is to a decreased frequency of defaecation with straining and/or harder stools [36]. Dark red bleeding also occurs in up to 20% of patients [4,6,7,35,36] and painless (implying non-haemorrhoid–associated) rectal bleeding occurs in 80% of patients in the community and general practice [7,36]. This means that many patients with rectal bleeding from benign conditions in the community have what, at present, are considered higher risk symptoms.

3. The Basis of the Current Selection Process for Referral of Patients for Investigation

It is likely that at least some patients and GPs decide whether to seek investigation in hospital by adopting watch-and-wait strategies [47] that are based on the assumption that most benign conditions get better whereas symptoms from cancer persist. In general practice, "treat, watch-and-wait" strategies [47] in conjunction with "safety-netting" [48] are an integral and safe part of the diagnostic process, and are the keystones of the GP's gatekeeper role (Figure 1.3).

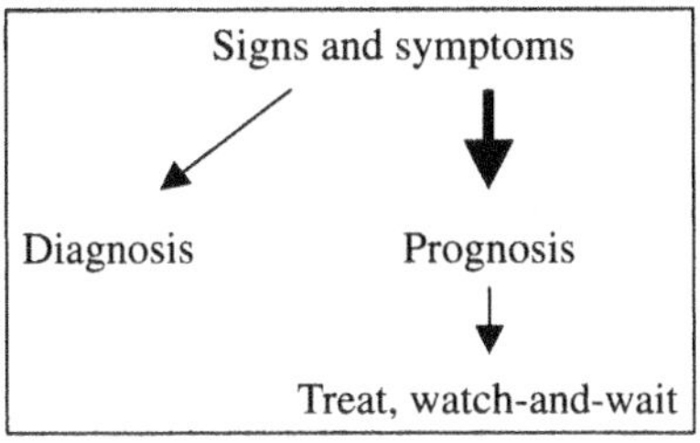

FIGURE 1.3. Diagnosis in primary care: the importance of "treat, watch-and-wait" policies. Reproduced from Sackett DL, Haynes RB, Guyatt GH, Tugwell P. *Clinical Epidemiology—A Basic Science for Clinical Medicine.* 2nd ed. Boston: Little Brown & Co; 1991: 4.

The gate-keeper role saves the majority of patients with transient symptoms unnecessary investigations, which conserves hospital resources for more rapid investigation and treatment of patients with serious disease. It is crucial that the new paradigm for the management of rectal bleeding supports the GP in this important role [27–29].

The question arises: Can the selection process between the patient/GP interface and the GP/hospital interface be improved and will it improve survival from colorectal cancer?

4. Will Prompt Referral and Earlier Diagnosis Improve Survival?

The term "early," used so often in discussions of cancer therapy, is generally applied inappropriately. Although "early" refers to a dimension in time, the usual evidence assessed in the designation of "early" comes mainly from anatomy not chronometry.

Alvan F. Feinstein, *Nature*, 1966 [49]

The diagnosis of early-stage cancer results in better survival, but this should not be confused with the assumption that diagnosis early after the onset of symptoms also improves survival. This assumption is one of the reasons for the drive to promptly investigate all patients with rectal bleeding [20] and for the introduction of the "Two-Week Standard" [26], which could discourage more pragmatic "treat, watch-and-wait" approaches [29,47,48].

The rationale for early referral of patients with rectal bleeding is based on the following unproven assumptions:

- A significant number of patients currently die as a result of an avoidable delay in diagnosis and treatment.
- Delays in referral are due to patients and GPs being poorly informed of the significance of the symptoms of bowel cancer, and that this can be corrected by public awareness campaigns and better referral guidelines for GPs.
- Earlier diagnosis during the symptomatic phase of the natural history of colorectal cancer will improve survival.

There is little evidence for these assumptions, but what is certain is that encouraging more patients to have investigation for rectal bleeding will further strain already limited resources. It is therefore important to determine what proportion of patients have delay in treatment, whether it has previously been possible to persuade appropriate patients to consult their GPs earlier, and for GPs to recognise higher risk patients for referral and to determine the size of the benefit that earlier symptomatic diagnosis might achieve.

4.1. What Proportion of Patients Have Prolonged Delays in Treatment?

The mean time between the onset of symptoms and treatment of bowel cancer has remained constant at approximately 7 months for rectal cancers in different countries over many years [50–56]. It is particularly disappointing that up to 20% of patients with colorectal cancer have a delay in referral and treatment of more than 1 year, and many of these patients have rectal bleeding [9,54,55,57–66].

4.2. Are Delays Caused by Poorly Informed Patients and GPs, and Can This Be Improved?

The causes of delay in referral include patient embarrassment and fear of cancer [25,34,56,67] as well as a lack of knowledge of the symptoms of colorectal cancer [67]. The delays in referral have not changed over many years in spite of disease awareness campaigns and referral guidelines for doctors in primary care. It has also been suggested that the speed of referral may be affected by the biological nature of the cancer and its effect on the symptoms. If this is correct, it may be very difficult to modulate the speed of patient consultation and primary-care doctor referral.

4.3. What Is the Evidence That Earlier Diagnosis of Colorectal Cancer Improves Survival?

A few reports [68–73], mostly based on reviews of small numbers of cancer patients, often with historical controls, have suggested an improvement in survival with shorter delays in treatment. There are more reports of an inverse relationship, with delay in treatment being associated with better outcomes [50–55,58,64,65,74,75]. This paradoxical relationship is thought to be due to biological predeterminism [49,76,77], which suggests that some slow-growing cancers may produce low grade, nondisturbing symptoms resulting in delay in referral but with good outcomes, whereas some aggressive cancers may produce more severe, rapidly progressive, and worrying symptoms resulting in rapid referral but poor survival [40,76,77]. This para-

TABLE 1.1. The symptom iceberg.

Symptoms of rectal bleeding in the community
High prevalence: 17%–20% of the population each year
Only 15% visit their GP
Only 7% are at present investigated in hospital
More common in the younger age groups
Often associated with a change in bowel habit to decreased frequency and/or increased hardness of stool and straining
10%–20% have dark red bleeding

doxical effect makes it difficult to demonstrate the possible beneficial effect of earlier symptomatic diagnosis [50–55,57–66,70,74,78–85]. It is clear, however, that many patients die in spite of prompt treatment and substantial numbers survive in spite of delay so that the total number of patients that might benefit from earlier diagnosis could be small [50].

One study [86] determined the effect that delay in treatment had on survival after referral to hospital on the assumption that this would occur in a random fashion and would not be dependent on the biological nature of the cancer. However, this study still did not show that delay had an adverse effect on outcome, even in patients having hospital delays in treatment of over 5 months [86].

4.4. Conclusion on the Benefits of Earlier Symptomatic Diagnosis

Earlier symptomatic diagnosis may be difficult to achieve for many patients with bowel cancer, and even if this could be achieved, the overall improvement in survival is likely to be small [50,54–56,58,80,81,85]. This would require a considerable increase in resources for investigating increasing numbers of symptomatic patients.

5. When Does the Risk of Cancer Exceed the Risk of Investigation?

Most doctors are now accustomed to balancing the benefits of treatment with its risks [87,88]. They are less familiar with this sort of analysis when deciding whether to refer low-risk patients for investigation, even though

TABLE 1.2. Predictive value of rectal bleeding for cancer.

	Community	Hospital outpatients
Predictive value of rectal bleeding for cancer	1:705	1:17

it is now accepted that before introducing screening for colorectal cancer there should be some evidence of significant overall benefit. It is possible that younger patients with lower GI symptoms are at lower risk of cancer than older asymptomatic screened patients, and similar rules to those developed for screening should be applied when deciding at what stage investigating symptomatic patients will do more good than harm.

The various disadvantages that can occur during investigation are listed in Table 1.3.

In patients at very low risk of cancer, the question must be asked: Is the risk of having a cancer greater than the risk of investigation? Or, when is the small potential benefit of earlier symptomatic diagnosis in the very few with cancer outweighed by the disadvantage of investigation in the majority without cancer (Figure 1.4).

5.1. Summary of the Basis for Changing the Current Paradigm Governing the Management of Rectal Bleeding

- The high prevalence of rectal bleeding in the community establishes the need for a selective policy for its investigation.
- There is no evidence that short time lags before referral reduce the chances of survival from colorectal cancer.
- Investigations can harm people, and in patients at very low risk of cancer, any benefit from earlier diagnosis to the few with cancer may be outweighed by the disadvantage of investigations to those without cancer.

TABLE 1.3. Disadvantages of investigation.

Disadvantages of investigation
Unnecessary worry of investigation and fear of cancer[89,90]
Labelling[91]
Physical harm
• Colonoscopy[92,93]
Risk of perforation
Risk of death 1:17000
• Barium enema 1:57000 deaths[94]
• False positives/unnecessary operations
• False negatives/delayed diagnosis
Costs of investigation
• Patient and caregiver costs
Time off work
Travel costs
Consuming scarce resources
• Delay in investigation of those with cancer
• Opportunity costs
Medico-legal costs

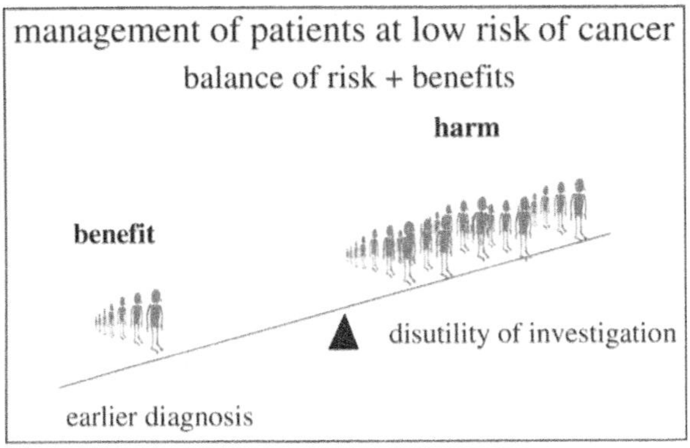

FIGURE 1.4. Management of patients at low risk of cancer.

These three fundamental points establish the need, safety, and pragmatism for new strategies to manage rectal bleeding based on careful "treat, watch-and-wait" policies [4] according to cancer risk. These are a natural and integral part of clinical diagnosis in all situations, particularly in primary care and are the keystones of the GP's "gate-keeper" role [29]. Public awareness campaigns for patients with rectal bleeding and referral guidelines for GPs must emphasise the value of these strategies, particularly for those patients at very low risk of cancer, and to establish appropriate periods of "wait" in "treat, watch-and-wait" policies according to cancer risk [29].

The key to a new paradigm governing the management of rectal bleeding therefore depends on the identification of patients at higher and low risk of cancer on the basis a simple history and examination [27–30].

6. Can Symptoms and Signs Be Used to Determine Cancer Risk in the Community and in Primary Care?

The challenge for providing advice for public awareness campaigns and the new referral guidelines is to identify criteria determining cancer risk that maintain high sensitivity for cancer, that is, include the majority of patients with cancer, with as little loss of specificity as possible, which means including a minority of patients with benign disease [27–30].

It is important to understand that "as sensitivity increases, a point is reached at which very small increases in sensitivity are accompanied by very large decreases in specificity, i.e., the number of false-positive results increases. An increase in the number of false-positive tests increases patient anxiety, the costs of '*investigation*' and the risk associated with unnecessary '*investigation*'" [95].

The implication of this is that there will be an exponential increase in the number of patients needing to be investigated to capture the last few cancer patients with less common symptom profiles.

6.1. The Common Age, Symptom, and Sign Profiles of Rectal Bleeding in Patients with Established Cancer

It is likely that the common age, symptom, and sign profiles of rectal bleeding in patients with established cancer will have higher predictive values than those occurring less commonly.

It is clear from many previous articles [9–11,53,54,60–63,65] that colorectal cancer presents with more than one symptom or one sign. For example, it is now clear that approximately 75% of cancer patients presenting with rectal bleeding also have a change in bowel habit, and another 20% have bleeding without anal symptoms or with a palpable anorectal mass [11,15,46]. This means that as little as 5% of cancer patients present with rectal bleeding, anal symptoms, no persistent change in bowel habit, and no palpable anorectal mass; the common symptom pattern in patients bleeding from piles [11,46].

6.2. The Symptom Patterns with the Highest Predictive and Diagnostic Values

6.2.1. Rectal Bleeding with a Change in Bowel Habit

Several studies in primary care [2,5–7] and in a surgical outpatient department [46] have shown that patients presenting with both rectal bleeding and a change in bowel habit have up to a 5 times greater risk of cancer as compared with patients presenting with rectal bleeding as a single symptom (Table 1.4).

6.2.2. Rectal Bleeding and No Perianal Symptoms

Two studies, one in primary care [7] and one in a surgical outpatient department [46], have shown that patients presenting with rectal bleeding and no anal symptoms have up to a 4 times greater risk of cancer compared with those patients presenting with anal symptoms (Table 1.4). This occurs in patients whether or not their rectal bleeding is associated with a change in bowel habit.

6.3. The Diagnostic Value of the Other Characteristics of Rectal Bleeding

6.3.1. Dark Red Bleeding

Three recent studies have shown dark red bleeding to have a predictive value of 9%–13% compared with 4%–8% for bright red bleeding [5–7,19] (Table 1.5).

TABLE 1.4. The predictive and diagnostic value of the symptom combinations of rectal bleeding.

Symptom	Study	Sensitivity	Specificity	LR	95% CI	PPV change in bowel habit	
						With	Without
Rectal bleeding with a change in bowel habit	Fijten[6]*	89%	78%	4.0	2.9–5.5	11%	0.4%
	Ellis[7]*	100%	58%	2.4	1.6–2.7	9%	0%
	Dodds[97]**	75%	65%	2.13	2.0–2.3	13%	3%
Symptom	**Study**	**Sensitivity**	**Specificity**	**LR**	**95% CI**	**PPV anal symptoms**	
						With	Without
Rectal bleeding without anal symptoms	Ellis[7]*	64%	78%	2.9	1.6–4.3	2%	11%
	Dodds[97]**	59%	73%	2.2	2.0–2.5	4%	13%

*Primary-care population.
**Hospital population.
LR, likelihood ratio (sensitivity/1-specificity); PPV, positive predictive value.

6.3.2. The Manifestation of Rectal Bleeding

The way rectal bleeding is noticed and bleeding of recent onset are either of no or little diagnostic value [7,19], although blood mixed with the stool has been shown to be of value in 2 studies [5,6] and of no value in 2 others [7,19]. Sudden, self-limiting, large-volume, fresh bleeding after defaecation can be very frightening and is a common reason for referral to a surgical outpatient clinic, but paradoxically is probably of diagnostic value in identifying patients at very low risk of cancer [7]. This is contrary to what many patients and GPs understandably feel.

6.3.3. Palpable Rectal Mass

Forty to eighty percent of rectal cancers, most of which present with rectal bleeding, have a palpable rectal mass [7,10,24,49,96]. This is a crucially

TABLE 1.5. The diagnostic value of dark red bleeding.

Symptom	Study	Sensitivity	Specificity	LR	95% CI	PPV color	
						Dark	Bright
Dark red Bleeding	Ellis[7]*	27%	88%	2.3	0.8–5.3	9%	4%
	Metcalf[5]*	37%	70%	1.25	0.5–3.2	11%	8%
	Chave[98]**	37%	83%	2.08	1.8–2.5	13%	5%

*Primary-care population.
**Hospital population.
LR, likelihood ratio (sensitivity/1-specificity); PPV, positive predictive value.

important physical sign for a small number of cancer patients presenting with rectal bleeding who otherwise have a low-risk symptom pattern, that is, rectal bleeding with anal symptoms without a change in bowel habit.

6.4. The Nature of the Change in Bowel Habit

The nature of the change in bowel habit in 80%–90% of patients with colorectal cancer is to increased frequency and/or looser stools [7,11,46]. It is likely that this type of change in bowel habit will have higher diagnostic value [97] than a change in bowel habit to decreased frequency and harder stools, which is extremely common in patients with rectal bleeding from benign disease in the community [32].

6.5. The Effect of Age on the Diagnostic Value of Rectal Bleeding

The prevalence of rectal bleeding in the community is highest in the 20–40 age group and decreases with age (Figure 1.1, Figure 1.2). In contrast, 85% of patients with colorectal cancer are over the age of 60 with less than 1% below the age of 40 [98]. This means that rectal bleeding is of much greater significance in patients over the age of 60 years [4–8,46].

In patients presenting to a surgical outpatient department [42], the prevalence of cancer varied from 50% in patients over 80 with the highest risk symptom profile (rectal bleeding with a change in bowel habit, no abdominal pain, and no perianal symptoms) to 1:888 in patients below the age of 50 with the lowest risk symptom profile (rectal bleeding without a change in bowel habit, with perianal symptoms, and no other significant diagnostic factors), a 444-fold difference in cancer prevalence [46] (Table 1.6).

7. New Management Strategies for Investigating Rectal Bleeding

These new data on the predictive values of age, symptom, and sign profiles of rectal bleeding suggest it is now sensible to discard the idea that all cancer patients presenting with rectal bleeding have nonspecific symptoms. In the future, different management strategies with different speeds of referral should be introduced on the basis of cancer risk assessment as determined by a simple history and examination (Table 1.7, Table 1.8).

Fast-track referral is appropriate for patients with higher risk criteria, but only after symptoms have persisted for 6 weeks [27–29]. For patients at low risk of cancer, longer "treat, watch-and-wait" policies are appropriate, both in the community, perhaps with help from a pharmacist, and also in primary care [27–29]. If these patients do need referral, this should be to a routine

TABLE 1.6. The effect of age on the prevalence of cancer in patients with rectal bleeding and other symptoms.

Age	Rectal bleeding (all patients)	Plus a change in bowel habit	Plus a change in bowel habit but no abdominal pain or anal symptoms	No change in bowel habit and no anal symptoms	No change in bowel habit with anal symptoms*
<39	1:268	1:73	1:26	1:148	0.633
40–49	1:83	1:32	1:9	1:122	1:255
50–59	1:26	1:13	1:6	1:62	1:178
60–69	1:10	1:6	1:3	1:13	1:100
70–79	1:8	1:6	1:3	1:8	1:47
≥80	1:5	1:4	1:2	1:6	1:18
Total number of patients	5442	2063	331	810	2544
Total number of cancers	347	261	97	49	16
Overall	1:16	1:8	1:3	1:17	1:159

*Not including patients with a palpable rectal or abdominal mass and those with iron-deficiency anaemia below 10 g.
Personal data from a study of 8000 surgical outpatients (Thompson MR, Swarbrick ET, Ellis BG, et al. In: Cunningham D, Topham C, Miles A, eds. *The Effective Management of Colorectal Cancer.* 2nd ed. London: Aesculapius Medical Press; 2000: 173).

TABLE 1.7. Management of rectal bleeding.

Old paradigm	New paradigm
Patients with colorectal cancer present with nonspecific rectal bleeding, and therefore all patients with this symptom over a certain age should have prompt and full colonic investigation.	There are large differences in the predictive value of rectal bleeding for cancer according to its association with other symptoms and signs and the age of the patient. Different management strategies with different speeds of referral should be adopted according to cancer risk so that patients with transient low-risk symptoms from benign disease avoid investigation.

TABLE 1.8. Criteria determining the management strategy [29].

Higher-risk symptoms

- Rectal bleeding with a *persistent* change in bowel habit to looser stools and/or increased frequency of defaecation for at least 6 weeks.
- Rectal bleeding *persistently* without anal symptoms in patients over the age of 60.

Low-risk symptoms

- Rectal bleeding *with* anal symptoms and *without* a change in bowel habit and *no* anal mass (or with a transient change in bowel habit, particularly to decreased frequency of defaecation, harder stools and straining).

TABLE 1.9. The three alternative methods for referral.

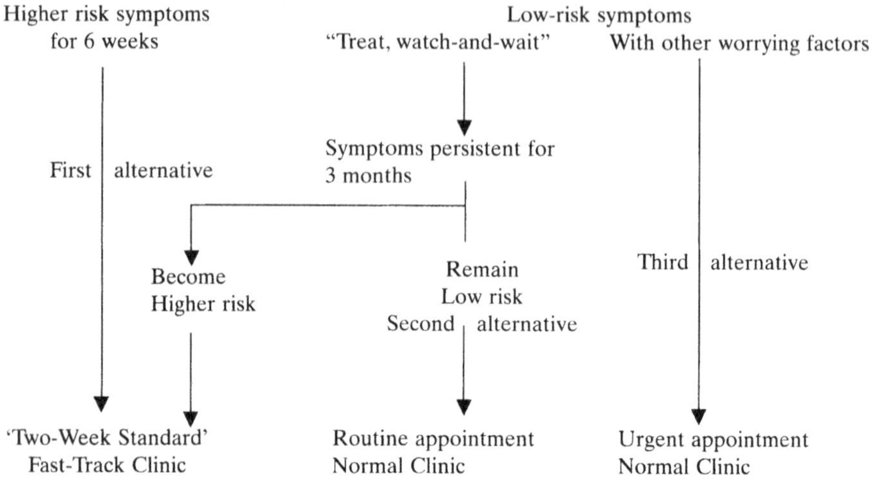

Reproduced with permission from Thompson MR, Heath I, Ellis BG, Swarbrick ET, Faultds Wood L, Atkin WS. Identifying and managing patients at low risk of bowel cancer in general practice. *BMJ.* 2003;327: 263–265.

clinic, where the waiting time will depend on the available resources and the numbers of patients referred with low risk symptoms (Table 1.9).

7.1. Management of Recurrent Rectal Bleeding Over Prolonged Periods of Time Following Negative Investigations

Some patients have recurrent bleeding [32] over long periods of time and may have had previous investigations in hospital. If patients have already had a flexible sigmoidoscopy within the previous 3 years, they can be safely managed by longer watch-and-wait strategies, but if these symptoms persist, even if they remain low-risk symptoms, they need to be re-referred to a routine clinic, and if flexible sigmoidoscopy is again normal, they may need examination by colonoscopy.

8. "Treat, Watch-and-Wait" Strategies for Patients at Low Risk of Cancer

Approximately 5%–10% of patients presenting with rectal bleeding from a colorectal cancer will present with low-risk symptoms and these patients will continue to be diagnosed in routine clinics. Careful "treat, watch-and-wait" management strategies are therefore needed in primary care to avoid excessive time lags before referral of these low-risk patients. This means that all patients with persistent symptoms, even if low risk, must eventually be investigated, and it is likely that the only long-term solution to the management of rectal bleeding is to develop more resources so that all patients referred are investigated promptly, not just those with higher risk symptoms.

"Treat, watch-and-wait" strategies must be with the agreement of the patient, who will need to understand the overall benefit to the majority of patients with transient symptoms of avoiding unnecessary investigations [29]. Patients who are not happy with this arrangement can still be referred routinely to a normal clinic, and others may be given written information about what constitutes higher risk symptoms so they can self-refer back at an earlier stage if these develop [48]. If patients are overly anxious with low-risk symptoms or in younger age groups with persistent higher risk symptoms (i.e., rectal bleeding without anal symptoms), there is a third alternative route for referral, an urgent appointment in a routine clinic [27–29]. This mode of referral must be kept to a minimum to ensure that all patients referred in this way are seen promptly.

There are therefore three alternative routes or speeds of referral dependent on cancer risk and the concern of the patient and the GP (Table 1.9).

9. Conclusion

The current lack of resources for investigating rectal bleeding means that the efficient management of patients without cancer is the key to the effective diagnosis of those with cancer.

The traditional assumption suggesting that all patients with rectal bleeding over the age of 40 years seeking medical advice should have prompt and full colonic investigation should now be reviewed. The high prevalence of rectal bleeding in the community, especially in patients below the age of 60 years, means that selection of patients for investigation may always be necessary, both because it is unlikely that at least in the near future there will be sufficient resources to meet the demand for its investigation, and because in younger patients at low risk the possible benefit to the very few with cancer from earlier symptomatic diagnosis may be outweighed by the harm of full colonic imaging for the great majority who do not have cancer. The key to better selection of patients for investigation, and therefore efficient as well as effective diagnosis of colorectal cancer in patients with rectal bleeding, is a clear understanding of the diagnostic value of symptom and sign profiles in determining cancer risk and how this is affected by age. This will enable higher risk patients to be identified, who should be encouraged to have prompt investigation and, just as important, those at very low risk who can initially self-care [45] or be managed by their GPs in primary care for more prolonged periods of time.

Every patient at low risk of cancer successfully managed in the community or in primary care will conserve the investigative resources for those at higher risk, who can then be seen, investigated, and treated more quickly. This strategy, even if it does not increase the overall survival of cancer patients, will ensure a higher quality of care for all patients, not just those with cancer. The greatest challenge for the new guidelines will be to construct safe "treat, watch-and-wait" policies for those patients at low risk to ensure that the few with cancer do not suffer excessive time lags before referral.

Every patient with low-risk symptoms and signs successfully treated in the community or in primary care may enable a patient with cancer to be seen and treated more quickly.

References

1. Cochrane AL. *Effectiveness and efficiency; random reflections on health services.* London: The Nuffield Provincial Hospitals Trust 1972. Printed by Burgess & Son (Abingdon Berks Limited).
2. Norreland N, Norreland H. Colorectal cancer and polyps in patients aged 40 years and over who consult a GP with rectal bleeding. *Fam Pract.* 1996;13: 160–165.
3. Chapuis PH, Goulston KJ, Dent OF, Tait AD. Predictive value of rectal bleeding in screening for rectal and sigmoid polyps. *Br Med J.* 1985;290:1546–1548.
4. Goulston KJ, Cook I, Dent OF, and General Practitioners and Specialists Associated with the Concord Hospital Gastroenterology Unit. How important is rectal bleeding in the diagnosis of bowel cancer and polyps? *Lancet* 1986; 2:261–265.
5. Metcalf JV, Smith J, Jones R, Record CO. Incidence and causes of rectal bleeding in general practice as detected by colonoscopy. *Br J Gen Pract.* 1996;46: 161–164.
6. Fijten GH, Starmans R, Muris JWM, Schouten HJA, Blijham GH, Knottnerus JA. Predictive value of signs and symptoms for colorectal cancer in patients with rectal bleeding in general practice. *Fam Pract.* 1995;12:279–286.
7. Ellis BG, Jones M, Thompson MR. Rectal bleeding in general practice: who needs referral? *Colorect Dis.* 1999;1(suppl 1):23–24.
8. Wauters H, Van Casteren V, Buntinx F. Rectal bleeding and colorectal cancer in general practice: diagnostic study. *BMJ.* 2000;321:998–999.
9. McSherry CK, Cornell GN, Glenn F. Carcinoma of the colon and rectum. *Ann Surg.* 1969;169:502–509.
10. Shallow TA, Wagner FB, Colcher RE. Clinical evaluation of 750 patients with colon cancer. Diagnostic survey and follow-up covering a 15-year period. *Ann Surg.* 1955;142:164–175.
11. Ellis B, Baig MK, Cripps NPJ, et al. Common modes of presentation of colorectal cancer patients. *Colorect Dis.* 1999;1(suppl 1):24.
12. Chapuis PH, Dent OF, Fisher R, et al. A multivariate analysis of clinical and pathological variables in prognosis after resection of large bowel cancer. *Br J Surg.* 1985;72:698–702.

13. Armstrong-James D, Moss S, Bygrave S, Thompson MR. Colorectal cancer patients presenting with rectal bleeding have earlier stage tumours and longer pre-diagnosis history [abstract]. *Gut* 1997;40(suppl 1):A50. Abstract TH199.
14. Rafftery TL, Samson N. Carcinoma of the colon: a clinical correlation between presenting symptoms and survival. *Am J Surg.* 1980;46:600–606.
15. Tsavellas G, Pond C, Thompson MR. Colorectal cancer patients with rectal bleeding have earlier stage disease and better outcomes. *Colorect Dis.* 2000; 2(suppl 1):41.
16. Atkin WS, Morson BC, Cuzick J. Long-term risk of colorectal cancer after excision of rectosigmoid adenomas. *N Engl J Med.* 1992:326:658–662.
17. Dent OF, Goulston KJ, Zubrzycki J, Chapuis PH. Bowel symptoms in an apparently well population. *Dis Colon Rectum.* 1986;29:243–247.
18. Goulston K, Chapuis P, Dent O, Bokey L. Significance of bowel symptoms. *Med J Aust.* 1987;146:631–633.
19. Mant A, Bokey EL, Chapuis Ph, et al. Rectal bleeding. Do other symptoms aid in diagnosis? *Dis Colon Rectum.* 1989;32:191–196.
20. Keddie N, Hargreaves A. Symptoms of carcinoma of the colon and rectum. *Lancet* 1968;2:749–750.
21. Curless R, French J, Williams GV, James OFW. Comparison of gastrointestinal symptoms in colorectal carcinoma patients and community controls with respect to age. *Gut* 1994;35:1267–1270.
22. Byles JE, Redman S, Hennrikus D, Sanson-Fisher RW, Dickinson J. Delay in consulting a medical practitioner about rectal bleeding. *J Epidemiol Community Health.* 1992;46:241–244.
23. Holliday HW, Hardcastle JD. Delay in diagnosis and treatment of symptoms colorectal cancer. *Lancet* 1979:1:309–311.
24. MacArthur C, Smith A. Factors associated with speed of diagnosis, referral and treatment in colorectal cancer. *J Epidemiol Community Health.* 1984;38: 122–126.
25. McLennan I, Hill J. How can doctors diagnose colorectal cancer earlier? By increasing patient's awareness of the disease and investigating them promptly when they present. *BMJ.* 1993;306:1707.
26. Great Britain: Department of Health. London: *The new NHS—Modern Dependable.* Published by the Department of Health 1997. London: The Stationery Office; 1997. (Command paper Cm 3807)
27. www.acpgbi.org.uk
28. Referral guidelines for colorectal cancer. *Colorect Dis.* 2002;4:287–297.
29. Thompson MR, Heath I, Ellis BG, et al. Identifying and managing patients at low risk of bowel cancer in general practice. *BMJ.* 2003;327:263–265.
30. Selvachandran SN, Hodder RJ, Ballal MS, Cade D. Prediction of colorectal cancer by a patient consultation questionnaire and scoring system: a prospective study. *Lancet* 2002;360:278–283.
31. Pearse IH, Crocker LH. *The Peckham Experiment: A Study of the Living Structure of Society.* London: Scottish Academic Press Ltd; 1985.
32. Wadsworth MEJ, Butterfield WJH, Blaney R. *Health and Sickness, The Choice of Treatment. Perception of Illness and Use of Services in an Urban Community.* London: Camelot Press Ltd; 1971.
33. Hannay DR. *The Symptom Iceberg: A Study of Community Health.* London: Routledge & Kegan Paul; 1979.

34. Crossland A, Jones R. Rectal bleeding: prevalence and consultation behaviour. *BMJ.* 1995;311:486–488.
35. Talley NJ, Jones M. Self-reported rectal bleeding in a United States community; prevalence, risk factors, and health care seeking. *Am J Gastroenterol.* 1998; 11:2179–2183.
36. Thompson JA, Pond CL, Ellis BG, Beach A, Thompson MR. Rectal bleeding in general and hospital practice: the tip of the iceberg. *Colorect Dis.* 2000;2 :288–293.
37. Jones ISC. An analysis of bowel habit and its significance in the diagnosis of carcinoma of the colon. *Am J Proctol.* 1976;27:45–46.
38. Kewenter J, Haglind, Smith L. Value of a risk questionnaire in screening for colorectal neoplasm. *Br J Surg.* 1989;76:280–283.
39. Silman AJ, Mitchell P, Nicholls RJ, et al. Self-reported dark red bleeding as a marker comparable with occult blood testing in screening for large bowel neoplasms. *Br J Surg.* 1983;70:721–724.
40. Farrands PA, Hardcastle JD. Colorectal screening by a self-completion questionnaire. *Gut* 1984;25:445–447.
41. Chapuis PH, Goulston KJ, Dent OF, Tait AD. Predictive value of rectal bleeding in screening for rectal and sigmoid polyps. *BMJ.* 1985;290:1546–1548.
42. Dent OF, Goulston KJ, Zubrzychi J, Chapuis PH. Bowel symptoms in an apparently well population. *Dis Colon Rectum.* 1986;29:243–247.
43. Jones R, Lydeard S. Irritable bowel syndrome in the general population. *BMJ.* 1992;303:87–90.
44. Fijten G, Blijham GH, Knottnerus JA. Occurrence and clinical significance of overt blood loss per rectum in the general population and in medical practice. A review. *Br J Gen Pract.* 1994;44:320–325.
45. Jones R. Self care. *BMJ.* 2000;320:596.
46. Thompson MR, Swarbrick ET, Ellis BG, et al. Strategies for the efficient management of all patients with lower gastrointestinal symptoms to achieve effective diagnosis of colorectal cancer. In: Cunningham D, Topham C, Miles A, eds. *The Effective Management of Colorectal Cancer.* 2nd ed. London: Aesculapius Medical Press; 2000: 173.
47. Sackett DL, Haynes RB, Guyatt GH, Tugwell P. *Clinical Epidemiology—A Basic Science for Clinical Medicine.* 2nd ed. Boston: Little Brown & Co; 1991: 4.
48. Neighbour R. *The Inner Consultation. How to Develop an Effective and Intuitive Consulting Style.* Lancaster: MTP Press Limited; 1987.
49. Feinstein AR. Symptoms as an index of biological behaviour and prognosis in human cancer. *Nature.* 1966;209:241–245.
50. Baig MK, Whatley P, Thompson MR. Delays during stages of referral diagnosis and treatment of colorectal cancer: their relationship to mortality. *Colorect Dis.* 1999;1(suppl 1):3.
51. Copeland EM, Miller LD, Jones RS. Prognostic factors in carcinoma of the colon and rectum. *Am J Surg.* 1968;116:875–881.
52. Pescatori M, Maria G, Beltrani B, Mattana C. Site, emergency and duration of symptoms in the prognosis of colorectal cancer. *Dis Colon Rectum.* 1982; 25:33–40.
53. Mulcahy HE, O'Donoghue DP. Duration of colorectal cancer symptoms and survival: the effect of confounding clinical and pathological variables. *Eur J Cancer.* 1997;33:1461–1467.

54. Barillari P, de Angelis R, Valabrega S, et al. Relationship of symptom duration and survival in patients with colorectal carcinoma. *Eur J Surg Oncol.* 1989;15: 441–445.
55. McDermott F, Hughes E, Pihl E, Milne B, Price A. Symptom duration and survival prospects in carcinoma of the rectum. *Surg Gynecol Obstet.* 1981;153: 321-326.
56. Holliday HW, Hardcastle JD. Delay in diagnosis and treatment of symptomatic colorectal cancer. *Lancet* 1979;2:309–311.
57. Tamoney HJ Jr, Caldarelli RA. Cancer of the right colon. An analysis of 211 patients. *Dis Colon Rectum.* 1966;9:13–19.
58. McDermott FT, Hughes ESR Pihl E, Milnes BJ, Price AB. Prognosis in relation to symptom duration in colon cancer. *Br J Surg.* 1981;68:846–849.
59. Clarke AM, Jones ISC. Diagnostic accuracy and diagnostic delay in carcinoma of the large bowel. *NZ Med J.* 1970;71:341–347.
60. Jolly KD, Scott JP, MacKinnon MJ, Clarke AM. Diagnosis and survival in carcinoma of the large bowel. *Aust NZ J Surg.* 1982;52:12–16.
61. Turnbull PRG, Isbister WH. Colorectal cancer in New Zealand: a Wellington study. *Aust NZ J Surg.* 1979;49:365–367.
62. Bassett ML, Bennett SA, Goulston KJ. Colorectal cancer. A study of 230 patients. *Med J Aust.* 1979;1:589–592.
63. Schillaci A, Cavallaro A, Nicolanti V, Ferri M, Gallo P, Stipa S. The importance of symptom duration in relation to prognosis of carcinoma of the large intestine. *Surg Gynecol Obstet.* 1984;158:423–426.
64. Khubchandani M. Relationship of symptom duration and survival in patients and carcinoma of the colon and rectum. *Dis Colon Rectum.* 1985;28:585–587.
65. Polissar L, Sim D, Francis A. Survival of colorectal cancer patients in relation to duration of symptoms and other prognostic factors. *Dis Colon Rectum.* 1981; 24:364–369.
66. Wessex Colorectal Cancer Audit. Final Report on behalf of the Wessex Colorectal Cancer Working Group. October 2000. *South-West Cancer Intelligence Service.* Hampshire, U.K.
67. Hackett TP, Cassem NH, Raker JW. Patient delay in cancer. *N Eng J Med.* 1973;289:14–20.
68. Robinson E, Mohilever J, Zidan J, Sapir D. Colorectal cancer: incidence delay in diagnosis and stage of disease. *Eur J Cancer Clin Oncol.* 1986;22:157–161.
69. Rowe-Jones D, Aylett S. Delay in treatment in carcinoma of colon and rectum. *Lancet* 1965;2:973–976.
70. Welch CE, Burke JF. Carcinoma of the colon and rectum. *N Engl J Med.* 1962; 266:846; 211–9.
71. Rubin M, Zer M, Dintsman M. Factors influencing delay in treatment of cancer of rectum and colon in Israel. *Israel J Med Sci.* 1980;16:641–645.
72. Launoy G, Le Courtour X, Gignoux M, Pottier D, Dugleux G. Influence of rural environment on diagnosis, treatment and prognosis of colorectal cancer. *J Epidemiol Community Health.* 1992;46:365–367.
73. Clarke JP, Kettlewell MGW, Dehn TCB. Changing patterns of colorectal cancer in a regional teaching hospital. *Ann R Coll Surg Engl.* 1992;74:291–293.
74. Chapuis PH, Dent OF, Fisher R, et al. A multivariate analysis of clinical and pathological variables in prognosis after resection of large bowel cancer. *Br J Surg.* 1985;72:698–702.

75. Baig MK, Whatley P, Thompson MR. Does early diagnosis and prompt treatment of symptomatic colorectal cancer improve survival. *Gut* 1998;42(suppl 1): A93.
76. Macdonald I. Biological predeterminism in human cancer. *Surg Gynecol Obstet.* 1951;92:443–452.
77. Macdonald I. The individual basis of biologic variability in cancer. *Surg Gynecol Obstet.* 1958;106:227–229.
78. Ragland JJ, Londe AM, Spratt JS Jr. Correlation of the prognosis of obstructing colorectal carcinoma with clinical and pathologic variables. *Am J Surg.* 1971; 121:552–556.
79. Stubbs RS, Long MG. Symptom duration and pathologic staging of colorectal cancer. *Eur J Surg Oncol.* 1986;12:127–130.
80. Irvin TT, Greaney MG. Duration of symptoms and prognosis of carcinoma of the colon and rectum. *Surg Gynecol Obstet.* 1997:144:883–886.
81. Slaney G. Results of treatment of carcinoma of the colon and rectum. In: Irvine WT, ed. *Modern Trends in Surgery 3.* London: Butterworths; 1971:69–89.
82. Kyle SM, Isbister WH, Yeong ML. Presentation, duration of symptoms and staging of colorectal carcinoma. *Aust NZ J Surg.* 1991;61:137–140.
83. Ratcliffe R, Kiff RS, Kingston RD, Walsh SH, Jeacock J. Early diagnosis in colorectal cancer. Still no benefit? *J R Coll Surg Edinb.* 1989;34:152–155.
84. Dent OF, Chapuis PH, Goulston KJ. Relationship of survival to stage of the tumour and duration of symptoms in colorectal cancer. *Med J Aust.* 1983; 1:274–275.
85. Goodman D, Irvin TT. Delay in the diagnosis and prognosis of carcinoma of the right colon. *Br J Surg.* 1993;80:1327–1329.
86. Baig MK, Whatley P, Thompson MR. Delay in diagnosis and treatment of colorectal cancer of colorectal cancer: does it affect outcome? *Colorect Dis.* 1999:1(suppl 1):3.
87. Muir Gray JA. *Evidence-Based Healthcare: How to Make Health Policy and Management Decisions.* New York: Churchill Livingstone; 1997.
88. Sackett DL, Haynes RB, Guyatt GH, Tugwell P. *Clinical Epidemiology—A Basic Science for Clinical Medicine.* 2nd ed. Boston: Little Brown & Co; 1991: 283–302.
89. Marshall KG. Prevention. How much harm? How much benefit? 3. Physical psychological and social harm. *Can Med Assoc.* 1996;155:169–170.
90. Haynes RB, Sackett DL, Taylor DW, Gibson ES, Johnson AL. Increased absenteeism from work after detection and labelling of hypertensive patients. *N Engl J Med.* 1978;299:741–744.
91. MacDonald LA, Sackett DL, Haynes RB, Taylor DW. Labelling in hypertension: a review of the behavioural and psychological consequences. *J Chron Dis.* 1984;37:933–942.
92. Williams CB. Colonoscopy. *Br Med Bull.* 1986;42:265–269.
93. Waye JD, Kahn O, Auerbach ME. Complications of colonoscopy and flexible sigmoidoscopy. *Gastrointest Endosc Clin N Am.* 1996;6:343–377.
94. Blakeborough A, Sheridan MB, Chapman AH. Complications of barium enema examinations: a survey of UK consultant radiologists 1992 to 1994. *Clin Radiol.* 1997;52:142–148.
95. Muir Gray JA. *Evidence-Based Healthcare: How to Make Health Policy and Management Decisions.* New York: Churchill Livingstone; 1997:39.

96. Staniland JR, Ditchburn J, De Dombal FT. Clinical presentation of diseases of the large bowel. A detailed study of 642 patients. *Gastroenterology* 1976:70: 22–28.
97. Chave H, Flashman K, Senapati A, Cripps NPJ, Thompson MR. Characteristics of the change in bowel habit in patients with colorectal cancer. *Colorect Dis.* 2000;2(suppl 1):1–2.
98. Cancer Research UK. Large Bowel Cancer Factsheet. April 2004. *Cancer Research UK*. London.

2
Screening for Colorectal Cancer

John H. Scholefield and Susan J. Ritchie

1. Introduction

Colorectal cancer is the third most-common malignancy in the United Kingdom; there are approximately 32,000 new cases and 17,000 deaths in the United Kingdom per annum. Colorectal cancer is equally prevalent in men and women, usually occurring in later life (60–70 years of age). Prognosis is dependant upon stage of disease at presentation. For the majority of patients with lymph-node involvement at presentation, median survival is around 40% [1]. Although the incidence and mortality of colorectal cancer have remained static for the last 40 years, there is a recent trend showing a slight decline in incidence and mortality in both the United Kingdom and the United States. This decrease in mortality may reflect a trend towards earlier diagnosis, perhaps as a result of increased public awareness of the disease [1].

Surgery remains the mainstay of treatment for colorectal cancer, but early diagnosis of the disease provides an opportunity to improve outcome. Early diagnosis of colorectal cancer makes it more likely that the tumour can be completely removed and thereby improves the chance of cure.

2. Why Screen for Colorectal Cancer?

The vast majority of colorectal cancers result from malignant change in polyps (adenomas) occurring in the lining of the bowel. The best available evidence suggests that only 10% of 1-cm adenomas undergo malignant change after 10 years. The incidence of adenomatous polyps in the colon increases with age, and although adenomatous polyps can be identified in up to 20% of the population, most of these are small and unlikely to undergo malignant change. The vast majority (90%) of adenomas can be removed at colonoscopy. Other types of polyps occurring in the colon, such as metaplastic (alternatively known as hyperplastic) polyps, are usually small and have much lower malignant potential than adenomas.

Colorectal cancer (Figure 2.1) is a common condition with a known premalignant lesion (adenoma). There is a relatively long time course for malignant transformation from adenoma to carcinoma and outcomes are markedly improved by early detection of adenomas and early cancers. Thus, there is great potential for reducing the mortality from this disease by detecting adenomas and early cancers through screening asymptomatic individuals.

The single greatest risk factor for the development of colorectal cancer is old age. Over 90% of colorectal cancers occur in the over-60 age group. Because it takes approximately 10 years for a 1-cm adenoma to become a carcinoma, screening needs to begin 10 years before this peak incidence of carcinomas; most experts agree that screening should target those over 50 years of age. There is agreement that there is little point in screening individuals over 75 years of age, as their life expectancy is limited and the potential gain from the screening process decreases. However, as average life expectancy is increasing, this figure may need to be revised [2].

3. Which Test(s) for Population Screening?

Because bowels are a taboo subject for most people, public awareness of the symptoms of bowel cancer is generally poor. A recent survey revealed that only 30% of the British population were aware that cancer of the bowel

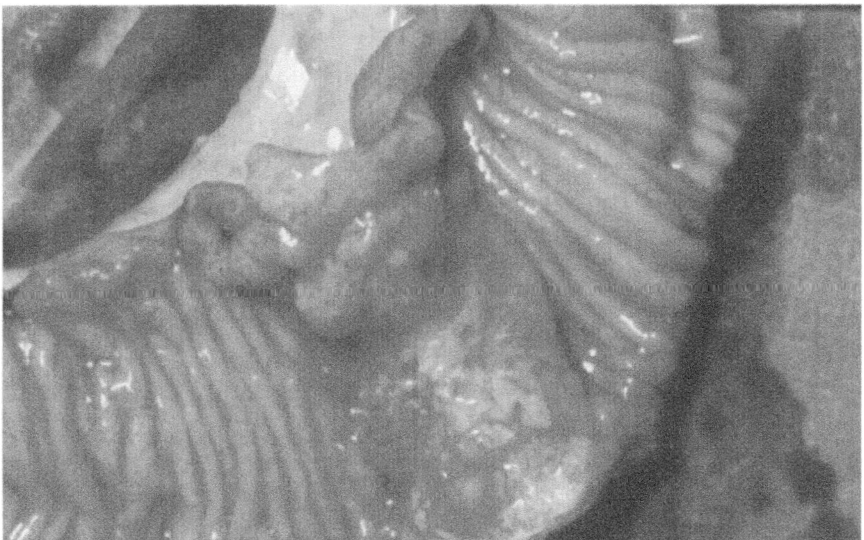

FIGURE 2.1. A colonic carcinoma. (Reproduced from ABC of Colorectal Screening; JH Scholefield, *Br Med J.* 2000;321:1004–1005, with permission from the BMJ Publishing Group.)

occurred. Such ignorance increases the difficulties of early detection. In addition, the symptoms of bowel cancer may initially be similar to those of more benign lesions, adding to the difficulty of early diagnosis.

In order for a screening test to be applicable to large populations it has to be inexpensive, reliable, and acceptable. Ideally it should also be simple to perform and amenable to rapid interpretation. Many different screening tests have been evaluated in order to diagnose colorectal cancer at an early stage. Perhaps the simplest and least expensive is the symptom questionnaire, but this has proved predictably insensitive and only becomes reliable when the tumour is relatively advanced. Digital rectal examination will detect only 10% of colorectal cancers (those within the reach of a gloved finger) and rigid sigmoidoscopy will generally only detect those cancers distal to the rectosigmoid junction (around 30% of colorectal cancers). Both digital rectal examination and rigid sigmoidoscopy suffer from the further limitation that they are unpleasant and invasive.

Flexible sigmoidoscopy has the capacity to detect 70% of colorectal cancers, as it examines the whole of the left colon and rectum. A strategy to provide a single flexible sigmoidoscopy for adults between 55 and 65 years of age aimed at detecting adenomas would probably be the most likely option. Although flexible sigmoidoscopy is more expensive than rigid sigmoidoscopy, it is generally more acceptable to patients because it is less uncomfortable and has much higher yield than the rigid instrument. Many nurses are now trained to perform flexible sigmoidoscopy, making potential screening programs using this modality more cost effective. A multicentre trial of this population-screening strategy has recently been completed and the results have not yet been published.

In a population-screening program, the proportion of the population who take up the offer of the screening test is crucial. It seems that compliance with flexible sigmoidoscopy is likely to be around 45%, and of these 6% will subsequently require full colonoscopy [3]. The effect this will have on the incidence and mortality from colorectal cancer is uncertain. The outcome of this large multicentre trial will provide much needed information, but mortality data will not be available until 2006.

Some enthusiasts in the United States have advocated colonoscopy as the ideal screening test for colorectal cancer. While colonoscopy (Figure 2.2) is the gold standard for examination of the colon and rectum, it is expensive and very dependant on the expertise of the endoscopist. In addition, the need for full bowel preparation, sedation, and the small risk of colonic perforation make it unacceptable for population screening. Colonoscopy is, however, the investigation of choice for screening high-risk patients.

Barium enema, like colonoscopy, examines the whole colon and rectum. Although barium enema is cheaper and has a lower complication rate than colonoscopy, it is invasive, exposes the individual to a sizeable radiation dose, and requires full bowel preparation. Whereas colonoscopy may be therapeutic, barium enema does not allow removal or biopsy of lesions.

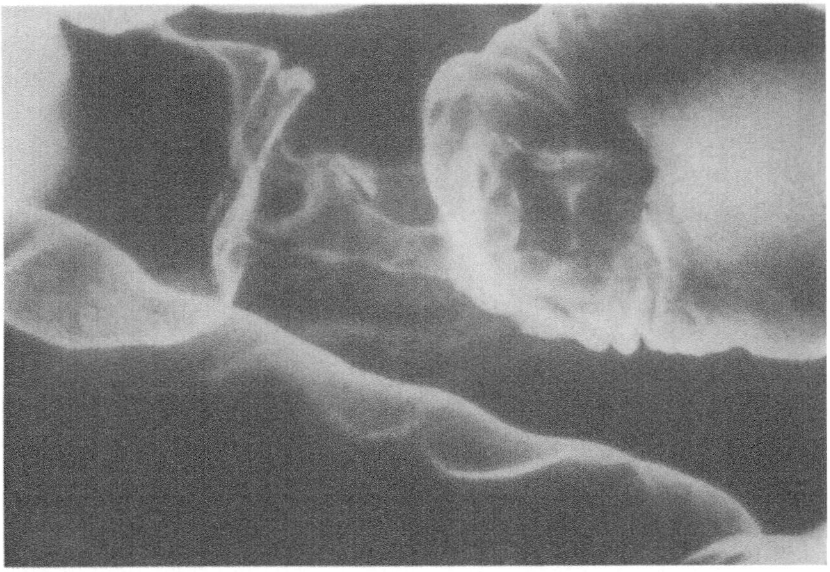

FIGURE 2.2. A double-contrast barium enema showing a carcinoma in the sigmoid colon. (Reproduced from ABC of Colorectal Cancer; JH Scholefield, *Br Med J.* 2000;321:1004–1005, with permission from the BMJ Publishing Group.)

Although there are pockets of enthusiasm for the use of double-contrast barium enema as a screening tool (mainly in the United States), its disadvantages seem to preclude it from use in population screening. There are no population-screening studies using barium enema and no trials in progress.

Computed tomographic (CT) colography (a.k.a., virtual colonoscopy) is a relatively new radiological technique that in the future may find a role in population screening for colorectal cancer. Although this technique requires full bowel preparation, very expensive CT scanners, and computing facilities, it is minimally invasive and views of the whole colon can be obtained within 5 minutes. Preliminary data suggest that this technique has an acceptable sensitivity for large polyps and cancers. As yet there are no published trials of CT colography in population screening but this is surely only a matter of time. CT colography has the potential to be cost effective and to reduce the need for colonoscopy in population screening. There is concern about the dose of radiation each patient receives; each patient is required to have one prone and one supine scan per investigation. The radiation dose involved in this type of investigation may become less of a problem as magnetic resonance (MR) colography is developed [2].

Faecal occult blood (FOB) tests are the most extensively studied screening tests for colorectal cancer. These tests detect hematin from partially digested blood in the stool. The overall sensitivity of FOB tests for colorectal neoplasia is only 50%–60%, though their specificity is high (around 95%) for polyps and cancers. A further drawback of this test is that ingested animal hemoglobin and peroxidase-containing vegetables (parsnips, broccoli, and cauliflower) may cause false-positive results.

In screening studies using FOB tests, individuals are usually invited to take 2 samples from each of 3 consecutive stools. Compliance tends to be around 50%–60% but with population education this could be improved. Individuals with more than 4 positives in 6 tests (around 2%) need colonoscopy. While normal blood loss from the gut is around 1 mL/d, haemoccult will detect blood loss in excess of 10 mL/d.

Several large randomised studies have shown that FOB screening is feasible and three studies have shown that FOB screening reduces the mortality from colorectal cancer [4–7]. In the Nottingham study, for every 100 haemoccult-positive individuals, 12 had cancer and 23 had adenomatous polyps. The detected cancers tended to be at an earlier stage than those presenting symptomatically (26% Dukes A screen detected vs. 11% Dukes A in controls) [5]. The downside of FOB screening at present is its relatively low sensitivity, which means that some cancers will be missed on each round of screening. The Nottingham data suggest that screening every 2 years only detects 72% of cancers. This could be improved by testing annually [8]. Future screening programs may use newer immunological FOB tests that can reduce the number of false-positive results by detecting only human hemoglobin. More specific stool-based tests looking for DNA mutations in shed cells from the colonic lining may also prove to be a valuable screening tool, but this technology is still in its infancy and its full potential remains uncertain.

4. Who Should Be Screened?

There is a broad spectrum of risk for colorectal cancer. Although 19% of the population will develop adenomatous polyps (Figure 2.3), only 5% will develop colorectal cancer. This equates to a 1 in 35 lifetime risk for colorectal cancer. Most of these cancers will occur in people between 65–75 years of age, but the peak incidence for adenomas is slightly earlier at 55–65 years of age. Thus, population screening for colorectal cancer should probably target the age group starting at 55 years of age and ending at 75 years of age. In addition, there are some individuals in the population who will have inherited a much higher susceptibility to colorectal cancer (Figure 2.4). Population screening for colorectal cancer is not adequate for those at highest risk. Those individuals who have inherited a well-recognised single gene disorder such as familial adenomatous polyposis or hereditary

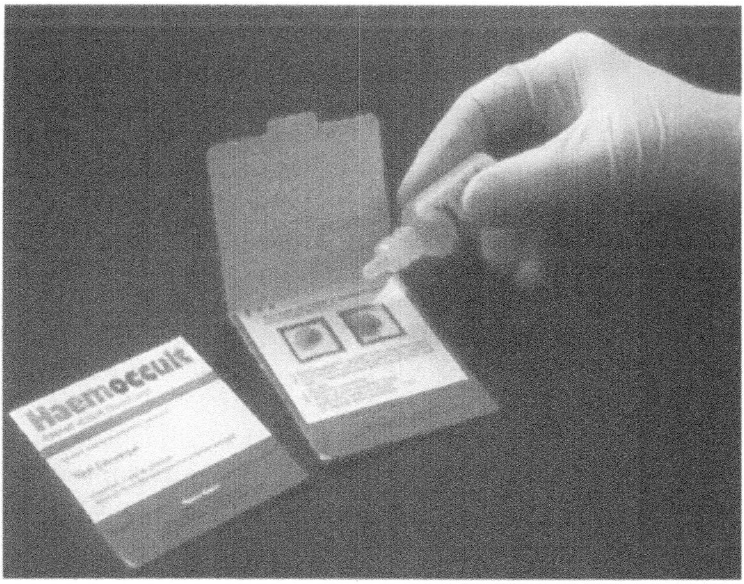

FIGURE 2.3. Developing a Haemoccult test. (Reproduced from ABC of Colorectal Cancer; JH Scholefield, *Br Med J.* 2000;321:1004–1005, with permission from the BMJ Publishing Group.)

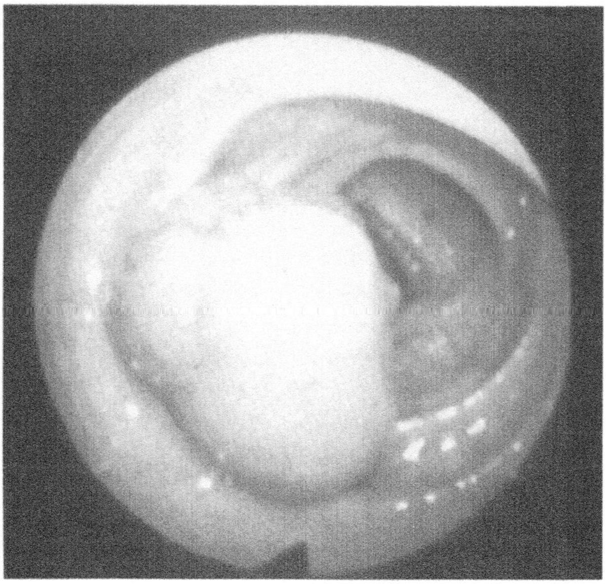

FIGURE 2.4. Colonoscopic view of an adenoma. (Reproduced from ABC of Colorectal Cancer; JH Scholefield, *Br Med J.* 2000;321:1004–1005, with permission from the BMJ Publishing Group.)

non-polyposis colorectal cancer may well develop colorectal cancers before the age of 50 and therefore screening for these high-risk individuals needs to be tailored to their individual risk pattern. Such individuals may also be at risk for cancers at other sites and screening for ovarian, breast, and endometrial cancers may be appropriate in some of these cases [9,10]. Individuals and families with these conditions need careful risk assessment and the optimal screening strategy may require multidisciplinary care, best coordinated by clinical geneticists.

5. Cost Effectiveness of Screening

In order for screening for colorectal cancer to be acceptable to healthcare providers it must be shown to be cost effective. Data from the Nottingham study show that the cost per cancer detected was less than £2700 and that FOB screening for colorectal cancer costs around £1000 per life year saved [11–13]. This is similar to models for breast cancer screening. By comparison, screening by barium enema or colonoscopy at 5-year intervals would cost £1500 and £3000, respectively, per life year saved. A single flexible sigmoidoscopy would cost around £1500 per life year saved [14].

These models all suffer from a number of uncertainties. Of these, the one which causes greatest concern to those considering funding screening programs is the cost of cancers missed by the screening process and the occurrence of complications following colonoscopy in asymptomatic individuals.

6. Ethical Dilemmas in Population Screening for Colorectal Cancer

In any population-screening program there is a major concern that the vast majority of the population have no symptoms and are at relatively low risk for the condition. By definition population screening exposes a large number of individuals to the screening process. Therefore, the screening process must be as simple as possible, have high sensitivity and specificity, and be reliable and safe.

A major concern in the introduction of a screening program is the potential for harm to those who have positive test results but turn out not to have colorectal cancer. The positivity rate in the Nottingham study was 2% using haemoccult; using a more sensitive test would increase the proportion of people needing colonoscopy. Thus, any screening program can be assumed to need to colonoscope a minimum of 2% of the screened population [5]. The potential harm includes psychological stress related to having a positive test and having to undergo invasive investigations, waiting for results, etc. While the evidence available suggests that this stress is transient, it may affect compliance with the program. The physical harm of the screening process relates mainly to the complications of colonoscopy. Although perforation and haemorrhage are rare (around 1 in 1000 procedures for each), these figures begin to assume worrying proportions when one considers that a national screening program might generate 10,000 extra colonoscopies per annum. A high standard of colonoscopy is crucial to minimising complications and maximising yield from the screening process [8].

7. Population Screening—The Current Situation

7.1. National

A national pilot program for colorectal cancer screening began in Warwickshire (England) and Grampian (Scotland) in 2000. These pilots are using a FOB test similar to that used in the Nottingham study. The initial data from these studies is very immature and all that can be said so far is that people do seem to be willing to do the tests and that compliance appears similar to the Nottingham study at around 50%. A flexible sigmoidoscopy study has been completed but mortality data are unlikely to be available until 2006 [18]. The pilot data from this study is available and show that flexible sigmoidoscopy is an effective screening tool and that people are prepared to have this invasive test. The yield of polyps and cancers is higher than for FOB testing but the colonoscopy rate is also three times higher and this is a concern. The introduction of any screening program using FOB or flexible sigmoidoscopy will necessitate an improvement in the resources available for colonoscopy.

7.2. International

No country has yet adopted a national screening program for colorectal cancer. The United States has suggested yearly FOB tests for people over 50 and flexible sigmoidoscopy every 3 years. Many insured patients get more frequent screening, but the uninsured get none! In Europe, Germany has tried to introduce a screening program but has run into enormous difficulties with its administration. Australia is developing a screening program and may be the first country with a national program in place.

8. Population Screening—The Future

Research into serum- and stool-based tests for colorectal cancer screening is being undertaken. Sidransky and others have identified genetic mutations in stool from patients with colorectal cancer, but translating these findings into a screening test applicable to populations is proving difficult. The development of chip technology provides the capability to screen for many thousands of gene mutations from a single sample of blood or stool and adds a new dimension to screening for all types of cancer.

Noninvasive methods of imaging the colon such as MR colography may also revolutionise the screening process by reducing the need for colonoscopy. The development of stool labeling may allow computer software to subtract stool from scans and thereby obviate the need for bowel preparation prior to this type of imaging.

9. Genetic Risk Assessment for Colorectal Cancer: Screening Based on Family History

Centers across the country have been designing protocols for efficient risk assessment, for recommending appropriate DNA studies, and for endoscopy and prophylactic surgery. A lack of consistency in some of these areas has caused confusion and anxiety in families, general practitioners, and hospital specialists.

It has been estimated that in 20% or more of individuals with colorectal cancer, there may be a genetic predisposition. Among these, familial adenomatous polyposis, caused by germline mutations in the *APC* gene, accounts for less than 1% of cases and hereditary non-polyposis colorectal cancer (previously called Lynch Syndrome) accounts for 2%–3%. These individuals have inherited a high risk for colorectal cancer [15,16]. In the remainder of colorectal cancers (>95%), the genetic predisposition is much less clear-cut than in familial adenomatous polyposis or hereditary non-polyposis colorectal cancer, and is likely to be due to gene mutation and polymorphism of low penetrance (yet to be identified). These individuals are in the moderate- and low-risk groups. The role of environmental triggers and other modifier genes in these groups remains to be determined.

10. High-Risk Groups

10.1. Familial Adenomatous Polyposis (FAP)

Familial adenomatous polyposis was the first inherited bowel cancer syndrome to be described. It is autosomal dominant with almost full penetrance. Affected individuals usually have distinctive appearances of the colon and rectum, with hundreds of adenomas. Left untreated, the risk of colorectal cancer is thought to be 100%. However, this is not only a disease of the large bowel; upper GI malignancies will develop in around 10% of affected individuals. Desmoid tumours, as well as osteomas (particularly of the jaw) and epidermoid cysts may also be a part of this condition (sometimes called Gardner's syndrome).

Annual screening by sigmoidoscopy should start in the early teens in an at-risk individual and those affected require discussion about options for prophylactic colectomy/proctocolectomy and continued endoscopic surveillance.

The gene for FAP was mapped to 5q in 1987 and cloned in 1991. Mutations can be identified in the vast majority of families. This has also enabled further elucidation of the phenotype, for example, there is an attenuated form with fewer polyps in which the mutations tend to be in the 3′ end of the gene [17]. In this variant, there are usually fewer than 100 polyps and the average age of onset of colorectal cancer is 10–20 years later. With appropriate screening, reduction in mortality and morbidity in FAP families has been demonstrated. Depending on the family experience and wishes, prenatal diagnosis has become an option.

10.2. Hereditary Non-polyposis Colorectal Cancer (HNPCC)

Hereditary non-polyposis colorectal cancer is also dominantly inherited (penetrance is around 85%–90%). Fewer polyps are present than in FAP and the average age for developing colorectal cancer is the early 40s. Two thirds of the cancers occur in the right side of the colon, distinctly different from that seen in FAP and the general population. Adenocarcinomas can occur elsewhere in the body; the endometrium is the most frequent site. Several studies suggest that endometrial cancer is as likely as colorectal cancer in HNPCC families. Other associated cancers include gastric, renal, ovarian, ureteric, and brain.

The clinical diagnosis of HNPCC can be difficult and a set of diagnostic criteria were drawn up in Amsterdam in 1991. It is now realised that these criteria were too strict and excluded many cases, particularly those involving endometrial cancer. The criteria have now been modified (Table 2.1).

Screening for HNPCC requires examination of the entire colon by colonoscopy or barium enema; the predominance of right-side tumours makes it imperative that colonoscopy is complete in this condition. Colonic surveillance should start at 25 years of age and be repeated every 2–3 years until the age of 70 (Table 2.2).

Table 2.1. Modified Amsterdam criteria.

At least 3 colorectal or HNPCC-associated cancers.
One of 3 affected relatives is a first-degree relative of the others.
The cancers affect 2 or more generations within a family.
At least one of the cancers diagnosed before 45 years of age.
FAP has been excluded.

TABLE 2.2. Inherited risk of colorectal cancer.

Risk group	Family history	Action
Low risk	1 FDR >45 y	No screening
	2 FDR >70 y	No screening
Low-to-moderate risk	2 FDR average 60–70 y	Single colonoscopy at 55 y
Moderate risk	1 FDR <45 y	Colonoscopy every 5 y from 5 y prior to index case
	2 FDR average 50–60 y	Colonoscopy every 5 y beginning at 35 y—refer to genetic screening
High-to-moderate risk	2 FDR average <50 y	Colonoscopy every 3–5 y beginning at 30–40 y (see family history)—refer to genetic screening
	3 FDR (Amsterdam negative)	Colonoscopy every 3–5 y beginning at 30 y (see family history)—refer to genetic screening + Gynecological screening for women
High risk	3 FDR (Amsterdam positive)	Colonoscopy every 2–3 y beginning at 30–40 y (see family history)—refer to genetic screening
	FAP	Annual sigmoidoscopy / genetic screening

FDR, first-degree relative.
Endoscopic screening should cease in most cases after 75 years of age, but depends on the individual's health and comorbidities.

It may be justifiable to colonoscope more frequently than every 2–3 years in families in which interval cancers have occurred. Evidence from the Dutch Registry has demonstrated that such screening reduces the incidence of colorectal cancer in this group and is cost effective [9,10].

Female members of these families are advised to have gynaecological surveillance that may take the form of annual pipelle sampling of the endometrium and ultrasound of the ovaries. If there are individuals in the family with associated gastric or renal tumours, screening for these is also required.

DNA mutation analysis can be fruitful in this condition; for example, if a mutation in one of the mismatch repair genes (most commonly MLH1 & MSH2) is identified, 50% of family members will test negative and can be reassured that they do not need endoscopic screening. This greatly reduces the need for endoscopic and gynaecological surveillance in these families. Six mismatch repair genes have been identified so far with hundreds of mutations in each gene possible. Nearly all the tumours from HNPCC families (vs 12%–16% of sporadic colorectal cancer) show microsatellite instability or replication error positivity on molecular testing. This measure of genetic instability, suggesting that a mismatch repair gene mutation may be present, can be a useful prelude to mutation testing in some families where the history is borderline for HNPCC.

Other rare but related conditions should be considered in some families, for example, Muir-Torre syndrome with characteristic skin lesions

(HNPCC variant) and Turcot's Syndrome with cerebellar medulloblastomas occurring in association with FAP, or glioblastomas in association with HNPCC.

11. Moderate-Risk Group

This is a larger group than the high-risk group and consists of those who have more than 1 affected relative (or one under 45 years of age) but do not fulfil the Amsterdam criteria (Table 2.1). The recommendation for screening depends on the number of affected relatives, how closely related they are, and the age of onset (Table 2.2). Application of these criteria depends on a detailed family history, which may often be incomplete. It is often necessary to obtain consent and request the records of living relatives or obtain confirmation from the relevant cancer registry about those who are deceased. Indeed this is an essential part of the process because in 10%–15% of cases the diagnosis reported by the relative turns out to be incorrect, thus compromising the risk assessment and recommendation for lifelong screening.

Colonoscopy every 5 years is adequate for these individuals once a normal colon has been demonstrated. Ages for commencing (5 years before age of onset of the youngest family member) and ceasing (>75 years of age) such surveillance are controversial, and should be discussed with the individual after taking into account any comorbidities.

At present, no informative molecular genetic tests are helpful in this group but there is probably some value in storing DNA from affected members for future testing.

12. Low-Risk Group

Some slight variation can be found across the United Kingdom about the exact definition of the low-risk group. In general, this includes those with no family history, those with only 1 affected relative over 45 years of age or 2 affected relatives over 70 years of age (Table 2.2). The risk would exceed the population risk in these last two groups (1:17 as opposed to 1:35), but not enough to warrant regular screening by colonoscopy. Although referral of low-risk individuals is a questionable use of resources, these referrals can provide reassurance and can give advice about diet, lifestyle, and bowel symptoms of which to be aware.

These worried-well relatives are generally referred via their general practitioner for a surgical or genetic outpatient appointment. Over one third of referrals to our own clinic are assessed as low risk according to their family history and are therefore not suitable for regular endoscopic screening. Ultimately, training should be provided for doctors or nurses in taking family history and doing risk assessment so that these low-risk individuals need not be referred to hospital.

13. The Need for a Multidisciplinary Approach

Collaboration between colorectal surgeons, primary-care staff, and geneticists is essential in order to agree on criteria for the different risk groups outlined above. In order to keep track of all family members and ensure their different screening needs are met, an efficient database with administrative support is required and is essential for the continuation and development of the service.

The Clinical Genetics Service is ideally placed to coordinate such a program and liase with other departments, especially when multisystem screening is required. They can also counsel people in high-risk groups about the possibility of genetic testing and the implications for them and their families.

Presymptomatic (or predictive) mutation testing in FAP and HNPCC is a relatively recent option, but this is an area in which geneticists have some experience in counselling for other conditions. It should not be assumed that at-risk people will avail themselves of the test even if a mutation was detected in an affected family member. Knowledge about the presence of a particular genetic change may have implications for such things as insurance, employment, or mortgage applications. This is covered as part of the pretest counseling. While one could argue that those who have the screening tests are behaving responsibly and may be reducing their risk of developing a cancer, their prospective employers or insurers may not see it in this way. Frequently, people do not want a numerical risk figure but just want to know if they are at sufficiently increased risk to warrant regular screening. The timing of predictive genetic testing must be chosen with care; for example, a recent bereavement or an age much younger than screening tests are applicable may be contraindications to predictive genetic testing. Advice can be given to them and their general practitioner to activate such tests again at the appropriate time.

14. Summary

Population screening for colorectal cancer using FOB tests is feasible and there is increasingly compelling evidence to show that such programs can save lives at a cost similar to that of the existing breast-cancer–screening program.

A single flexible sigmoidoscopy presents a promising alternative to FOB testing, but conclusive data will not be available for another 5 to 7 years. In order to be able to undertake such a program in the United Kingdom there would need to be a considerable investment in colonoscopy facilities and expertise.

Several countries, including the United States, have instituted screening programs utilising one or both of these modalities. Whether the United Kingdom follows will be determined by political decisions.

A more intensive screening approach for those with a strong family history of colorectal cancer (high- and moderate-risk groups) is being adopted in many centers, with colonoscopy being the most appropriate examination.

A multidisciplinary approach to family-history–based screening is the way to stratify individuals to appropriate risk groups and to provide the best possible service with the limited resources available.

References

1. Eurocare 2. *IARC Scientific Publications.* 1999;51:1–572.
2. Ransahoff D. Screening for colorectal cancer. *N Engl J Med.* 2002;346:40–44.
3. Atkin W. Screening for colorectal cancer: the heart of the matter. *Gut* 1999;45: 480–481.
4. Mandel JS, Bond JH, Church TR. Reducing mortality from colorectal cancer by screening for fecal occult blood. *N Engl J Med.* 1993;328:1365–1371.
5. Hardcastle JD, Chamberlain JO, Robinson MHE. Randomised controlled trial of faecal occult blood screening for colorectal cancer. *Lancet* 1996;348: 1472–1477.
6. Kronborg O, Fenger C, Olsen J, Jorgensen OD, Sondergaard O. Randomised study of screening for colorectal cancer with faecal-occult-blood test. *Lancet* 1996;348:1467–1471.
7. Towler B, Irwig L, Glasziou P. A systematic review of the effects of screening for colorectal cancer using the faecal occult blood test, haemoccult. *BMJ.* 1998; 317:559–565.
8. Robinson M, Hardcastle J, Moss S, et al. The risks of screening: data from the Nottingham randomised controlled trial of faecal occult blood screening for colorectal cancer. *Gut* 1999;45:588–592.
9. Vasen HFA. High incidence of interval cancers in HNPCC. An update of the Dutch HNPCC registry. Paper presented at: 10th Annual ICG-HNPCC Meeting; June 1998; Portugal.
10. Jarvinen HJ, Mecklin JP, Sistonen P. Screening reduces colorectal cancer rate in families with hereditary nonpolyposis colorectal cancer. *Gastroenterology* 1995; 108:1405–1411.
11. Hardcastle JD, Chamberlain JO, Robinson MH, et al. Randomised controlled trial of faecal occult blood screening in colorectal cancer. *Lancet* 1996;348: 1472–1477.
12. Mandel JS, Bond JH, Church TR, et al. Reducing mortality from colorectal cancer by screening for faecal occult blood. *N Engl J Med.* 1993;328:1365–1371.
13. Winawer SJ, Schottenfield D, Felhinger BJ. Colorectal cancer screening. *J Natl Cancer Inst.* 1991;83:243–253.
14. Atkin WS, Hart A, Edwards R. Uptake, yield of neoplasia, and adverse effects of flexible sigmoidoscopy screening. *Gut* 1998;42:560–565.

15. Cannon-Albright LA, Thomas TC, Bishop DT, Skolnick MH, Burt RW. Characteristics of familial colon cancer in a large population database. *Cancer* 1989; 64:1971–1975.
16. Dunlop MG, Farrington SM, Carothers AD, et al. Cancer risk associated with germline DNA mismatch repair gene mutations. *Hum Mol Genet.* 1997;6:105–110.
17. Friedl W, Meuschel S, Caspari, et al. Attenuated familial adenomatous polyposis due to a mutation in the 3′ part of the APC gene. *Hum Genet.* 1996; 97:579–584.
18. UK Flexible Sigmoidoscopy Screening Trial Investigation. Single flexible sigmoidoscopy screening to prevent colorectal cancer: baseline finding of a UK multicentre randomised trial. *Lancet* 2002;359:1291–1300.

3
Familial Colorectal Cancer

Sunil Dolwani and Julian R. Sampson

1. Introduction

Epidemiological studies suggest that at least 15% of colorectal cancers arise in individuals with an inherited predisposition to the disease [1]. A much smaller proportion of cases, fewer than 5%, can be accounted for by mutant genes that are associated with a small number of well-defined mendelian syndromes, notably familial adenomatous polyposis (FAP) and hereditary non-polyposis colorectal cancer (HNPCC). In these settings colorectal cancer risk is very high, but proactive management of the extended family can substantially improve the prognosis for those at risk. This is best achieved through a coordinated approach involving genetic counselling and testing, surveillance, and prophylactic or early surgical intervention.

Often, a family history is reported that is consistent with an inherited predisposition to colorectal cancer but this cannot be attributed to a specific mendelian syndrome or to a specific gene or genes. Currently undefined genetic variants that are associated with more modest increases in risk of colorectal cancer are likely to play a role in many of these families. Although genetic testing is not possible in this setting, the family history of cancers and the ages at which they were diagnosed can be assessed, enabling an estimation of the future risk of colorectal cancer in currently unaffected family members. Such risk estimates provide a rational basis for decisions regarding surveillance.

The potential benefits of a systematic approach to risk assessment are much clearer for colorectal cancer than for many other common cancers as the large bowel is readily accessible for direct endoscopic inspection, the natural history usually involves a well-defined adenoma-carcinoma sequence, and the prognosis is highly stage dependent. However, there is still a paucity of high-quality data to inform the development of surveillance protocols in all but the highest risk groups and considerable local variation in the availability of resources for surveillance. Consequently clinical management of those with a family history of colorectal cancer is often inconsistent.

2. Family History: Awareness and Models for Management

Recommendations for colorectal cancer screening that include risk stratification according to family history criteria have been suggested in the United Kingdom [2]. However, questionnaire surveys have revealed wide variation in both awareness and clinical practice among healthcare professionals. For example, the majority of gastroenterologists report routinely obtaining a family history of colorectal cancers and related conditions such as polyps from their patients, but there is little consistency in the surveillance that they recommend on the basis of this information [3,4]. Furthermore, even a recent survey found that less than half of specialists were clear about the availability and role of mutation testing for FAP and HNPCC, and 28% reported that they never discussed these issues with their patients [4].

In the United Kingdom and many European countries, systems for obtaining accurate family histories, categorising risk, and, where appropriate, coordinating genetic testing and surveillance have been developed through clinical genetics services. For the highest risk families these processes are often formalised via genetic registers. Ideally, genetic registers should provide comprehensive cover for a geographically defined population and comprise (computerised) pedigree-based records that link genetic testing to ongoing surveillance and management. This approach minimises the danger of at-risk family members missing out on recruitment into surveillance programmes when they reach an appropriate age or of their being lost to follow-up. Conversely, other family members can be reassured following normal results on genetic testing, avoiding the costs to both patient and health services of unnecessarily increased surveillance. For families in which a specific genetic cause or syndrome cannot be identified, risk assessment is based on collation of accurate family history data. Although this is time consuming, it usually enables reassurance for the worried well (when risks are low or only marginally elevated) and the offer of appropriate advice or surveillance where risks are increased significantly.

3. Inherited Syndromes Predisposing to Colorectal Cancer

3.1. Familial Adenomatous Polyposis

Historically, the autosomal dominant disorder familial adenomatous polyposis (FAP) has accounted for less than 1% of all colorectal cancers. Familial adenomatous polyposis has a prevalence of around 1 in 8000 [5]. However, colorectal cancer occurs at an early age in patients with FAP unless they are treated by prophylactic colectomy. Effective proactive management of the extended family is therefore extremely important. The hallmark of the syndrome is the development of hundreds to thousands of colonic adenomas (Figure 3.1). These are visible endoscopically from a mean age of 16 years but may be identified in much younger children or may only appear in middle age [6]. By 35 years of age, approximately 95% of (mutant) gene carriers have multiple adenomas detectable at colonoscopy. Without colectomy, colorectal cancer is virtually inevitable and occurs at a mean age of 39 years in untreated patients.

3.1.1. Clinical Features and Diagnosis

Traditionally, FAP has been diagnosed in all individuals with over 100 colorectal adenomas. The adenomas are typically tubular, sessile, and distributed throughout the large bowel. Polyps can also occur elsewhere, particularly in the gastric fundus (where they are usually hamartomatous and occur in approximately 50% of cases) or gastric antrum (where they are usually adenomatous and occur in approximately 10% of cases). However, the risk of development of gastric cancer appears to be only slightly increased [7]. The small bowel is also frequently involved, most commonly in the second or third part of the duodenum (50%–90% of cases) and in

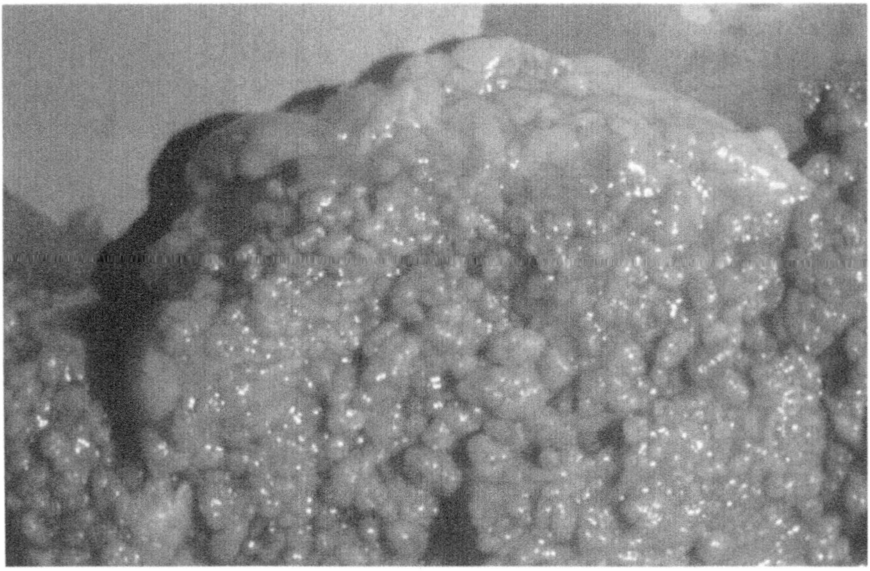

FIGURE 3.1. Macroscopic appearance of the colon in classical familial adenomatous polyposis. The specimen shows dense carpeting of the colonic mucosa with thousands of adenomas.

the periampullary region. There is no clear association between the density of colonic polyps and of upper gastrointestinal polyps. A classification system for duodenal polyps based on their number, size, histology, and degree of dysplasia has been developed [8]. A variety of other organs and tissues can be involved, including the liver (hepatoblastoma), bone (osteomas, particularly in the mandible), teeth (various abnormalities of dentition including absent or supernumerary teeth, cysts, and odontomas) and skin (epidermoid cysts and fibromas). Congenital hypertrophy of retinal pigment epithelium (CHRPE) is found in some families and was used to aid identification of gene carriers prior to the development of DNA testing [9]. These are flat, pigmented lesions of the retina that do not normally cause visual problems. The presence of 2 or more CHRPEs is rare in the general population and the presence of 4 or more is highly indicative of gene carriage in the context of a family history of FAP [10]. Approximately 10% of children and adults with FAP develop desmoid tumours [11]. These are clonal proliferations of myofibroblasts producing locally invasive fibrous tumours that that do not metastasize. Desmoids form predominantly within the abdomen, retroperitoneal tissues, or the abdominal wall, but they may also occur extra-abdominally. They may compress vital organs or complicate abdominal surgery, as they are very vascular. There is a marginal increase in the incidence of tumours of the endocrine glands in FAP, particularly papillary carcinoma of the thyroid.

3.1.2. Genetics and Genotype–Phenotype Correlation

Familial adenomatous polyposis is transmitted as an autosomal dominant trait with complete penetrance but striking variation in expression. A parent with FAP has a 50% chance of passing the disorder to each of his or her offspring. Familial adenomatous polyposis and its variants, attenuated FAP (AFAP) and Gardner's syndrome (FAP with florid extracolonic manifestations), arise from mutations of the adenomatous polyposis coli (*APC*) gene located on the long arm of chromosome 5 [12]. Approximately 70% of FAP families have unique or very infrequent mutations of this gene. A small number of recurrent mutations (e.g. codons 1061 and 1309) account for the remainder [12,13]. Virtually all disease-causing mutations create premature stop codons resulting in truncation of the predicted protein product. Studies of the large (311 kDa) APC protein have revealed multiple functional domains and roles in a variety of cellular functions linked to carcinogenesis. These include regulation of the Wnt signalling pathway, cell adhesion, cell cycle control through interaction with hDLG, chromosome segregation, and apoptosis [14–16]. The location of the inherited (germline) mutation in the *APC* gene has considerable bearing on the clinical manifestations of the disease, including polyp number and the age at which polyposis is manifest, mean age at development of colorectal cancer, and the risk of various extracolonic features. Attenuated familial adenomatous polyposis is associated with smaller numbers of macroscopic polyps (often under 100) and later onset of polyps and cancer (Figure 3.2). It is caused by mutations at the extreme 5′ or 3′ ends of the gene or by mutations in the alternatively spliced region of exon 9 [17,18]. In classical FAP, the greatest numbers of colorectal polyps are seen in patients with germline mutations close to codon 1309 [19] (Figure 3.3). CHRPEs are almost always absent when the mutation occurs 3′ to exon 9 and present where the mutation occurs more 5′ [20]. Extracolonic features such as desmoids, osteomas, and severe gastric and duodenal disease are more commonly associated with mutations between codons 177 and 452 [21]. Intrafamilial variability in FAP may be considerable [22] but disease severity appears to be more similar between first-degree than second-degree relatives, suggesting that modifying genes at other loci may play a role in determining the phenotype. It has also been suggested that functional polymorphisms of the normal *APC* allele may play a role in determining disease severity.

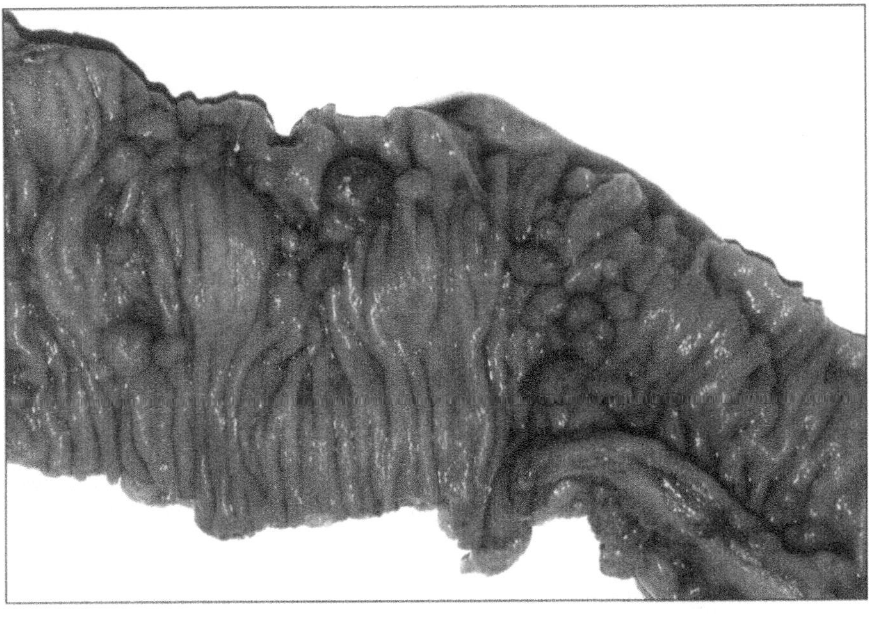

FIGURE 3.2. Macroscopic appearance of the colon in a case with multiple colorectal adenomas. Multiple adenomas are visible, but do not carpet the colonic mucosa. In all, the patient had some 50 adenomas. Similar findings may be seen in attenuated familial adenomatous polyposis and in MYH polyposis, but the underlying cause is often unclear. (Courtesy of Dr N.W. Williams.)

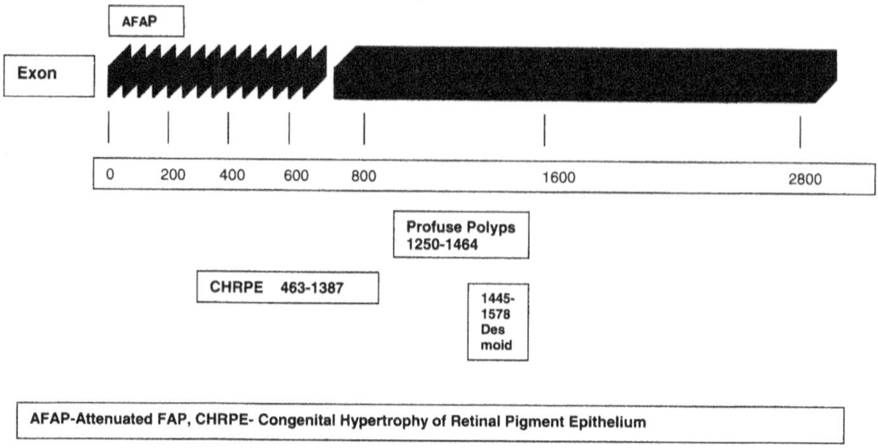

FIGURE 3.3. Correlation of position of germline *APC* mutation with phenotypic manifestations of FAP. Black boxes represent the exons of the *APC* gene (exons 1–14 are relatively small and exon 15 is extremely large). The scale refers to amino-acid residue number in the full-length APC protein. The positions of boxes indicating specific aspects of the FAP phenotype (AFAP, CHRPE, profuse polyposis, and desmoid disease) correspond to the positions of associated truncating mutations relative to the predicted APC protein.

3.1.3. Management

The diagnosis of FAP in the first (index) case in a family should prompt investigation of at-risk members of the extended family and mark the beginning of an ongoing commitment to their proactive management. This role is normally fulfilled by specific polyposis registries that are organised at regional and sometimes national level and to which all affected families should be offered referral. Predictive genetic testing by direct mutation analysis or, when no mutation is identified, by genetic linkage analysis now forms the cornerstone of proactive management for the extended family. It is informative in the vast majority of cases. Diagnosis of FAP in the index case is normally followed by genetic counseling and testing of adult family members and subsequently by genetic testing of further family members once they reach secondary (high) school age. Those who do not carry the mutant *APC* gene can be reassured that neither they nor their offspring are at risk and that no special surveillance will be required. Gene carriers are offered information on the transmission and natural history of FAP, surveillance by annual or biennial colonoscopy, and checks for extracolonic manifestations of FAP (Table 3.1).

There are several reasons for offering genetic testing and counselling between 11 and 14 years of age. First, although colorectal cancer is very rare before 20 years of age in those with FAP, it has been reported occasionally in younger patients [23]. Second, by completing genetic testing at this age, the initial surveillance colonoscopies can be undertaken in a paediatric rather than an adult setting in adolescent gene carriers. Third, it is operationally much easier to see youngsters prior to their leaving the nuclear family. Furthermore, psychological studies have shown that children of early-secondary–school age understand and adapt well to their genetic status and its implications for their subsequent clinical management [24].

Once adenomas develop, surgical options are discussed and definitive elective surgery can be planned. The timing of prophylactic surgery for patients with FAP entails liaison between gastroenterologists, pathologists, and colorectal surgeons and sometimes requires coordination with the educational or career demands of the patient. Surgical options include proctocolectomy with ileoanal pouch formation, colectomy and ileorectal anastomosis, and panproctocolectomy with permanent ileostomy. After colectomy and ileorectal anastomosis, the rectum must be kept under surveillance for life because the risk of cancer in the retained rectum is 12%–29% [25,26]. After restorative proctocolectomy, the anorectal cuff should also be kept under surveillance for life [2].

The risk of FAP-associated extracolonic cancers is of increasing importance as the risk of colorectal cancer is now largely avoided. In particular, the overall lifetime risk of periampullary cancer is 3%–4%, and is likely to become higher [27]. Despite this, the place of upper gastrointestinal surveillance remains controversial. Endoscopic resection of duodenal

TABLE 3.1. Surveillance protocols for family history of colorectal cancer.

Diagnostic group	Gastrointestinal screening procedure	Age at initial screen	Screening interval
FAP and variants	Genetic testing, colonoscopy + OGD	Early teens; colonoscopy age 25 years	Annual, dependant on findings
Juvenile polyposis and Peutz-Jegher's syndrome	Genetic testing, colonoscopy + OGD	Early teens	Annual
HNPCC gene carriers or 50% risk in Amsterdam criteria families or >2 FDR with colorectal cancer	Genetic testing, colonoscopy + OGD	Early 20s or 5 years prior to earliest colorectal cancer in family; gastroscopy age 50 or 5 years prior to earliest gastric cancer in family	Colonoscopy and gastroscopy every 2 years
2 FDR with colorectal cancer	Colonoscopy	At first consultation or age 35–40 years, whichever is later	If initial colonoscopy clear, repeat at 55 years

FDR, first-degree relative; OGD, oesophago-gastro-duodenoscopy.

adenomas is associated with recurrence within 1 year in most cases, while definitive surgery is associated with significant morbidity and mortality. Epigastric pain or obstructive jaundice may suggest periampullary carcinoma and should always be investigated promptly.

Nonsurgical treatments for FAP are currently under investigation. Regression of colorectal and duodenal adenomas has been observed in patients treated with nonsteroidal anti-inflammatory drugs and COX-2 inhibitors, probably though a pro-apoptotic mechanism [28–30]. The results from a number of clinical trials investigating the impact of long-term use of these drugs in FAP are awaited.

3.1.4. Nontruncating Variants of the *APC* Gene and Inherited Colorectal Cancer Risk

Although the role of inherited truncating mutations of *APC* is well established in FAP and AFAP, the possibility that more subtle variants (such as missense mutations) might have functional consequences and predispose to colorectal adenoma and carcinoma has only been investigated more recently.

3.1.4.1. I1307K (3920 T to A)

The point mutation T to A at position 3920 within the *APC* gene has been demonstrated in 6% of all Ashkenazi Jews and about 28% of those with a personal and family history of colorectal cancer. The variant does not appear at a significant frequency in other populations. Rather than altering the function of the APC protein, this mutation changes the local gene sequence from the normal A_3TA_4 to an A_8 tract and apparently leads to hypermutability in the region between APC codons 1296 and 1317. Results from a number of studies indicate that *APC* I1307K carriers have a modestly elevated risk (relative risk 1.7) of developing colorectal cancer.

3.1.4.2. E1317Q (3949 G to C)

Lamlum et al. [31] screened 164 unrelated patients with multiple (3–100) colorectal adenomas for germline variants of *APC* using the mutation detection technique of fluorescent single-strand conformation polymorphism (SSCP) and identified the missense variant E1317Q in 7. By contrast, only 2 of 503 controls showed the same change ($P < .001$, relative risk 11.17). In an earlier study, the same variant was found in 4 out of 116 patients with multiple colorectal adenomas or colorectal cancer and 0 out of 80 controls ($P < .001$) [32]. However, we have also noted E1317Q as an apparently incidental finding in a family with a truncating mutation located more 5′ in *APC* and the variant has also been reported coincidentally in a family with autosomal recessive *MYH* polyposis [33]; further studies are required to confirm whether *APC* E1317Q represents a true colorectal adenoma-carcinoma predisposition allele [34].

3.2. Hereditary Non-polyposis Colorectal Cancer (HNPCC)

3.2.1. Genetics

Hereditary non-polyposis colorectal cancer is an autosomal dominant disorder that predisposes to colorectal and other cancers. Traditionally, HNPCC has been defined on the basis of family-history criteria, initially the Amsterdam criteria and more recently the revised criteria of the International Collaborative Group or ICG (Table 3.2). The disorder is now better defined on the basis of the causative genetic defects. These are inherited mutations in five DNA mismatch repair (MMR) genes, *hMLH1, hMSH2, hPMS1, hPMS2, GTBP/hMSH6*, and possibly also in a sixth, *MSH3*. Mutations in *hMSH2* and *hMLH1* account for the majority of reported HNPCC cases [35]. Families with *GTBP/hMSH6* mutations are being recognised increasingly, while *hPMS1* and hPMS2 appear to be involved only rarely [36]. A wide variety of inherited mutations occur within the MMR genes including both truncating and missense changes. Caution must be exercised before assuming that rare variants are truly pathogenic and can be used for predictive genetic testing. The protein products of the MMR genes form complexes that are involved in repair of alterations in copy number at microsatellite sequences (short repetitive sequences that are scattered throughout the genome) and repair of DNA base mismatches [37,38]. Because of the role of the genes in repair of microsatellite copy number mutations, HNPCC-associated tumours exhibit a distinct pattern of genetic instability termed microsatellite instability (MSI; Figure 3.4). MSI becomes manifest after a somatic mutation or epigenetic silencing has inactivated the second allele of the MMR gene that is mutated in the germline. Mutations within microsatellite sequences then accumulate rapidly with each round of cell division. Although most of these mutations have no phenotypic effect, some arise within tumour suppressor genes and their secondary inactivation is considered to be a key mechanism underlying tumour initiation and progression in HNPCC.

Only a minority of families that fulfil the ICG family history criteria for HNPCC actually harbour a demonstrable germline mutation in one of the MMR genes. A larger proportion exhibit MSI, indicating that some muta-

TABLE 3.2. Amsterdam criteria II [International Collaborative Group] for the diagnosis of HNPCC.

Three or more relatives with histologically verified HNPCC-associated cancer (colorectal, endometrial, small bowel, ureter, or renal pelvis).
One of 3 affected relatives is a first-degree relative of the others.
FAP excluded.
Colorectal cancer involving at least 2 generations.
One or more cancer cases diagnosed before the age of 50.

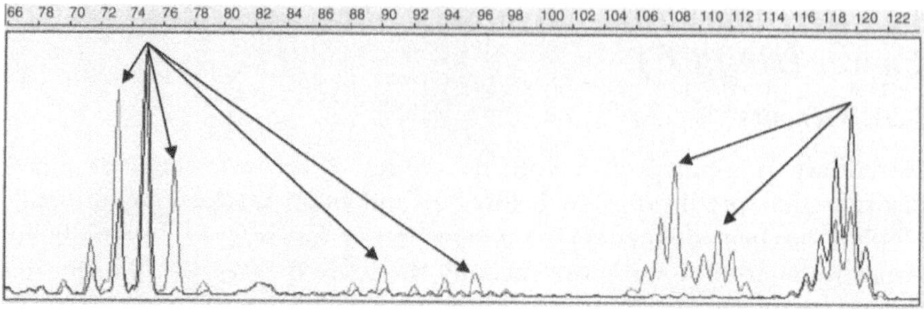

FIGURE 3.4. Microsatellite instability in DNA from an HNPCC-associated colorectal cancer. The traces show genotypes for the markers ACTC (left) and BAT26 (right). Arrows link a constitutional allele for each marker to the novel derivative alleles that are present only in the tumour material. The cancer was from a patient with an inherited mutation in the *hMLH1* gene. (Courtesy of Dr Ian Frayling.)

tions remain undetected by current approaches or that further HNPCC-determining loci exist. Different mechanisms of tumour predisposition are likely to be operating in ICG criteria families in which the tumours are MSI negative and assays for MSI can be helpful in distinguishing these groups of families. In addition, some 15% of sporadic colorectal cancers and a proportion of many other cancers exhibit MSI. This is usually the result of somatic biallelic inactivation of one of the MMR genes and this is often mediated via promoter methylation [39].

3.2.2. Clinical Features and Diagnosis

Hereditary non-polyposis colorectal cancer is probably more prevalent than FAP but is unlikely to account for more than a small percentage of all colorectal cancers [40,41]. It is characterised by colorectal cancers that present at an early age (mean 42 years) [42], with significantly more right-side cancers than is seen in sporadic cases and with significantly more synchronous or metachronous cancers. Polyps (adenomas) may occur but are not a prominent feature and the presence of more than 10 adenomas makes the diagnosis of HNPCC very unlikely. Hereditary-non-polyposis-colorectal-cancer–associated colorectal cancers are usually poorly differentiated and mucinous. They often show signet-ring cell formation and a heavy lymphocytic infiltrate. The prognosis for HNPCC-associated colorectal cancer appears to be significantly better than that for colorectal cancer in general, and this may reflect, at least in part, a better response to chemotherapy with 5-flourouracil [43].

Extracolonic cancers are also frequent in HNPCC and include those of the endometrium, ovary, stomach, small bowel, hepatobiliary tract, ureter, and renal pelvis (Table 3.3). Although the original Amsterdam family history criteria for HNPCC included only colorectal cancers, the revised ICG criteria that are now in common use make allowance for some of the other cancers that constitute the HNPCC spectrum.

Males with MMR gene mutations are at greater risk (to the age of 70) than females of developing any cancer (91% vs 69%) and their risk of developing colorectal cancer is also greater than in females [44]. In females the risk of endometrial cancer is particularly high and a family history fulfilling the ICG criteria and including both endometrial and colorectal cancers is a very strong predictor of an inherited MMR gene mutation [45]. The Muir-Torre syndrome is a variant of HNPCC characterised by the combination of HNPCC-associated cancers and cutaneous sebaceous tumours (sebaceous adenomas and carcinomas and keratoacanthomas) [46]. Turcot syndrome is characterised by colorectal cancer in association with primary brain tumours, particularly glioblastoma multiforme [47] and can be associated with inherited MMR gene mutations. However, some families described as having Turcot syndrome have multiple colonic adenomas and brain tumours and have been found to have germline *APC* mutations.

3.2.3. Management

In the clinical setting, the ICG criteria serve to select those families in which a MMR mutation is likely to be found. However, inherited mutations in the MMR genes may also be identified in patients with colorectal cancer who have less suggestive family histories, including a small proportion of apparently sporadic early-onset colorectal cancer cases. Screening of incident colorectal cancer cases using assays for MSI or immunohistochemical staining for the protein products of the MMR genes in colorectal tumour specimens may facilitate the identification of likely HNPCC cases from the majority of non-HNPCC cases (Figure 3.5). However, these measures have been implemented in only a small proportion of centres. The ICG has recommended that at least 5 microsatellite markers (Bat25, Bat26, D2S123, D5S346, and D17S250) should be assayed to assess MSI and that tumours should be classified as high level (MSI-H), where over 30% of markers show instability, low level (MSI-L), where some but less than 30% of markers show instability; or microsatellite stable, where none show instability.

TABLE 3.3. Cancer risk and age at diagnosis in HNPCC.

Cancer	Lifetime risk for mutation carriers	General population risk	Median age at diagnosis (y)
Colorectal	70%–82%	2%–4%	42
Endometrial	42%–60%	1.5%	49
Gastric	13%	<1%	54
Hepatobiliary	2%	<1%	54
Urinary tract	4%	<1%	60
Ovarian	12%	1%	47
Small intestine	1%–4%	<1%	49

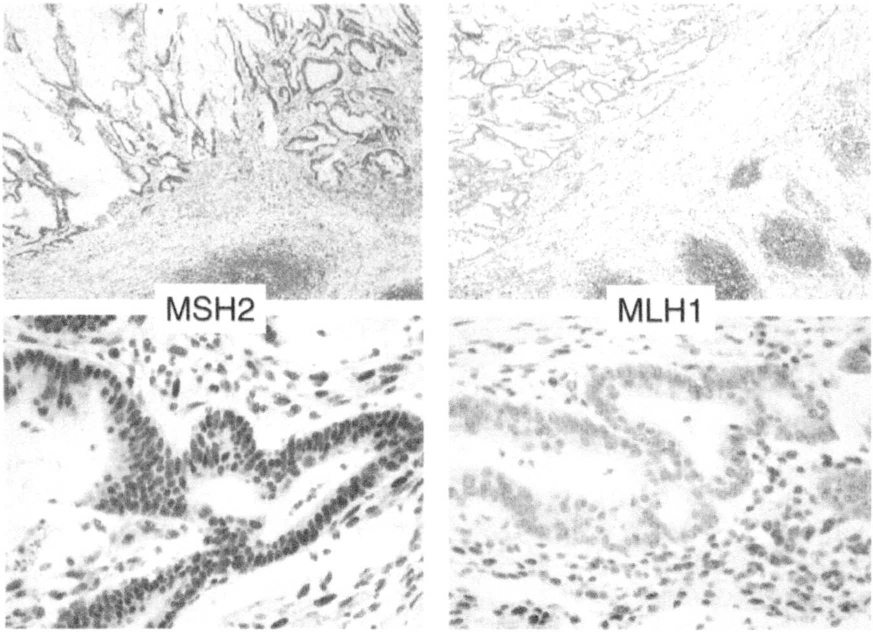

FIGURE 3.5. Immunohistochemical staining for the MSH2 and MLH1 proteins in a mucinous HNPCC-associated colorectal cancer. MSH2 protein (upper- and lower-left panels at low and high magnification, respectively) is abundant in tumour cells and stains strongly. By contrast, MLH1 protein (right) is deficient in tumour cells. Deficiency of protein staining does not, of itself, confirm HNPCC. In an HNPCC patient these appearances would be the result of an inherited mutation affecting one allele of *MLH1* together with somatic inactivation of the second allele in the tumour itself. In a sporadic case of colorectal cancer, these appearances would be the result of two somatic events (mutational or epigenetic) leading to biallelic inactivation of MLH1. Confirmation of HNPCC would therefore require the characterisation of an inherited MLH1 mutation in the constitutional DNA of the patient. (Courtesy of Dr Mark Arends.)

hMLH1- and *hMSH2*-associated tumours are usually MSI-H while *hMSH6* tumours are often MSI-L.

All families with definite or likely HNPCC should be offered registration with clinical genetics services [48] so that family members can receive information on risk, genetic testing, and surveillance for colorectal and other cancers. Verification of pedigree information is an important function of these services as self-reported family histories are often inaccurate [48]. Among families with identified MMR gene mutations, a proactive approach to extended family management based on predictive genetic testing is possible, similar in principle to family management for FAP. Among families fulfilling ICG criteria but without identified mutations, predictive genetic testing by linkage analysis is not usually possible because of locus heterogeneity and the availability of only a limited number of living affected relatives. In this situation, colonoscopic surveillance should be offered to the offspring and siblings of affected individuals and sometimes to a linking but unaffected parent. We suggest biennial total colonic surveillance starting at 21 years of age and continuing to at least 75 years of age (Table 3.1). Incomplete colonoscopy in skilled hands should be followed by a completion barium enema soon after the failed colonoscopy. Less frequent colonoscopy has been associated with an increased risk of interval cancers [49], consistent with an accelerated progression through the adenoma-carcinoma sequence in HNPCC compared to sporadic colorectal tumours. Others have suggested that colonoscopic surveillance only needs to be initiated at 25 years of age [48]. However, because a small proportion of HNPCC-associated colorectal cancers do occur earlier than this and the resource implications of offering earlier surveillance to this group are small, we believe that commencing surveillance at an earlier age is justified.

The efficacy of colonoscopic surveillance in HNPCC was supported by a 15-year follow-up study of 3-yearly colonoscopy in HNPCC gene carriers [50]. Colorectal cancer was identified in 18% of screened cases compared to 41% of unscreened control gene carriers and there were significantly less deaths in the screened group ($P = .003$). It is important that those who stand to benefit from surveillance are not discouraged from participating in genetic testing to clarify their status for fear of genetic discrimination, for example, by health or life insurance companies [51]. An informed debate is required to reach pragmatic solutions and avoid potential genetic discrimination in a range of settings, from employment to insurance and migration. Policy in relation to these issues is still developing and shows considerable international variation.

Surveillance colonoscopy will often identify premalignant adenomas in HNPCC gene carriers and these can usually be dealt with colonoscopically. However, colectomy and ileorectal anastomosis has been recommended for HNPCC patients found to have proximally located cancers as 45% will develop a metachronous second cancer after more limited resection [52]. The risk of cancer of the rectum (around 10%) persists after colectomy and ileorectal anastomosis and continuing surveillance is required [53]. Prophylactic colectomy is not normally considered in HNPCC.

Increasingly, surveillance for extracolonic tumours is being offered to members of likely or proven HNPCC families, although the evidence for this leading to a reduction in morbidity and mortality is poor. Biennial upper gastrointestinal endoscopy commencing at 50 years of age, or 5 years before the earliest gastric cancer case in the family has been suggested in families with a high proportion of gastric cancers [54]. Screening for HNPCC-associated gynaecological cancers in females carrying MMR gene mutations (and those at risk in ICG criteria families without identified mutations) is still under evaluation. Many centres now offer annual transvagninal ultrasound, CA125 measurement, and endometrial biopsy or hysteroscopy from 35 years of age. The effectiveness of these screening strategies is unproven and existing data does not suggest that they provide significant protection from ovarian cancer. Many women in this situation therefore opt for prophylactic hysterectomy and bilateral salpingo-oophorectomy after completion of their families.

3.3. Hamartomatous Polyposis Syndromes

Although rare, the hamartomatous polyposis syndromes have been the focus of considerable genetic research in recent years. This has yielded a number of causative genes. The recognition of these syndromes is important for the appropriate management of patients and their families as they are transmitted as autosomal dominant traits characterised by high penetrance and significant colorectal cancer risk.

3.3.1. Peutz-Jeghers Syndrome

Peutz-Jeghers syndrome (PJS) is defined by the presence of hamartomatous polyps of the small intestine, colon, and rectum that have distinctive histomorphology, including smooth muscle arborisation within the stroma, together with mucocutaneous melanin pigmentation. Polyp numbers vary from 0 to less than 100. Although the distinctive hamartomas are the characteristic lesion, other polyp types may be found, including hyperplastic polyps and adenomas. The risk of colorectal cancer is thought to be 10%–20% [55]. In about one third of cases inactivating mutations can be identified in the gene *STK11* (*LKB1*) [56]. The condition is rare and probably accounts for less than .01% of all colorectal cancers [48]. There appears to be an increased risk of gastric malignancy in PJS, probably in the region of 5%–10%, and of breast cancer in affected females [57]. The small-bowel polyps may lead to paediatric presentation with acute obstruction, but small-bowel cancer is rare. Surveillance protocols have been suggested, based on what is known of the natural history of PJS [48]. These include endoscopy of the upper and lower gastrointestinal tracts, small-bowel imaging (every 3 years), and full blood count (annually) from the early teenage years and annual breast, testicular, and pelvic examination and ultrasound and biennial mammography from the early 20s. However, these measures are of unproven benefit.

3.3.2. Juvenile Polyposis Syndrome

Juvenile polyposis syndrome (JPS) is an aetiologically heterogeneous autosomal dominant disorder characterised by the presence of multiple colorectal polyps with typical hamartomatous features on histopathological examination. Polyps may also occur in the stomach or small intestine. Isolated juvenile polyps are relatively common in youngsters (around 1%

of the population) but JPS is rare (probably not more than 1 in 10000). Juvenile polyposis syndrome is normally defined by the presence of at least 5 polyps with typical histology (dilated cystic glands, infiltration of the lamina propria by inflammatory cells, and abundant stroma) or at least 1 typical polyp in the context of a positive family history. At least 50% of cases are sporadic and are thought to represent new mutations at JPS loci. There may be an excess of congenital malformations and dysmorphic features among JPS cases. Patients may present with bleeding, anaemia, or shedding of colonic polyps via the rectum during the first decades of life, or they may present later with colorectal cancer. The risk of colorectal cancer is probably 30%–50% [58]. Inherited mutations in either the *Smad4 or BMPRa1* gene have been identified in patients and families with sporadic and dominantly transmitted JPS [59], but mutational and linkage studies indicate the presence of other as yet undefined JPS genes. The products of the established JPS genes play roles in the transforming growth factor β (TGF β) pathway. Where a causative mutation is identified, management of at-risk family members can be simplified by genetic testing. Otherwise, the parents and siblings of children with JPS and the offspring of adults with JPS should all be offered colonoscopic surveillance for polyps and cancer every 2 to 3 years, with more frequent review if polyps are detected.

3.3.3. Cowden Syndrome

Hamartomatous polyps of the gastrointestinal tract are also seen in Cowden syndrome (CS), an autosomal dominant disorder characterised by mucocutaneous hamartomas (particularly trichilemmomas) and a high risk of thyroid and breast cancer. Cowden syndrome is caused by inherited mutations in the *PTEN* tumour suppressor gene. Although colorectal cancer has been reported in CS, the risk does not appear to be greatly elevated [60].

3.4. MYH Polyposis

Very recently, mutations in the *MYH* gene on chromosome 1p have been associated with an autosomal recessive trait characterised by multiple colorectal adenomas and a high risk of colorectal cancer. Most patients have 10 to several hundred of adenomas and have been considered previously to have FAP or AFAP on clinical and pathological grounds [33,61]. The distinction of MYH polyposis from FAP/AFAP is important, as, until now, these families have been managed on the assumption of genetic dominance with an implied 50% risk for the offspring of affected cases. By contrast, the risks in MYH polyposis are extremely low for the offspring of affected patients, but 25% for their siblings. Genetic testing for MYH polyposis now enables accurate genetic counselling and appropriate targeting of surveillance for these families. The *MYH* gene is a homologue of the *E. coli* gene

MutY that plays a key role in base excision repair (BER) of DNA damage [62]. The BER pathway has a principal role in the repair of mutations caused by reactive oxygen species that are generated during aerobic metabolism. The MYH protein excises adenine bases that are misincorporated (instead of cytosine) opposite 8-oxo-7,8-dihydro2′deoxyguanosine (8-oxo-dG), a highly mutagenic product of oxidative damage to guanine [63]. Initial reports suggest that the Y165C and G382D mutations account for most Caucasian cases with MYH polyposis while the E466X mutation may be particularly important in patients from the Indian subcontinent [33,61]. Diagnostic strategies based on allele-specific assays may therefore streamline testing for MYH polyposis. Gene carriers should be managed by colonoscopic surveillance and most will require prophylactic surgery as for FAP/AFAP.

4. Estimating and Managing Risk in the Absence of a Defined Genetic Cause

In the United Kingdom (and the United States), the population lifetime risk of developing large-bowel malignancy is approximately 1:25 [64]. The risk is at least doubled for those with an affected first-degree relative. Risks increase further when multiple family members are affected and when colorectal cancer is diagnosed at an early age (Table 3.4). The risk of colorectal cancer is also increased for siblings and parents of patients with adenomatous polyps (relative risk 1.78, increasing to 2.59 if the adenoma is diagnosed before 60 years of age) [65]. The strong correlation between family history and risk is now widely appreciated among both the public and health professionals and this is leading to a rapid increase in use of colonoscopic surveillance for the worried well. The resource implications of ubiquitous screening in this group are immense. Recent recommendations in the United Kingdom [2] have focused on targeting high-risk groups such as those at increased familial risk, but advice to the worried well at lower risk must be explained clearly. Colorectal cancer is so common that its occurrence in some worried individuals who do not fall within screening

TABLE 3.4. Familial colorectal cancer risk.

Risk factor	Relative risk
One first-degree relative with colorectal cancer	2.25 (2.00–2.53)
Parent with colorectal cancer	2.26 (1.87–2.72)
Sibling with colorectal cancer	2.57 (2.19–3.02)
More than 1 first-degree relative with colorectal cancer	4.25 (3.01–6.08)
Relative diagnosed with colorectal cancer before age 45	1.87 (2.40–6.22)
One first-degree relative with colorectal adenoma	1.99 (1.55–2.55)

Adapted from Johns L, Houlston R. *Am J Gastroenterol.* 2001;96:2992–3003.

guidelines is inevitable. Referral to clinical genetic services for verification of family history and risk assessment can help to ensure that resources for colonoscopic surveillance are appropriately targeted. A more inclusive approach to surveillance has been recommended in the United Sates [66], where population level screening at or after age 50 with flexible sigmoidoscopy or colonoscopy has been advocated. Elsewhere recommendations for screening vary considerably. As ever, the spectre of defensive practice driven by medico-legal concerns lurks in the shadow of clinical uncertainty [67].

5. Predisposition to Colorectal Cancer and Chronic Ulcerative Colitis

The lifetime risk of colorectal cancer is markedly increased in individuals with chronic ulcerative colitis (UC) with a reported incidence of between 5.5% and 21% after 20 years of disease, primarily in patients with pancolitis [68]. The presence of UC may increase the genetic risk for an individual based on family history of colorectal cancer. Risk factors that have been implicated in the development of cancer in UC include extensive colonic involvement, long disease duration, early age at disease onset, and presence of primary sclerosing cholangitis.

6. Familial Colorectal Cancer—The Path Ahead

Almost all colorectal cancer susceptibility alleles identified so far are rare but highly penetrant. They account for a significant proportion of colorectal cancers that occur in the context of mendelian transmission, very early age-at-onset, or association with additional phenotypic features. However, most cases attributable to inherited factors do not occur in these settings, but in the context of a limited family history and without additional phenotypic manifestations. The recent delineation of autosomal recessive MYH polyposis confirms that recessive colorectal cancer predisposition genes should not be overlooked. Most recessively determined colorectal cancers would occur as apparently sporadic disease but, until recently, genetic studies have focussed largely on families showing dominant transmission and have assumed that the causative genes will behave as tumour suppressors. The contribution to be made by subtle functional variants in genes that have, until now, been considered mainly in the context of high penetrance traits demands further investigation. Currently only the uncommon *APC* missense variants I1307K and E1317Q have been investigated extensively in this regard. The majority of colorectal cancers that are attributable to inherited predisposition are likely to result from frequent alleles of low penetrance, acting either alone or in combination. These may include functional polymorphisms in genes responsible for metabolism of carcinogens, the antitumour immune response, or DNA repair, for example.

Determining the roles of such alleles at a population level represents a major challenge for the future. Using this knowledge for individual risk determination will not be simple. Different variants are likely to be of importance in different populations and the validation of risks associated with combinations of many variants will be a daunting task. Optimists look forward to a time when simultaneous assay for numerous susceptibility alleles (e.g., using DNA chip technology) will enable accurate computation of individualised risks on which to base screening protocols. Pessimists despair of the potential complexity of inherited predisposition to colorectal cancer and the constraints that are imposed by limited resources for surveillance. Immediate priorities include the implementation of genetic testing for mendelian colorectal cancer syndromes with appropriate evaluation and stratification of familial risk in the nonmendelian setting so that surveillance resources can be allocated accordingly. Meanwhile, the wealth of new knowledge provided by the human genome project will be used to identify further colorectal cancer predisposition genes. This will lead to progressive refinement of individualised risk estimation.

References

1. Dunlop MG. Colorectal cancer genetics. *Semin Cancer Biol.* 1992;3:131–140.
2. Cairns S, Scholefield JH. Guidelines for colorectal cancer screening in high risk groups. *Gut* 2002;51(suppl 5):V1–V2.
3. Sharma VK, Vasudeva R, Howden CW. Colorectal cancer screening and surveillance practices by primary care physicians: results of a national survey. *Am J Gastroenterol.* 2000;95:1551–1556.
4. Batra S, Valdimarsdottir H, McGovern M, Itzkowitz S, Brown K. Awareness of genetic testing for colorectal cancer predisposition among specialists in gastroenterology. *Am J Gastroenterol.* 2002;97:729–733.
5. Bisgaard ML, Fenger K, Bulow S, Niebuhr E, Mohr J. Familial adenomatous polyposis (FAP): frequency, penetrance, and mutation rate. *Hum Mutat.* 1994;3:121–125.
6. Burn J, Chapman PD, Eastham EJ. Familial adenomatous polyposis. *Arch Dis Child.* 1994;71:103–105.
7. Offerhaus GJ, Giardiello FM, Krush AJ, et al. The risk of upper gastrointestinal cancer in familial adenomatous polyposis. *Gastroenterology* 1992;102:1980–1982.
8. Spigelman AD, Williams CB, Talbot IC, Domizio P, Phillips RK. Upper gastrointestinal cancer in patients with familial adenomatous polyposis. *Lancet* 1989;2:783–785.
9. Bertario L, Bandello F, Rossetti C, et al. Congenital hypertrophy of retinal pigment epithelium (CHRPE) as a marker for familial adenomatous polyposis (FAP). *Eur J Cancer Prev.* 1993;2:69–75.

10. Chapman PD, Church W, Burn J, Gunn A. Congenital hypertrophy of retinal pigment epithelium: a sign of familial adenomatous polyposis. *BMJ.* 1989;29: 353–354.
11. Gurbuz AK, Giardiello FM, Petersen GM, et al. Desmoid tumours in familial adenomatous polyposis. *Gut* 1994;35:377–381.
12. Mandl M, Paffenholz R, Friedl W, Caspari R, Sengteller M, Propping P. Frequency of common and novel inactivating APC mutations in 202 families with familial adenomatous polyposis. *Hum Mol Genet.* 1994;3:181–184.
13. Beroud C, Soussi T. APC gene: database of germline and somatic mutations in human tumors and cell lines. *Nucleic Acids Res.* 1996;24:121–124.
14. van Es JH, Giles RH, Clevers HC. The many faces of the tumor suppressor gene APC. *Exp Cell Res.* 2001;264:126–134.
15. Seidensticker MJ, Behrens J. Biochemical interactions in the wnt pathway. *Biochim Biophys Acta.* 2000;1495:168–182.
16. Neufeld KL, Zhang F, Cullen BR, White RL. APC-mediated downregulation of beta-catenin activity involves nuclear sequestration and nuclear export. *EMBO Rep.* 2000;1:519–523.
17. Friedl W, Meuschel S, Caspari R, et al. Attenuated familial adenomatous polyposis due to a mutation in the 3′ part of the APC gene. A clue for understanding the function of the APC protein. *Hum Genet.* 1996;97:579–584.
18. Samowitz WS, Thliveris A, Spirio LN, White R. Alternatively spliced adenomatous polyposis coli (APC) gene transcripts that delete exons mutated in attenuated APC. *Cancer Res.* 1995;55:3732–3734.
19. Nugent KP, Phillips RK, Hodgson SV, et al. Phenotypic expression in familial adenomatous polyposis: partial prediction by mutation analysis. *Gut* 1994;35: 1622–1623.
20. Bunyan DJ, Shea-Simonds J, Reck AC, Finnis D, Eccles DM. Genotype-phenotype correlations of new causative APC gene mutations in patients with familial adenomatous polyposis. *J Med Genet.* 1995;32:728–731.
21. Wallis YL, Macdonald F, Hulten M, et al. Genotype-phenotype correlation between position of constitutional APC gene mutation and CHRPE expression in familial adenomatous polyposis. *Hum Genet.* 1994;94:543–548.
22. Houlston R, Crabtree M, Phillips R, Crabtree M, Tomlinson I. Explaining differences in the severity of familial adenomatous polyposis and the search for modifier genes. *Gut* 2001;48:1–5.
23. Caspari R, Friedl W, Mandl M, et al. Familial adenomatous polyposis: mutation at codon 1309 and early onset of colon cancer. *Lancet* 1994;343:629–632.
24. Michie S, Bobrow M, Marteau TM. Predictive genetic testing in children and adults: a study of emotional impact. *J Med Genet.* 2001;38:519–526.
25. De Cosse JJ, Bulow S, Neale K, et al. Rectal cancer risk in patients treated for familial adenomatous polyposis. The Leeds Castle Polyposis Group. *Br J Surg.* 1992;79:1372–1375.
26. Nugent KP, Phillips RK. Rectal cancer risk in older patients with familial adenomatous polyposis and an ileorectal anastomosis: a cause for concern. *Br J Surg.* 1992;79:1204–1206.
27. Spigelman A, Phillips R. Surveillance of the duodenum in patients with familial adenomatous polyposis. *Gut* 1998;4:144–145.
28. Bresalier RS. Chemoprevention comes to clinical practice: COX-2 inhibition in familial adenomatous polyposis. *Gastroenterology* 2000;119:1797–1798.

29. Oshima M, Murai N, Kargman S, et al. Chemoprevention of intestinal polyposis in the Apcdelta716 mouse by rofecoxib, a specific cyclooxygenase-2 inhibitor. *Cancer Res.* 2001;61:1733–1740.
30. Dobbie Z, Muller PY, Heinimann K, et al. Expression of COX-2 and Wnt pathway genes in adenomas of familial adenomatous polyposis patients treated with meloxicam. *Anticancer Res.* 2002;22:2215–2220.
31. Lamlum H, Al Tassan N, Jaeger E, et al. Germline APC variants in patients with multiple colorectal adenomas, with evidence for the particular importance of E1317Q. *Hum Mol Genet.* 2000;9:2215–2221.
32. Frayling IM, Beck NE, Ilyas M, et al. The APC variants I1307K and E1317Q are associated with colorectal tumors, but not always with a family history. *Proc Natl Acad Sci USA*. 1998;95:10722–10727.
33. Al Tassan N, Chmiel NH, Maynard J, et al. Inherited variants of MYH associated with somatic G:C→T:A mutations in colorectal tumors. *Nat Genet.* 2002;30:227–232.
34. Popat S, Stone J, Coleman G, et al. Prevalence of the APC E1317Q variant in colorectal cancer patients. *Cancer Lett.* 2000;149:203–206.
35. Eshleman JR, Markowitz SD. Mismatch repair defects in human carcinogenesis. *Hum Mol Genet.* 1996;5:1489–1494.
36. Akiyama Y, Sato H, Yamada T, et al. Germ-line mutation of the hMSH6/GTBP gene in an atypical hereditary nonpolyposis colorectal cancer kindred. *Cancer Res.* 1997;57:3920–3923.
37. Lazar V, Grandjouan S, Bognel C, et al. Accumulation of multiple mutations in tumour suppressor genes during colorectal tumorigenesis in HNPCC patients. *Hum Mol Genet.* 1994;3:2257–2260.
38. Konishi M, Kikuchi-Yanoshita R, Tanaka K, et al. Molecular nature of colon tumors in hereditary nonpolyposis colon cancer, familial polyposis, and sporadic colon cancer. *Gastroenterology* 1996;111:307–317.
39. Moslein G, Tester DJ, Lindor NM, et al. Microsatellite instability and mutation analysis of hMSH2 and hMLH1 in patients with sporadic, familial and hereditary colorectal cancer. *Hum Mol Genet.* 1996;5:1245–1252.
40. Aaltonen LA. Molecular epidemiology of hereditary nonpolyposis colorectal cancer in Finland. Recent results. *Cancer Res.* 1998;154:306–311.
41. Lin KM, Shashidharan M, Thorson AG, et al. Cumulative incidence of colorectal and extracolonic cancers in MLH1 and MSH2 mutation carriers of hereditary nonpolyposis colorectal cancer. *J Gastrointest Surg.* 1998;2:67–71.
42. Pensotti V, Radice P, Presciuttini S, et al. Mean age of tumor onset in hereditary nonpolyposis colorectal cancer [HNPCC] families correlates with the presence of mutations in DNA mismatch repair genes. *Genes Chromosomes Cancer.* 1997;19:135–142.
43. Gryfe R, Kim H, Hsieh ET, et al. Tumor microsatellite instability and clinical outcome in young patients with colorectal cancer. *N Engl J Med.* 2000;342: 69–77.
44. Dunlop MG, Farrington SM, Carothers AD, et al. Cancer risk associated with germline DNA mismatch repair gene mutations. *Hum Mol Genet.* 1997;6: 105–110.
45. Planck M, Rambech E, Moslein G, et al. High frequency of microsatellite instability and loss of mismatch-repair protein expression in patients with double

primary tumors of the endometrium and colorectum. *Cancer* 2002;94:2502–2510.
46. Cohen PR, Kohn SR, Kurzrock R. Association of sebaceous gland tumors and internal malignancy: the Muir-Torre syndrome. *Am J Med.* 1991;90:606–613.
47. Hamilton SR, Liu B, Parsons RE, et al. The molecular basis of Turcot's syndrome. *N Engl J Med.* 1995;332:839–847.
48. Dunlop MG. Guidance on gastrointestinal surveillance for hereditary nonpolyposis colorectal cancer, familial adenomatous polypolis, juvenile polyposis, and Peutz-Jeghers syndrome. *Gut* 2002;51(suppl 5):V21–V27.
49. Vasen HF, Nagengast FM, Khan PM. Interval cancers in hereditary nonpolyposis colorectal cancer [Lynch syndrome]. *Lancet* 1995;345:1183–1184.
50. Jarvinen HJ, Aarnio M, Mustonen H, et al. Controlled 15-year trial on screening for colorectal cancer in families with hereditary nonpolyposis colorectal cancer. *Gastroenterology* 2000;118:829–834.
51. Lapham EV, Kozma C, Weiss JO. Genetic discrimination: perspectives of consumers. *Science* 1996;274:621–624.
52. Church JM. Prophylactic colectomy in patients with hereditary nonpolyposis colorectal cancer. *Ann Med.* 1996;28:479–482.
53. Rodriguez-Bigas MA, Vasen HF, Pekka-Mecklin J, et al. Rectal cancer risk in hereditary nonpolyposis colorectal cancer after abdominal colectomy. International Collaborative Group on HNPCC. *Ann Surg.* 1997;225:202–207.
54. Aarnio M, Mecklin JP, Aaltonen LA, Nystrom-Lahti M, Jarvinen HJ. Life-time risk of different cancers in hereditary non-polyposis colorectal cancer [HNPCC] syndrome. *Int J Cancer.* 1995;64:430–433.
55. Giardiello FM, Offerhaus JG. Phenotype and cancer risk of various polyposis syndromes. *Eur J Cancer.* 1995;31A:1085–1087.
56. Hemminki K, Li X. Familial colorectal adenocarcinoma from the Swedish Family-Cancer Database. *Int J Cancer.* 2001;94:743–748.
57. Boardman LA, Pittelkow MR, Couch FJ, et al. Association of Peutz-Jeghers-like mucocutaneous pigmentation with breast and gynecologic carcinomas in women. *Medicine (Baltimore).* 2000;79(5):293–298.
58. Howe JR, Mitros FA, Summers RW. The risk of gastrointestinal carcinoma in familial juvenile polyposis. *Ann Surg Oncol.* 1998;5:751–756.
59. Woodford-Richens K, Bevan S, Churchman M, et al. Analysis of genetic and phenotypic heterogeneity in juvenile polyposis. *Gut* 2000;46:656–660.
60. Eng C. Genetics of Cowden syndrome: through the looking glass of oncology. *Int J Oncol.* 1998;12:701–710.
61. Jones S, Emmerson P, Maynard J, et al. Biallelic germline mutations in MYH predispose to multiple colorectal adenoma and somatic G:C→T:A mutations. *Hum Mol Genet.* 2002;11:2961–2967.
62. Ohtsubo T, Nishioka K, Imaiso Y, et al. Identification of human MutY homolog [hMYH] as a repair enzyme for 2-hydroxyadenine in DNA and detection of multiple forms of hMYH located in nuclei and mitochondria. *Nucleic Acids Res.* 2000;28:1355–1364.
63. Hayashi H, Tominaga Y, Hirano S, McKenna AE, Nakabeppu Y, Matsumoto Y. Replication-associated repair of adenine:8-oxoguanine mispairs by MYH. *Curr Biol.* 2002;12:335–339.
64. Dunlop MG. Colorectal cancer. *BMJ.* 1997;314:1882–1885.

65. Bishop DT, Hall NR. The genetics of colorectal cancer. *Eur J Cancer.* 1994; 30A:1946–1956.
66. American Gastroenterological Association medical position statement: hereditary colorectal cancer and genetic testing. *Gastroenterology* 2001;121:195–197.
67. Lynch HT, Paulson J, Severin M, Lynch J, Lynch P. Failure to diagnose hereditary colorectal cancer and its medicolegal implications: a hereditary nonpolyposis colorectal cancer case. *Dis Colon Rectum.* 1999;42:31–35.
68. Eaden JA, Maybery JF. Guidelines for screening and surveillance of asyptomatic colorectal cancer in patients with inflammatory bowel disease. *Gut* 2002; 51(suppl 5):V10–V12.

4
Advances in the Medical Treatment of Crohn's Disease

SARA MCCARTNEY and MICHAEL J.G. FARTHING

1. Introduction

Crohn's disease is a chronic inflammatory condition of the gastrointestinal tract arising in genetically susceptible individuals as a result of either an appropriate immunological response to a luminal antigen or an inappropriate or prolonged immunological response to the normal microflora of the gut. Specific targeting of this response with immunomodulatory regimens is likely to prove the way forward in the management of Crohn's disease, rather than relying on blanket immunosuppression with its associated side effects (Table 4.1).

There is little doubt that further development of treatment strategies is necessary. The incidence of Crohn's disease has risen steadily in most of the regions where repeated studies have been carried out. Annual incidence figures from both Europe and North America lie mostly between 2 and 6 per 100,000 [1–3]. Interestingly, over the last 2 decades the incidence figures in the under-16 age group have shown a more dramatic increase, from a mean of 1.3 cases per 100,000 from 1983 to 1988, to a mean of 3.1 per 100,000 between 1989 and 1993 [4]. As disease prevalence and chronicity increase, so does the awareness of the inadequacy of current therapy. This inadequacy drives forward the search for new approaches to treatment. This is particularly important because standard therapies fail to induce remission in approximately 30% of patients and there is a lack of efficacious maintenance regimens.

In this chapter we discuss both the current role and the new developments in the use of established treatments such as 5-aminosalicylate (5-ASA) drugs and corticosteroids that remain the mainstay of management of Crohn's disease. In addition, we will explore when and how to use the newer immunomodulatory drugs and biological therapies for steroid-efractory or steroid-dependent disease or when surgery is inappropriate (Table 4.2). Early trials, however, indicate spontaneous remission rates of up to 30% in Crohn's disease.

Table 4.1. Targets for new therapy in Crohn's disease.

Drug target	Agent evaluated	Efficacy to date	Current position/ indication/comments
Differentiation of CD4+ T-helper lymphocytes into Th1 and Th2	Anti–interferon-γ antibody	Efficacy in animal models, human trials underway	Results awaited
	Anti–interleukin-12 antibody	Human dose-finding studies in progress	Results awaited
	Interleukin 10	No benefit in placebo-controlled trials	Try alternative methods of administration
Lymphocyte trafficking	Anti-α4 integrin antibody (natalizumab)	Significant clinical response in RCT	Phase III and maintenance trials underway
	Anti-$\alpha 4\beta 7$ integrin antibody	Placebo-controlled dose-finding trials in progress	Results awaited
	Anti-sense ICAM-1 (Isis 2302)	No benefit in 2 large RCTs	Trial ensuring high serum dose underway
Tumour-necrosis-factor mediated	Chimeric anti–tumour necrosis-factor antibody (infliximab)	Efficacious,increasingly widely used, maintenance benefit	Refractory or fistulating disease
	Humanised anti–tumour necrosis-factor antibody (CDP571)	Placebo-controlled trials show benefit	Large placebo-controlled phase III studies underway
		RCT failed to show benefit	
	Tumour-necrosis-factor receptor fusion protein (etanercept)	Benefit shown in small dose-finding study	Large placebo-controlled phase II study in progress
	p55 tumour-necrosis-factor–binding protein (onercept) CNI-1493	Benefit in uncontrolled pilot study	Larger RCT necessary
	Thalidomide	Efficacious in uncontrolled pilot studies	Significant fistula closure
Miscellaneous	Interferon β-1a	Positive pilot study	Phase-IIb trial planned
	Granulocyte macrophage-colony–stimulating factor	Positive pilot studies	Suggest benefit in fistulating disease
	Interleukin 11	Negative phase-IIa dose-response study	Phase III trial halted after interim analysis

RCT, randomised controlled trial.

TABLE 4.2. Comparative features of efficacious drugs in Crohn's disease.

Feature	Corticosteroids	Azathioprine/6-MP	Methotrexate	Infliximab
Indication	Acute severe Crohn's disease	Steroid-sparing agent first-line treatment for repeat flares	Steroid/azathioprine-refractory, Azathioprine intolerant Crohn's disease	Fistulating disease, bridge to methotrexate therapy in drug refractory patients
Speed of action	24–72 h	8–12 wk	8 wk	2–4 wK
Ease of administration	Oral	Oral	Intramuscualr injection	Intravenous infusion
Toxicity	Well-documented short- and long-term side effects	Nausea, myelosuppression, pancreatitis	Hepatic fibrosis, pulmonary fibrosis/pneumonitis, myelosuppression	HACA formation, anaphylaxis, tuberculosis activation, potential stricturing
Cost	Inexpensive	Inexpensive	Inexpensive, but may be expensive to administer	Expensive
Use in pregnancy	Yes, if essential; risk of adrenal suppression in high dose	Yes, if essential; good safety profile but relatively limited data	Contraindicated	Very limited data, no guidelines at present.
Risk of malignancy	No increase	Probable small overall increase in risk	Low or absent, little data in inflammatory bowel disease	Early reports of increased lymphomas, further data awaited
Use in maintenance of remission	No	Yes	Yes	Yes, further results awaited

HACA, human anti-chimeric antibody.

2. Update on Established Treatment

2.1. The New Corticosteroids

Corticosteroids, in the form of intravenous hydrocortisone or oral prednisolone, remain one of the traditional mainstays of treatment for acute exacerbations of Crohn's disease due to their efficacy and speed of action. Prolonged use is limited by their adverse effects and there is an increasing vogue to avoid them altogether. There appears to be no difference between equivalent doses of methylprednisolone, prednisolone, and hydrocortisone, although intravenous administration does offer benefit in refractory cases. Most gastroenterologists treat moderate to severe Crohn's disease with a starting dose of 40 mg/d prednisolone or 0.5–1 mg/kg body weight. In severe disease or when absorption is likely to be impaired, 50–100 mg hydrocortisone intravenously 4 times daily is an effective dose. These doses can be tapered fairly rapidly depending on clinical response, although there are limited data available on the optimal rate of reduction. As steroids have no role in maintaining remission [5], they should be completely withdrawn or, if necessary, used as a bridge while an immunomodulatory drug such as azathioprine is introduced.

The newer, orally administered corticosteroids are designed to increase intraluminal drug concentrations but limit systemic availability either through high-affinity receptor binding or by undergoing extensive hepatic metabolism. Budesonide utilises an additional pH-dependent mechanism. By coating the drug with acrylic resin (Eudragit®, Roehm), which dissolves at pH 6 or 7, delivery to the terminal ileum and colon is enhanced. As a result, only about 10% of the absorbed drug reaches the systemic circulation. Greenberg et al. assessed the efficacy of 3 mg, 9 mg, and 15 mg of budesonide in 258 patients with active ileal or ileocaecal Crohn's disease [6]. This identified 9 mg as the optimal dose in terms of maximal efficacy with minimal adrenal suppression. Fifty-one percent of patients entered remission on 9 mg of budesonide daily (defined as a fall in the CDAI to less than 150), compared to 43% receiving 15 mg and 33% receiving 3 mg. When an initial dose of 9 mg of budesonide was compared directly to 40 mg of prednisolone in tapering dose in 176 patients, both drugs were efficacious in inducing remission in 53% and 66% of patients, respectively. However, the prednisolone group did have significantly reduced CDAI scores, although this was accompanied by a significant reduction in the morning plasma cortisol concentration, suggesting a higher level of systemic absorption, and, thus, steroid-related side effects [7].

There appears to be a good argument for switching patients with steroid-dependent ileocecal Crohn's disease to budesonide in view of the reduced glucocorticoid side effects [8], although it remains of unproven benefit in specific situations such as limiting growth impairment in paediatric Crohn's disease [9]. It is clear, however, from recent meta-analyses that oral budesonide, like prednisolone, is not effective as maintenance therapy in preventing relapses of Crohn's disease and should not be prescribed as such [10].

More recent trials have focused on comparing budesonide 9 mg daily to mesalamine 2 g twice daily for treatment of mild-to-moderate Crohn's disease. The remission rates were significantly better in those receiving budesonide than mesalamine, 69% versus 45% ($P = .001$) and although the morning cortisol levels were reduced in one third of the patients on budesonide, this did not reach statistical significance [11]. The addition of antibiotics to budesonide failed to show any benefit for patients with ileal disease although there is some possible benefit in the setting of colonic disease [12].

In current clinical practice budesonide is a useful, safe drug for treating moderately active Crohn's disease, but severe attacks are still probably best managed with the traditional corticosteroids despite their higher incidence of adverse effects. Drug development continues in this area of highly topically active but systemically inert preparations and it is likely further preparations will become available.

2.2. *Azathioprine and 6-Mercaptopurine*

These drugs have been used for many years as steroid-sparing agents and in refractory or recurrent disease. Azathioprine is metabolised almost completely to 6-methylmercaptopurine (6-MP) and subsequently by thiopurine methyltransferase (TPMT) to 6-MP or to active 6-thioguanine nucleotides. The main development in managing patients on these drugs is the measurement of TPMT levels to ensure they can adequately metabolise the drug. Myelosuppression is much more common in patients who are heterozygotes for TPMT deficiency and almost invariable for those homozygotes. The therapeutic dose can therefore be pushed to higher levels in nonresponders with high TPMT levels, but needs to be carefully monitored or avoided in those with low and absent levels, respectively. Studies from the 1980s confirm efficacy in induction of remission, reduction in steroid requirement, benefit in maintenance of remission, and an increase in fistula closure rate [13–15], and these findings have been endorsed by recent meta-analyses [16,17]. A recent trial has shown that the addition of 6-MP to a corticosteroid regimen at the start of therapy in children with moderate-to-severe Crohn's disease significantly reduces both the need for steroids and improves maintenance of remission [18]. It remains unclear, however, whether continued treatment with azathioprine rather than 5-ASA preparations after surgery is appropriate particularly when the disease is felt to be cleared [19]. A pragmatic approach is to reassess the disease 6 months postoperatively and to commence treatment if there is evidence of clinical or endoscopic recurrence.

2.3. Cyclosporin

Although of proven benefit in acute severe ulcerative colitis, the experience of using cyclosporin has been less promising in refractory Crohn's disease. Of a series of randomised, double-blind placebo-controlled trials, only one [20] shows a significant benefit (50% clinical improvement vs 32% in controls, $P = .032$) while the others show no benefit or actual deterioration in symptoms [21,22]. Questions have been raised regarding dosing regimens and routes of administration. These variables could perhaps be optimised but at present, in view of the toxicity and relapse rate, there is little clinical indication to use cyclosporin outside of a formal trial setting.

2.4. 5-ASAs in Crohn's Disease

As 5-ASA acts primarily on intestinal epithelial cells, it is likely to be more efficacious in the treatment of mucosal inflammation such as in ulcerative colitis rather than the transmural disease found in Crohn's. Sulphasalazine is the original and cheapest of the alternatives and shows comparable efficicacy to the newer preparations. However, most of the alternatives are perceived to have fewer side effects, although sulphasalazine does remain the drug of choice in patients with significant associated arthropathy. Most of the evidence shows that 5-ASA drugs are more useful in remission of ulcerative colitis than Crohn's disease. High-dose mesalazine in the form of Pentasa® (Ferring A/S Corp) 4 g/d has been shown to decrease the rate of relapse after surgical resection for small-bowel Crohn's disease [23]. The effects were limited to small-bowel disease only and no benefit was noted in ileocolonic disease. As the therapeutic effects are primarily achieved by high intraluminal drug concentrations, formulations with less systemic absorption are likely to offer benefit while minimising side effects. 5-Aminosalicylate in a dose of 3 g/d has also been compared to a fairly modest 50 mg 6-MP [24] in the postoperative setting. However, while endoscopic relapse was reduced in the group receiving 6-MP, clinical relapse was the same in both groups though significantly lower with either drug than in the placebo group.

One newly emerging benefit of all 5-ASA treatments is their role in colorectal cancer prophylaxis and although the case is better established in ulcerative colitis, patients with total Crohn's colitis may also experience significant risk reductions [25].

2.5. Antibiotics

While the immune defect in Crohn's disease remains uncertain, a gene for the disease was identified encoding NOD2/CARD 15, a protein involved in the recognition of microbes and the subsequent signalling that triggers the immune response, thus linking enteric bacteria to the development of disease. Metronidazole is well established in the treatment of Crohn's disease, particularly in association with fistulating perianal disease [26,27]. Unfortunately, prolonged usage tends to be limited by the development of peripheral neuropathy.

The combination of metronidazole and ciprofloxacin appears to have a synergistic effect and is highly efficacious in patients with colonic disease in particular [28]. In the postoperative setting, Rutgeerts et al. showed modest benefit at 1 year when the equivalent of 400 mg metronidazole was taken 3 times daily for 3 months following surgical resection [29]. The same group studied ornidazole postoperatively and again showed significantly reduced clinical and endoscopic recurrence of disease (although with a high incidence of peripheral neuropathy). These reductions were shown in both endoscopic (at 3 months and 12 months) and clinical recurrence at 12 months, although significantly more patients dropped out in the treatment group and the benefits were not sustained for more than 1 year [30].

Specific antituberculous regimens have been assessed following publication of data showing the presence of *Mycobacterium paratuberculosis* DNA in surgical resection samples of 65% of patients with Crohn's disease compared with 12.5% of normal controls [31]. The results are equivocal; a 2-year outcomes analysis of 46 patients treated with rifabutin in combination with a macrolide antibiotic (clarithromycin or azithromycin) indicated a response in terms of reduction in the steroid requirement, Harvey-Bradshaw CDAI, and improvement in inflammatory parameters particularily in those with widespread disease [32]. A double-blind trial of 51 patients showed improvements in those who had both streptomycin and rifabutin compared to those receiving streptomycin alone, although it was of note that treatment with conventional therapies continued throughout the trial period. Contrary to this, a controlled trial assessing 111 patients who received 2 years of treatment with antituberculous chemotherapy showed no clinical benefit either immediately after completion of treatment or after further follow up 3 years later [33]. The net result is that these regimens have not been used extensively outside the trial setting, although within that context do appear to be remarkably well tolerated. Thus, in view of the disappointing results in the randomised controlled trials, there seems to be little evidence to recommend the use of these multidrug regimens outside the setting of a randomised controlled trial.

3. The New Therapies

3.1. Biological Therapies

These radical new therapies include monoclonal antibodies, therapeutic peptides, nucleic-acid–based therapies such as antisense oligonucleotides and cell- and gene-based therapies. They have developed as a result of an increased understanding of immunological mechanisms in inflammation. The Th1 response seen in Crohn's disease is characterised by initial increased expression of IL-2, IL-12, and IL-18, followed by an increase in the production of TNFα, IL-1β, and NF-KB. To a lesser extent, a simultaneous increase is seen in Th2-mediated anti-inflammatory cytokines such as IL-10 and TGFβ. Therefore, in Crohn's disease the pro-inflammatory cytokines represent suitable targets for therapy. However the biologicals have several notable disadvantages including restricted administration via nonoral routes, the potential for immunogenicity, and considerable expense.

Inhibition of TNFα by a variety of approaches is currently the most proven clinically useful of these treatments for refractory Crohn's disease. TNFα has been measured in increased concentrations in both normal and inflamed mucosa from patients with Crohn's disease, suggesting an early key role in the inflammatory cascade. In addition, transgenic animal models engineered to overexpress TNFα develop a granulomatous enteropathy and arthritis, and blockade of TNFα is efficacious in treating inflammation in a number of animal models of inflammatory bowel disease [34,35]. Initial antigen binding to receptors on lymphocytes triggers further lymphocyte amplification and differentiation with resultant cytokine synthesis. As a result, increasing levels of circulating TNFα bind to transmembrane TNFα receptors and via NFkB activation initiate further pro-inflammatory cytokine production. Subsequent activation of other inflammatory pathways results in stimulation of the arachidonic acid pathway including up-regulation of cyclooxygenase 2 (COX-2) and inducible nitric oxide synthase (iNOS), up-regulation of adhesion molecules, and ligation of the death receptor TNFRI leading to increased apoptosis. TNFα is integral to the control of lymphocyte trafficking, resulting in the recruitment of inflammatory cells from the systemic circulation to the site of inflammation. These effects are largely via the increased expression of adhesion molecules including intercellular adhesion molecule-1 (ICAM-1), vascular cell adhesionmolecule-1 (VCAM-1), and mucosal-addressin cellular adhesion molecule-1 (Mad-CAM-1), along with integrins and selectins. Limitation of the effects of these adhesion molecules may prove therapeutic by reducing lymphocyte attraction and cell transmigration to the gut mucosa. Monoclonal antibodies in the form of infiximab and CDP571, the soluble TNFα receptor fusion protein etanercept, soluble TNFα receptor onercept, the MAPKinase inhibitor CNI-1493, and thalidomide all act to limit TNFα production and secretion while inhibitors of lymphocyte trafficking limit the subsequent inflammatory response. The efficacy and therapeutic potential of these agents will be discussed in more detail.

3.1.1. Infliximab

Infliximab is a genetically engineered murine-human chimeric antibody comprised of 75% human and 25% murine protein. It is thought to act by neutralising both soluble and transmembrane TNFα, in addition to causing lysis of TNFα-producing cells by complement fixation, antibody-dependent cytotoxicity, and apoptosis of T-lymphocytes.

Successful initial open-label studies led the way for a placebo-controlled trial of infliximab at doses ranging from 5–20 mg/kg [36]. By 4 weeks, 48% of patients had responded to 5 mg/kg of infliximab with higher doses being less efficacious with a 25% response and only 4% of the placebo patients achieving remission. Remission was defined as reduction in the Crohn's Disease Activity Index [37] to <150 points. Nonresponders were subsequently treated with 10 mg/kg of infliximab in an open-label study. Finally, responders from both studies were randomised at 12 weeks into a further study involving re-treatment at 8 weekly intervals. Fifty-three percent of these patients maintained remission to week 44 (compared with 20% on placebo), however, many subsequently relapsed between weeks 44 and 48 suggesting that the benefit is sustained for approximately 8 weeks [38]. Results from a larger re-treatment study have recently been reported in 573 patients following an initial open dose of 5 mg/kg of infliximab. Three hundred and thirty-five patients (59%) responded to initial treatment and were subsequently randomised to either placebo infusions, infliximab at 5 mg/kg for 2 induction doses (2 and 6 weeks) then 5 mg/kg every 8 weeks (group II), or infliximab with the same induction regimen but 10 mg/kg every 8 weeks (group III). The primary end-point was patients in remission at week 30, again defined by a CDAI of less than 150. Twenty-two percent of the placebo group versus 39% of group II and 46% of group III achieved clinical remission. These results were highly statistically significant with *P* values of .003 and .001, respectively. In addition, the study demonstrated that the 3-dose induction regimen was superior at inducing remission than a single induction dose (40% vs 28%) and that closure of Crohn's disease fistulas was maintained more effectively in re-treated patients [39]. In summary, patients with Crohn's disease initially responding to a 5 mg/kg dose of infliximab are more likely to be in remission at weeks 30 and 54, to discontinue corticosteroids, and to maintain their response for a longer period of time, if infliximab treatment is maintained every 8 weeks. A number of other trials have also confirmed the efficacy of infliximab therapy and in addition emphasised its usefulness in fistulating disease [40,41]. Several questions continue to remain unanswered such as the long-term safety of infliximab as a steroid-sparing agent and its efficacy in ulcerative colitis.

One of the major disadvantages of this treatment is the development of human antichimeric antibodies (HACAs) which may lead to loss of efficacy and an increase in the percentage of infusion reactions. The reported level of antibody formation in clinical trials is relatively low at 13% [42], but this seems highly dependent on the assay used as other studies report much more significant levels with cumulative frequencies of 36%–68% [43,44]. Infusion reactions, usually consisting of urticaria, dyspnoea, and hypotension, occurred in 17% of trial patients compared with 7% of placebo [42]. The frequency of HACA formation may be reduced in patients either on immunomodulatory therapy or receiving corticosteroids [45]. More worryingly, delayed hypersensitivity reactions with symptoms including myalgia, arthralgia, fever, pruritis, oedema, urticaria, sore throat, and headache are reported in 25% of re-treated patients after treatment free periods of between 2 and 4 years [46]. In addition there is concern regarding increased formation of antinuclear antibodies (ANAs) and anti–double-stranded DNA antibodies with occasional development of the features of drug-induced lupus [47]. Although most of this data is currently available in abstract form, many units are now treating patients with a single intravenous dose of hydrocortisone prior to receiving their infliximab infusion.

Infection particularly with tuberculosis, and, to a lesser extent, listeriosis, histoplasmosis, and aspergillosis remains a major concern following infliximab therapy. There were 70 reported cases of tuberculosis following treatment with infliximab, 48 of these occurring after 3 or less infusions, which was much higher than the reported frequency of other opportunistic infections. Current recommendations include screening for latent tuberculosis with tuberculin skin testing followed by chest X-ray in those with a positive skin test [48,49]. Patients with a history of tuberculosis must be reassessed and treated appropriately prior to starting infliximab therapy.

Long-term follow up of patients receiving infliximab is required before the risk of increased malignancy can be fully ascertained. Currently the risk appears relatively low, although recently a total 26 cases of lymphoma were reported to the United States Food and Drug Administration of which 81% were non-Hodgkin's lymphoma [50]. The interval between initiation of therapy with etanercept (18 cases) or infliximab (8 cases) and the development of lymphoma was very short, with a median time of 8 weeks and in 2 instances withdrawal of the drug was sufficient to precipitate lymphoma regression.

Infliximab is currently not recommended during pregnancy mainly due to a lack of sufficient safety data. However, it has been used extensively in paediatric Crohn's disease including in maintenance regimens in the United States without obvious complication, although again results of longer-term studies in this patient group are awaited.

3.1.2. CDP571

CDP571 is a genetically engineered humanised IgG4 antibody specific for human TNFα. It consists of approximately 95% human protein and only 5% murine protein and in theory less immunogenic than infliximab. The mechanism of action is likely to be neutralisation of soluble and transmembrane TNFα. Stack et al. reported the first randomised controlled trial of CDP571 showing that following a single dose of 5 mg/kg there was a significant decrease in Crohn's disease activity at 2 weeks compared to placebo in 1997 [51]. In a larger study of 169 patients with moderate-to-severe Crohn's disease, patients were randomised to receive a single dose of CDP571 either at 10 or 20 mg/kg; patients were then re-treated with 10 mg/kg at 8 weekly intervals. At 2 weeks, 54% of patients receiving 10 mg/kg had a clinical response (drop in CDAI of >70 points) compared to 37% response in those receiving 20 mg/kg, and a placebo response of 27%. There was also a trend towards a greater rate of remission in treated patients at 24 weeks and an increased rate of fistula closure, but the only results to reach statistical significance were in placebo-treated patients compared with those receiving 10 mg/kg of CDP571 [52]. Another study on 71 patients with steroid-dependent Crohn's disease treated with 20 mg/kg CDP571 at baseline and 10 mg/kg at 8 weeks found 44% of patients maintained remission and successfully discontinued steroids compared with 22% receiving placebo [53]. Further studies are awaited to confirm efficacy in acute disease, its use as a steroid-sparing agent, and the appropriateness of maintenance regimens.

Anti-idiotype antibody formation, infusion reactions, and the development of anti–double-stranded DNA antibodies all occurred but to a lesser degree than following infliximab use, as might be expected. Drug induced lupus, non-Hodgkin's lymphoma, and delayed hypersensitivity reactions have not been reported but this may simply reflect the limited clinical use of CDP571 to date.

3.1.3. Etanercept

Etanercept is a genetically engineered human soluble TNFα receptor fusion protein that acts by neutralising soluble TNFα. As there is no murine element, theoretically it should be less immunogenic than either infliximab or CDP571. It has been used widely and successfully in rheumatoid arthritis but the experience in Crohn's disease is much more limited. A pilot study on 10 patients with active Crohn's disease receiving 25 mg of etanercept by subcutaneous injection twice weekly for 12 weeks reported a clinical response (decrease in CDAI of >70 points) in 6 of the 10 patients [54]. A larger randomised placebo-controlled trial involving 43 patients subsequently failed to demonstrate any benefit and raised the question as to whether higher or more frequent dosing than is currently used in the rheumatoid population was required [55].

3.1.4. Onercept

Onercept is a recombinant human TNF-binding protein (TBP-1). Like etanercept it is wholly of human origin and therefore should have little immunogenicity. The mechanism of action has not been fully elucidated but is likely to relate to neutralisation of soluble TNFα.

Preliminary studies indicated that in 12 patients treated with 50 mg of TBP-1 subcutaneously 3 times a week for 2 weeks, 5 of 6 patients showed a clinical response and 4 of 6 patients achieved remission. The lower dose tested (11.7 mg) was not efficacious. The drug was well tolerated and no antibodies were found at the end of follow up, confirming it to be nonimmunogenic. Once more, larger, longer term studies are required [56].

3.1.5. Thalidomide

Thalidomide is not a biologic therapy per se but because of its anti-TNFα action it is most appropriate to include it in this section.

The mechanism of action appears to be by selective reduction in TNFα production by lipopolysaccharide- (LPS) stimulated monocytes [57] as a result of enhanced degradation of TNFα mRNA. Thalidomide also has the additional effect of inhibiting IL-12. Despite being a relatively weak TNFα inhibitor (at high drug concentrations, total inhibition of TNFα production by inflammatory cells is not achieved), efficacy has been reported in a wide range of conditions including erythema nodosum leprosum, Behcet's syndrome, aphthous stomatitis complicating HIV, and pyoderma gangrenosum. Several small open-label pilot studies, including one in paediatric patients, have shown benefit in steroid-dependent or refractory Crohn's disease [58]. Vasiliauskas et al. report response rates of 67% and remission rates of 0%–33% using 50–100 mg daily in patients with active inflammatory Crohn's disease [59]. Ehrenpreis et al. used a higher dose of 200–300 mg daily in patients with active inflammatory and fistulising disease and reported fistula closure in 80% and a 50% clinical response rate [60].

The serious adverse effects of thalidomide are well publicised and patients must practice either abstinence or strict birth control. It is recommended that women undergo regular pregnancy testing and use 2 forms of contraception. Other side effects include sedation—present in nearly all patients—symptomatic neuropathy (present in around 20%), and skin rashes. In the light of this and the fact that the results of controlled clinical trials are not yet available, thalidomide is currently a therapy that should be restricted to either severe refractory complications such as pyoderma gangrenosum and resistant oral ulceration or a clinical trial setting.

3.1.6. CNI-1493

Like thalidomide, this drug is also not strictly a biologic but because of its action in inhibiting the production of TNFα has been included in this section. The efficacy of monoclonal antibodies against TNFα has led to interest in identifying other means of reducing TNFα activity. Mitogen-activated protein kinases (MAPKs) are signal-transducing enzymes that regulate cellular processes including gene expression and cell proliferation [57,61]. Animal studies suggest an anti-inflammatory role for MAPK inhibition following work indicating LPS-induced TNFα production could be limited by inhibition of the MAPK signalling cascade.

CNI-1493 is a guanylhydrazone that inhibits the phosphorylation of p38 MAP kinase and c-Jun N-terminal kinase (JNK). CNI-1493 has been shown to inhibit macrophage formation and the production of a number of pro-inflammatory cytokines including TNFα.

Previous studies in melanoma and renal cancer using IL-2 indicated the drug was well tolerated and inhibited the IL-2–stimulated increase in TNFα. Furthermore, in a pilot study in patients with moderate-to-severe psoriasis there was a marked response to therapy.

Hommes et al. report successful results using CNI-1493 in patients with moderate-to-severe Crohn's disease [62]. Twelve patients with severe Crohn's disease were randomised to receive either 8 or 25 mg/m^2 of CNI-1493 daily for 12 days. The clinical endpoints included safety, the CDAI, Inflammatory Bowel Disease Questionnaire (IBDQ), the Crohn's Disease Endoscopic Index of Severity (CDEIS), and C-reactive protein levels (CRP). A clinical response was defined as a reduction in CDAI of >25% and >70 points and remission defined as reduction in CDAI to below 150. No serious adverse effects were noticed and by 4 weeks 67% of patients had responded with 25% achieving remission. Four months following the start of treatment one half of the patients were in remission and 58% had shown a response. There was no difference noted in the response rates between the treatment groups. In addition, closure of fistulas was noted in 4 out of 5 patients, steroid reduction was achieved in 89% of patients, and arthropathy had resolved in the 5 patients who were symptomatic at the outset.

Further study is required as this is an uncontrolled pilot study. It does, however, indicate that inhibition of inflammatory MAPKs may result in significant clinical improvement. In addition the drugs are orally active, relatively cheap, and small doses only are likely to be required so certainly warrant further investigation.

3.1.7. Other Approaches Involving Cytokine Manipulation

3.1.7.1. IL-10

The genetically engineered IL-10 knock-out mouse develops progressive patchy intestinal inflammation when reared in a normal environment. Administration of IL-10 to these animals prior to the development of the enterocolitis will prevent inflammatory bowel disease and attenuate already established disease. These observations, along with evidence that IL-10 reduces production of IL-10 and IFN-γ by T-helper type 1 cells and IL-12 production by macrophages, lead to interest in developing a therapeutic recombinant IL-10. An initial dose-response study suggested benefit in 46 patients with medically refractory Crohn's disease [63], but larger placebo-controlled dose-response trials could not confirm these findings [64,65]. Alternative methods of administering IL-10 may result in higher levels within the colonic mucosa such as the use of bacteria genetically engineered to produce IL-10 but it has yet to be seen if these are either efficacious or appropriate for human use [66].

3.1.7.2. Anti–IL-12

IL-12 is both a pro-inflammatory and regulatory cytokine. It acts via the IL-12 receptor on naive T cells to induce differentiation into Th1 cells stimulating increased production of IFN-γ. Antibodies to IL-12 have been shown to abrogate experimental colitis induced by TNBS when administered either early or late following disease induction [67,68]. Human phase II dose-finding studies are currently underway.

3.1.7.3. IFN-γ and Anti–IFN-γ

Interferon-γ is a pro-inflammatory cytokine produced by Th1 cells. In theory, antibodies to IFN-γ should be therapeutic but it has not been shown to be particularly efficacious in ameliorating experimental colitis in animal studies [69]. Human trials are currently underway. Interferon-γ might be predicted to exacerbate Crohn's disease, however, in practice this does not actually appear to be the case [70].

3.1.7.4. Anti–IL-18

Interleukin-18 is produced by intestinal epithelial cells and lamina propria cells from patients with Crohn's disease; its main action is to augment IFN-γ production. Animal model studies suggest efficacy of both anti–IL-18 antibodies and administration of an adenovirus expressing IL-18 antisense mRNA [71].

3.1.7.5. Anti–IL-2 Receptor Antibodies

No controlled trials have been carried out but a small pilot study suggests daclizumab, a humanised anti–IL-2 receptor (CD25) antibody is helpful in refractory ulcerative colitis [72], but whether it will be useful in Crohn's disease remains unclear.

3.1.8. Inhibition of Lymphocyte Trafficking

To date, the main therapeutic targets identified to inhibit lymphocyte trafficking include anti-sense to the intercellular adhesion molecule-1 (ICAM-1) and monoclonal antibodies to either α4 integrin that is expressed on lymphocytes or α4β7 integrin that acts in conjunction with other adhesion molecules to facilitate leucocyte migration.

Anti-ICAM-1 antisense oligonucleotide (ISIS-2302) acts as a substrate for nuclease Rnase-H with resultant reduction in ICAM-1 expression. This limits the effects of ICAM-1 in promoting inflammation by reducing leucocyte migration from the intravascular space. In addition, the role of

ICAM-1 in facilitating cytotoxic T-cell, natural killer cell, and neutrophil-mediated damage of target cells should in theory be attenuated.

An initial randomised controlled trial included 20 patients with active steroid-refractory Crohn's disease treated with either 13 intravenous infusions of ISIS-2302 or placebo over 26 days. Seven of 15 patients treated with ISIS-2302 achieved remission compared to only 1 of the 5 patients receiving placebo. In the majority of cases, the response appeared to last up to 6 months. [73].

Unfortunately these promising results have not been confirmed by further trials. In one trial, 75 patients with steroid-refractory Crohn's disease were randomised to receive 1 of 4 treatment courses of subcutaneous ISIS-2302 (0.5 mg/kg for 2 days, 1 week, 2 weeks, 4 weeks) or placebo. The primary end-point of remission without steroids at week 13 was attained by just 3.3% of the patients [74]. Similarly, a larger randomised controlled trial involving 299 patients with active disease treated with intravenous ISIS-2302 at 2 mg/kg 3 days a week for either 2 or 4 weeks or placebo failed to demonstrate efficacy [75].

The remission rate in treated patients at 20% was similar to that of the placebo group at 18.8%. However patients who achieved high serum concentrations of ISIS-2302 (a small subgroup of obese females) showed increased rates of remission.

A recent study [76] to evaluate safety, pharmacokinetics, and clinical efficacy of ISIS-2302 at 250–350 mg in 22 patients with active Crohn's disease has shown overall remission rates (defined as a CDAI <150) were 41% but reached 53% in patients who received more than 3 of the intended 12 infusions. There was a trend to more rapid remission in the cohort receiving 350 mg and the disease response was most durable in the 300-mg group. Although results of this trial suggest that a dose of 300–350 mg achieves adequate drug exposure, there was no placebo cohort, limiting any accurate assessment of efficacy.

Unfortunately, despite the studies reported to date further large-scale trials with an adequate dosing regime still remain necessary to show conclusive benefit.

Natalizumab (Antegren®, Biogen Idec) is a recombinant IgG4 humanised anti-α4 integrin monoclonal antibody that is 95% human IgG4 and 5% murine. Its mode of action is via high-affinity binding to α4 integrin, thus inhibiting further interactions with VCAM-1 and Mad-CAM-1, resulting in reduced leucocyte homing to inflamed gut mucosa. Initial studies involving the cotton-top tamarin showed that the spontaneous development of colitis could be prevented by blocking α4 integrin with monoclonal antibodies.

In the larger of the two reported placebo-controlled trials with natalizumab, 244 patients with moderate-to-severe Crohn's disease were randomised into 4 treatment groups [77]. These consisted of either a single 3 mg/kg dose, 2 3 mg/kg doses at a 4-week interval, 2 6 mg/kg doses at a 4-week interval, or placebo. By 6 weeks, 29% of patients receiving the single dose 3 mg/kg dose, 46% receiving 2 doses at 3 mg/kg, and 31% receiving the higher dose of 6 mg/kg had a CDAI score of <150 points, indicating remission compared to 27% of patients receiving placebo. This was statistically significant for the group receiving 2 doses of 3 mg/kg at 6 weeks, but interestingly not for the group receiving the higher dose (although significant benefit was seen at the other time points). The numbers achieving a clinical response (reduction in CDAI of at least 70 points) were higher at 71% against 38% in the placebo group and significant clinical responses were seen in all 3 groups who received the active drug. There were no serious adverse events attributable to natalizumab and the short-term efficacy appears comparable to that of infliximab. Antibody formation was reported in 7% of patients but was only associated with an infusion reaction in one case.

A smaller trial assessed 30 patients randomised to either a single intravenous infusion of natalizumab at a dose of 3 mg/kg or placebo [78]. This showed a benefit by week 2 in terms of a reduction in CDAI by 45 points in the treatment group but not in those receiving placebo ($P = .02$). Clinical remission (CDAI score of <150 points) occurred in a larger proportion of patients receiving natalizumab than in placebo (39% vs 8%, respectively), but this did not reach statistical significance.

In addition, a pilot study using natalizumab in patients with active ulcerative colitis has recently reported positive results [79].

A recombinant IgG1 humanized monoclonal antibody comprising mouse anti-human $\alpha4\beta7$ integrin monoclonal antibody grafted to human IgG1 (LDP-02) has shown some promise in studies in both animal models and in patients with active ulcerative colitis [80,81]. Currently, larger placebo-controlled dose-finding trials are in progress in active Crohn's disease.

In view of the positive findings in pilot and short-term studies, further randomised placebo-controlled trials appear necessary to define longer-term benefit and safety both of natalizumab and orally available α_4-integrin inhibitors.

3.1.9. Miscellaneous

Inhibitors of NF-κB may prove efficacious in treating Crohn's disease by limiting transcription of promoters of pro-inflammatory cytokines. Animal studies appear promising but obviously human studies are required.

Interest in targeting T-helper cells has arisen as a result of case reports of either complete remission of Crohn's disease or stabilisation of symptoms in patients with HIV infection [82]. cM-T412, a murine-human (25% : 75%) chimeric monoclonal antibody to CD4 has been studied in 2 small phase-1 trials involving patients with either Crohn's disease or ulcerative colitis. Both studies have response rates of around 75% and CD4 counts decreased significantly compared to baseline. Although no opportunistic infections were reported in either study, there were concerns relating to long-term side effects from prolonged CD4 lymphopenia. Both MAX.16H5 and BF-5 monoclonal antibodies to CD4 have shown efficacy in phase-1 trials in inflammatory bowel disease, although the numbers were small in both studies [83,84].

A number of growth factors, including epidermal growth factor (EGF) and keratinocyte growth factor-1 (KGF-1), are currently under investigation in pilot studies in ulcerative colitis but have not yet been trialed in active Crohn's disease.

Other biological therapies under investigation in small, often uncontrolled, pilot studies include IFN-α-2a, IFN-β, human growth hormone, granulocyte colony stimulated factor (filgrastim), granulocyte-macrophage–colony stimulating factor (sargramostim), and IL-11 [42]. The available data regarding these treatments are insufficient and large randomised placebo-controlled trials are required to establish efficacy, some of which are currently underway. The most interesting preliminary reports are that filgrastim and sargramostim may be efficacious in fistulising Crohns disease, although the numbers studied were only 18 and 11 patients, respectively [85–87].

3.1.10. Conclusions

Of all the biological agents in development and at clinical trial, only infliximab is widely accepted as providing unequivocal clinical benefit. The success of the initial treatment regimen on both gut and extraintestinal symptoms of Crohn's disease combined with positive results from maintenance regimes is likely to result in more widespread and long-term usage. Some caution should remain, however, as this drug is expensive, antibody development may limit efficacy, and the implications to the immune system of repeated infusions over a number of years have not yet been fully evaluated.

Although a number of other pro-inflammatory cytokines have been targeted as discussed above and many have shown a significant response rate when compared to placebo, these have not in general exceeded 50%. In addition there are often further issues in terms of administration and side-effect profiles that make them unsuitable for general clinical use. It may prove that the way forward is to target the transcription factor NFκB as this plays a pivotal role in activating many of the genes involved in promoting cytokine expression, inducible enzymes, growth factors, and adhesion molecules. The activation of other transcription factors that act in conjunction with NFκB may also be important. The actions of activator protein-1 are controlled by MAP-kinase pathways. Blockade of these pathways in patients with active Crohn's disease appears a promising way to increase treatment specificity while limiting systemic side effects.

3.2. Methotrexate

Patients with either steroid-refractory or steroid-dependent Crohn's disease unsuitable for surgery, who cannot tolerate or do not benefit from azathioprine present a management problem. This group may comprise up to 20% of patients requiring immunomodulatory therapy and for these patients methotrexate has become second-line therapy.

Methotrexate has previously been shown to be efficacious in both psoriasis and rheumatoid arthritis [88,89]. The antiproliferative and cytotoxic effects of methotrexate are presumed to be due to reduction in DNA, RNA, and protein synthesis via inhibition of dihydrofolate reductase. Further, immunomodulatory properties at lower dosages may relate to inhibition of other folate-dependent enzymes and an increase in adenosine levels. In addition, increased regulation of pro-inflammatory cytokines and impairment of neutrophil chemotaxis may enhance the anti-inflammatory effects.

3.2.1. Evidence for Efficacy

In 1989, Kozarek et al. [90] published a non-randomised, open-label preliminary study of methotrexate in 21 patients with refractory inflammatory bowel disease, 10 of whom had previously failed azathioprine or 6-MP. Methotrexate was given as a 25 mg intramuscular injection weekly for 12 weeks and then switched to a tapering oral dose if an objective improvement was noted. Eleven of 14 patients with Crohn's disease and 5 of 7 with chronic ulcerative colitis responded as measured by the relevant disease activity indices. In addition, prednisolone requirements decreased significantly in both groups. Thirty-six percent of the patients with Crohn's colitis had colonoscopic evidence of healing, with normal histology in 28%. The same was not true of the ulcerative-colitis patients who continued to have macroscopic disease although histologic improvement was noted in 71%. Since then a number of uncontrolled and 5 randomised controlled trials have further clarified the role of methotrexate in inflammatory bowel disease.

The largest studies in the use of methotrexate to both induce and maintain remission come from Feagan et al. In 1995, they published the results of a double-blind, placebo-controlled study assessing the efficacy of weekly intramuscular methotrexate versus placebo in patients with chronically active steroid-refractory Crohn's disease [91]. Ninety-four patients received 25 mg of methotrexate for 16 weeks. When analysed, just under 40% of the treated patients were in clinical remission compared to 19% of the placebo group. The patients receiving methotrexate also required less prednisolone than the placebo group and experienced a significant reduction in their CDAI. However, 17% of patients in the methotrexate group had to withdraw due to side effects, primarily elevation in serum aminotransferase and nausea, as compared to only 2% of the placebo group. The same group of investigators subsequently addressed the issue of methotrexate in the maintenance of remission [92]. Seventy-six patients with Crohn's disease who had entered remission after a 16–24-week course of treatment with intramuscular methotrexate (25 mg weekly) were subsequently randomised to either placebo or 15 mg of intramuscular methotrexate for a further 40 weeks. Sixty-five percent of the patients receiving methotrexate remained in remission compared to 39% in the placebo group. Significantly less prednisolone was required to treat relapse in the patients receiving methotrexate. There were no serious adverse events and only 1 patient withdrew because of nausea; there were no recorded episodes of leucopenia or abnormalities of liver function. It must be noted, however, that this patient cohort represented a highly selected group in that they had all previously both responded to and successfully tolerated the higher dose.

Other randomised studies are limited by small patient numbers. One trial evaluated 28 patients with steroid-dependent Crohn's disease, of whom 13 received 15 mg of oral methotrexate weekly for up to 1 year and 15 placebo [93]. Forty-six percent of the treated patients experienced disease flares compared to 80% receiving placebo, but this was not statistically significant. The side effects were increased in the methotrexate group. A further study assessed dose response and included patients with both Crohn's disease and ulcerative colitis. Initial treatment with either 25 mg or 15 mg of methotrexate administered weekly by subcutaneous injection was assessed after 16 weeks, these doses were noted to be equally efficacious but disappointingly only 17% entered remission [94]. Comparing oral methotrexate (12.5 mg) to 6-MP (50 mg daily) and placebo indicate that methotrexate is reasonably efficacious at reducing abdominal pain, allowing a reduction in steroid dose and improving general well being even when administered orally. However, at a low dose it was no more effective at inducing remission than placebo [95]. Open studies have shown remission rates as high as 72% [96] with a significant reduction in steroid requirements in previously dependent patients, but the lack of blinding and randomisation leaves these open to criticism. Similar benefits are reported in paediatric patients [97].

3.2.2. Side-Effect Profile

Adverse events resulted in discontinuation of the drug at the 25 mg weekly dose in around 17% of patients. Weekly dosing rather than daily regimens appears to reduce risk of toxicity. Gastrointestinal toxicity is the most common side effect predominantly resulting in nausea diarrhea and stomatitis in approximately 5% of patients. Headache is also common but is generally fairly mild and dose related. Pneumonitis fortunately appears uncommon, affecting 1%–2% of patients, usually presenting with dyspnoea and cough and responding to a combination of methotrexate withdrawal and corticosteroids. A full blood count carried out initially weekly and then every 2 months is required to detect any bone-marrow depression. In addition, standard treatment regimens include regular folic acid administration to minimize haematological toxicity. The more clinically worrying issue of methotrexate-induced hepatotoxicity does not appear to be a problem at cumulative doses up to 5g [98]. Routine liver biopsy is not therefore recommended.

3.2.3. Future Questions

Issues continue to remain regarding the optimal dose and mode of administration. Although orally administered methotrexate appears well absorbed in patients with inflammatory bowel disease, including those with small-bowel disease [99], the largest successful trial administered methotrexate by intramuscular injection and many clinicians may feel reluctant to deviate from this procedure, especially in the context of possible malabsorption. Other questions remain unanswered, such as how rapidly the drug works, particularly in comparison with the purine analogues and for how long patients can be safely maintained on treatment. All long-term immunosuppression carries a theoretical risk of malignancy. Finally, teratogenicity limits methotrexate use in young women, whereas limited trial data indicate that azathioprine is relatively safe in pregnancy and breast feeding.

3.3. Dietary Therapy

3.3.1. Nutritional Therapies

Although the aetiology of Crohn's disease is not clearly elucidated, nutrition remains a central issue in both the pathogenesis and management of active disease. There are two important aspects of nutritional therapy to address in Crohn's disease. The first is to treat nutritionally related complications resulting from malnutrition and malabsorption and the second is the use of enteral nutrition as primary therapy for active intestinal inflammation. In addition, nutritionally related treatments may be extended to include the use of short-chain fatty acids, probiotics, and prebiotics.

Malnutrition is extremely common in patients with active Crohn's disease, with up to 75% experiencing weight loss associated with disease exacerbation although obviously the extent depends on both the severity and frequency of the symptoms. In children with Crohn's disease, approximately 85% present with weight loss at the time of initial diagnosis. These figures are a source of concern because of the consequences of protein-energy malnutrition, namely, reduced tolerance to blood loss, poor healing of wounds and fistulas, adverse surgical outcomes, and permanent linear growth retardation in children [100,101]. The cause of malnutrition is multifactorial although reduced oral intake is the predominant factor. This may occur as a result of anorexia, in part due to an increase in circulating levels of pro-inflammatory cytokines such as TNFα and IL-1, because eating exacerbates symptoms such as abdominal pain, vomiting, and diarrhoea, or as a result of dietary restrictions limiting overall calorie intake. It is generally accepted that although increased catabolic requirements and increased losses may contribute to the overall poor nutritional state they are exacerbating factors rather than causal. Malabsorption secondary to extensive inflammation or surgical resection (which may be complicated by bacterial overgrowth) may lead to a variety of vitamin and mineral deficiencies requiring specific identification and supplementation. Decreased bone mineral density with resultant osteopenia or osteoporosis presents a particular problem in Crohn's disease with up to 45% of patients being affected. The use of corticosteroids, reduced absorption of fat-soluble vitamins including vitamin D, and low body weight are all contributing factors and again need to be specifically addressed. There are premorbid differences in the dietary habits of patients with Crohn's disease, notably that they eat more carbohydrate, particularly in the form of sugar, than normal controls and in addition may describe a greater degree of food intolerance [102]. There certainly does not appear to be any clinical role for the use of reduced sugar diets in Crohn's disease [103].

3.3.2. Growth and Development

In children with Crohn's disease, failure to thrive, growth retardation, weight loss, and associated pubertal delay are common presenting symptoms. Once treatment is initiated (dietary, medical, or surgical) growth and weight gain often occur although final height may be reduced in these patients when compared to predicted end heights. The cause of growth retardation is multifactorial but limited protein and/or calorie intake is likely to be the most important. In addition, corticosteroids, although suppressing inflammation, have a detrimental effect on bone growth partly by promoting proteolysis and osteolysis; they should be avoided in growing children but if required should be used used on an alternate-day basis.

3.3.3. Total Parenteral Nutrition as Treatment for Crohn's Disease

Complete bowel rest and the use of exclusive total parenteral nutrition (TPN) reduces intestinal inflammation and disease activity in 80%–95% of patients with active Crohn's disease. Patients with fistulating disease appear to fare less well with a lower rate of both initial and maintained remission (58%–61% in nonfistulous disease vs 36% in fistulous disease at 1 year) [104]. In this trial TPN offered benefit even in steroid-refractory disease. In a more recent study looking at the effects of TPN (in addition to corticosteroids) on short-term outcome in acute attacks of ulcerative colitis and Crohn's colitis, the ulcerative colitis group did not show any benefits in terms of clinical remission or colectomy rate. In contrast, the patients with Crohn's disease receiving TPN showed marked improvement in both their inflammatory and nutritional parameters [105]. When TPN was compared to both an elemental diet and a polymeric diet in 28 patients with active Crohn's disease, the reduction in inflammation and early symptomatic improvement was most marked in those on TPN followed by those receiving the elemental diet. The polymeric diet performed less well although as none of these differences reached statistical significance firm conclusions cannot be drawn [106].

3.3.4. Enteral Nutrition as Primary Therapy for Crohn's Disease

In view of the detrimental long-term side effects of corticosteroids and the known or potential toxicities of the other available first- and second-line therapies for Crohn's disease, interest has focused on nutritional therapy as a safe and efficacious treatment of active disease. In addition, in particular circumstances such as pregnancy, an elemental diet provides a safe form of treatment with no risk of teratogenesis [107]. A number of trials have addressed the issue of elemental and semi-elemental formulas as treatment for active Crohn's disease comparing efficacy to that of steroid therapy. The mechanism of action of these diets is not fully understood but may relate to both decreased dietary antigens and bacterial load. Other pathways by which enteral diets may reduce mucosal inflammation include inhibition of the inflammatory response by reducing the number of cytokine producing cells, boosting immunosuppressive pathways, and promoting epithelial healing. As a result, the integrity of the intestinal barrier, as shown by a significant decrease in gut permeability, is improved [108].

Since the 1980s interest has arisen in the use of elemental feeds as primary therapy for active inflammatory bowel disease. Initial studies showed distinct benefits but were either uncontrolled or compared responses to those occurring while on a normal diet [109,110]. A controlled trial involving 21 acutely ill patients with exacerbations of Crohn's disease compared an elemental diet (Vivonex®, Novartis Nutritional) to prednisolone 0.75 mg/kg/day and assessment at 4 and 12 weeks showed equal improvement in each group [111]. There was insufficient power to demonstrate a difference in treatment efficacy. It is also difficult to achieve adequate blinding due to the nature of the treatment. Similar studies have yielded comparable results although the European Cooperative Study involving 55 patients showed prednisolone to be more effective regardless of initial disease activity or disease location [112].

A meta-analysis published in 1995 [113] specifically addressed the issue of the efficacy of steroids in comparison to nutritional therapies (both elemental and nonelemental formulas were assessed). The results were based on clinical remission in 413 patients with active Crohn's disease on an intention-to-treat basis. Almost 81% of patients treated with steroids achieved clinical remission compared to 56.8% of those receiving nutritional therapy (pooled odds ratio, 0.35; 95% CI, 0.23–0.53). Interestingly, once remission had been achieved the relapse rates at 12 months were similar at 65% for those on steroids compared to 67% in those on dietary treatment.

In spite of the findings of this meta-analysis there are many situations in which treatment with enteral feeding remains first line. Patients may be either unwilling to take corticosteroids or have steroid-refractory disease, the newer therapies may be poorly tolerated or limited by toxicity. In addition, there may be evidence that certain subgroups such as those with extensive small-bowel disease may fare better with dietary treatments, wheras those with fistulating or perianal disease, who suffer early relapse [114], should avoid it as therapy.

One of the factors that may adversely affect remission rates for nutritional treatments when assessed on an intention-to-treat basis is the difficulty involved in achieving patient compliance. Few studies have looked at the practical aspects involved in maintaining compliance; elemental feeds are often unpalatable and patients may find it difficult to abstain from their normal diet. Despite this the majority of patients (85%) can manage to sip feed with 15% requiring nasogastric feeding [115]. Nausea and postural hypotension are commonly reported within the first week of treatment but tend to abate. Vomiting was reported in 3 out of 89 patients and this appeared to be due to sensitivity to a particular formula. In the same study 65% of patients reported that they would have treatment with an elemental diet again. A percutaneous endoscopic gastostomy tube can be used in the absence of upper-gastrointestinal Crohn's disease to allow direct feeding and to overcome the problem of unpalatability.

Although from the data available it appears that in adult Crohn's disease steroid therapy is superior to exclusive enteral nutrition the same is not true of children. On review of the results from 5 randomised clinical trials in paediatric Crohn's disease involving a total of 147 patients, exclusive enteral nutrition was as efficacious as corticosteroids at inducing remission (relative risk for induction of remission, 95% CI, 0.67–1.34) [116]. The inclusion of findings from 2 further nonrandomised studies did not significantly affect this result. One caveat, however, is the limited power of the trials to demonstrate a benefit of either treatment, and it has been estimated that a minimum of 10 further studies comparable in size to the largest of the reported paediatric trials would be required to show a treatment superiority. This is logistically unlikely to happen and given the additional benefits of enteral nutrition in terms of improved growth and pubertal development without the deleterious side effects of steroids, enteral therapy is the most appropriate first-line treatment in children with active Crohn's disease.

The other major issue involves the composition of the diet. Initial studies used true elemental feeds based on amino acids and glucose but these were found to be unpalatable and patients preferred polymeric diets using whole protein and complex carbohydrate. In 5 trials involving 134 patients reviewed by Griffiths et al. there was no difference noted in the efficacy of elemental versus polymeric formulas (OR, 0.87; 95% CI, 0.41–1.83) [113]. Similarly, a more recent double-blind randomised trial comparing a polymeric diet to an elemental feed involving 21 patients found both diets to be equally effective [117]. These figures would tend to mitigate against the theory of reduced antigen exposure inducing remission but they were analysed on an intention-to-treat basis and the increased tolerability and therefore compliance with polymeric feeds may result in the similar levels of efficacy.

Although no differences in remission rates are noted with amino acid, peptide, or whole-protein–based diets, outcome may be altered by the fat composition of the diet. Changes in dietary fat have been postulated to modify ecoisanoid synthesis and other immunomodulatory processes. In addition it has been suggested on the basis of a meta-analysis of published studies that the beneficial effects of enteral nutrition are inversely related to the quantity of dietary long-chain triglycerides [113]. A double-blind trial in active Crohn's disease evaluated the effects of high versus low dietary concentrations of long-chain triglycerides in active Crohn's disease. These polymeric diets contained whole protein, complex carbohydrate, and had equal total fat content. Despite the low remission rates on an intention-to-treat basis, the patients receiving a higher concentration of long-chain triglycerides fared slightly better (33% vs 25%), although this result was not significant [118]. More recently, Gassull et al. randomised 62 patients with active Crohn's to receive either a polymeric diet high in oleate (79%) and low in linoleate (6.5%) (PEN1), an identical enteral diet except for the fat content which comprised 45% linoleate and 28% oleate (PEN2), or oral prednisolone at 1 mg/kg/day [119]. On an intention-to-treat basis, the remission rates were 20%, 52%, and 79%, respectively. Excluding patients who were noncompliant during the first week (per protocol analysis) remission rates were 27% for PEN1, 63% for PEN2, and 79% for steroids. Even after adjustment for confounding variables, PEN1 remained significantly associated with a poor response indicating that an excess of synthetic oleate in the diet may prevent the induction of remission in active Crohn's disease. In this study, however, there was no difference in the amount of long-chain triglycerides between diets suggesting that other properties of the predominant fat are also important. Interestingly, high concentrations of linoleate had previously been avoided as it was felt as a precursor to arachidonic acid, linoleate may lead to enhanced production of pro-inflammatory ecoisanoids such as leukotriene B4, thromboxane A2, and prostaglandin E2. The quantities of medium-chain triglycerides in nutrient formulas does not appear to exert a significant effect [120].

3.3.5. Fish Oils

Fish oil rich in n-3 polyunsaturated fatty acids (PUFAs) theoretically exert anti-inflammatory properties by diverting eicosanoid metabolism towards the less inflammatory leucotriene B5 and prostaglandin E2. There are also suggested benefits resulting from inhibition of cytokine production and reductions in platelet adhesion.

Published data are limited on the treatment of active disease. The introduction of a n-3 fatty-acid–rich diet combined with nutritional education was not noted to alter levels of disease activity although as expected, nutritional status improved [121]. An Italian study assessed the effects of an enteric-coated fish-oil preparation in the maintenance of remission in 78 patients with Crohn's disease deemed at high risk of relapse [122]. Patients were randomised to receive either 9 fish-oil capsules containing a total of 2.7 g of n-3 fatty acids or 9 placebo capsules daily. Compliance was good and only 4 out of the 39 patients in the treatment arm dropped out (because of diarrhoea). After 1 year of therapy, 59% of the patients receiving fish-oil remained in remission, compared to only 26% in the placebo group ($P = .003$). Subsequent logistic-regression analysis indicated that the likelihood of relapse was only affected by the fish-oil rather than confounding factors of smoking, surgery, or duration of disease.

3.3.6. Probiotics

Evidence that probiotics are useful therapy for inflammatory bowel disease is currently restricted to the treatment of pouchitis and potentially, ulcerative colitis [123]. In-vitro studies indicate that probiotics interact with immunocompetent cells at the mucosal interface and modulate local production of pro-inflammatory cytokines [124]. In a pilot study of 4 children with mild-to-moderate Crohn's disease treated with enteric-coated *Lactobacillus* GG for 6 months an improvement was noted in both clinical activity and in intestinal permeability [125]. However, a randomised, controlled trial involving adults with Crohn's disease assessed whether orally administered *Lactobacillus* could prevent or reduce the severity of postoperative disease recurrence failed to show a benefit. Forty-five patients were randomised to 12 billion colony-forming units of *Lactobacillus* GG, or identical placebo for 1 year. There were no significant differences in either the rate of endoscopic recurrence or the disease severity at 1 year [126]. This trial has however simply assessed 1 probiotic agent and it is not yet clear whether a particular bacteria or combination of bacteria is necessary to optimise the anti-inflammatory effect.

3.3.7. Exclusion and Microparticle Diets

Following remission achieved by an elemental diet those who return to normal eating often relapse; however, in some studies, patients have had prolonged remissions by taking exclusion diets. The foods excluded have been not sugar, but generally involve cereals, dairy products, and yeast. The nature of this treatment makes it difficult to assess in a double-blind study and the reports are therefore highly susceptible to both patient and observer bias.

Recently Lomer et al. investigated the theory that ultrafine and fine particles are adjuvants in antigen-mediated immune responses and as a consequence may cause inflammation. Twenty patients with active corticosteroid-treated ileal or ileocolonic Crohn's were randomised to receive a low microparticle diet (n = 10) or a control diet (n = 10) for a 4-month period. There was a significant and progressive decrease in the CDAI in the treatment group, with 7 attaining remission (CDAI at entry 392 ± 25 vs 145 ± 47 at month 4) in comparison to the control group where at month 4 the CDAI had returned to baseline levels and none were in remission [127].

This was a small study and larger numbers will be required to confirm a beneficial role but the findings could help explain the efficacy of elemental diets which are equally low in microparticles.

4. Conclusions

The last 10 years have proved to be a very exciting time for the development of new medical therapies for Crohn's disease. The traditional therapies of corticosteroids, 5-ASA, and azathioprine have been updated and hopefully are now safer with improved tolerability. Advances have been made in the use and understanding of nutritional therapies that are highly attractive as they treat active disease, have minimal side effects, and improve the patient's nutritional status. Early use of first-line immunosuppresion in the form of azathioprine or 6-MP with TMPT preassessment continues to reduce the need for long-term steroids and minimises bone-marrow toxicity. The reliance on steroids should further be reduced by the introduction of new treatments especially methotrexate and infliximab. These have been fairly extensively evaluated and are currently being used on a more widespread basis for refractory disease that may previously have required surgery. Whether these new, more aggressive therapies reduce the incidence of surgical complications such as the development of short-bowel syndrome remain to be seen. Finally, there are a number of therapies in pilot or phase-2 trials of which the nonbiological or small-molecule–based treatments appear particularly exciting.

References

1. Loftus EV Jr, Schoenfeld P, Sandborn WJ. The epidemiology and natural history of Crohn's disease in population-based patient cohorts from North America: a systematic review. Aliment Pharmacol Ther. 2002;16.
2. Gower-Rousseau C, Salomez JL, Dupas JL, et al. Incidence of inflammatory bowel disease in northern France (1988–1990). *Gut* 1994;35:1433–1438.
3. Munkholm P, Langholz E, Nielsen OH, Kreiner S, Binder V. Incidence and prevalence of Crohn's disease in the county of Copenhagen, 1962–87: a sixfold increase in incidence. *Scand J Gastroenterol.* 1992;27:609–614.

4. Cosgrove M, Al-Atia RF, Jenkins HR. The epidemiology of paediatric inflammatory bowel disease. *Arch Dis Child.* 1996;74:460–461.
5. Steinhart AH, Ewe K, Griffiths AM, Modigliani R, Thomsen OO. Corticosteroids for maintaining remission of Crohn's disease. *Cochrane Database Syst Rev.* 2001;3:CD000301.
6. Greenberg GR, Feagan BG, Martin F, et al. Oral budesonide as maintenance treatment for Crohn's disease: a placebo-controlled, dose-ranging study. Canadian Inflammatory Bowel Disease Study Group. *Gastroenterology* 1996; 110:45–51.
7. Rutgeerts P, Lofberg R, Malchow H, et al. A comparison of budesonide with prednisolone for active Crohn's disease. *N Engl J Med.* 1994;331:842–845.
8. Cortot A, Colombel JF, Rutgeerts P, et al. Switch from systemic steroids to budesonide in steroid dependent patients with inactive Crohn's disease. *Gut* 2001;48:186–90.
9. Kundhal P, Zachos M, Holmes JL, Griffiths AM. Controlled ileal release budesonide in pediatric Crohn disease: efficacy and effect on growth. *J Pediatr Gastroenterol Nutr.* 2001;33:75–80.
10. Simms L, Steinhart AH. Budesonide for maintenance of remission in Crohn's disease. *Cochrane Database Syst Rev.* 2001;1:CD002913.
11. Thomsen OO, Cortot A, Jewell D, et al. A comparison of budesonide and mesalamine for active Crohn's disease. International Budesonide-Mesalamine Study Group. *N Engl J Med.* 1998;339:370–374.
12. Steinhart AH, Feagan BG, Wong CJ, et al. Combined budesonide and antibiotic therapy for active Crohn's disease: a randomized controlled trial. *Gastroenterology* 2002;123:33–40.
13. Present DH, Korelitz BI, Wisch N, Glass JL, Sachar DB, Pasternack BS. Treatment of Crohn's disease with 6-mercaptopurine. A long-term, randomized, double-blind study. *N Engl J Med.* 1980;302:981–987.
14. Korelitz BI, Present DH. Favorable effect of 6-mercaptopurine on fistulae of Crohn's disease. *Dig Dis Sci.* 1985;30:58–64.
15. Markowitz J, Rosa J, Grancher K, Aiges H, Daum F. Long-term 6-mercaptopurine treatment in adolescents with Crohn's disease. *Gastroenterology* 1990;99:1347–1351.
16. Sandborn W, Sutherland L, Pearson D, May G, Modigliani R, Prantera C. Azathioprine or 6-mercaptopurine for inducing remission of Crohn's disease. *Cochrane Database Syst Rev.* 2000;2:CD000545.
17. Pearson DC, May GR, Fick G, Sutherland LR. Azathioprine for maintaining remission of Crohn's disease. *Cochrane Database Syst Rev.* 2000;2: CD000067.
18. Markowitz J, Grancher K, Kohn N, Lesser M, Daum F. A multicenter trial of 6-mercaptopurine and prednisone in children with newly diagnosed Crohn's disease. *Gastroenterology* 2000;119:895–902.
19. Cuillerier E, Lemann M, Bouhnik Y, Allez M, Rambaud JC, Modigliani R. Azathioprine for prevention of postoperative recurrence in Crohn's disease: a retrospective study. *Eur J Gastroenterol Hepatol.* 2001;13:1291–1296.
20. Brynskov J, Freund L, Rasmussen SN, et al. A placebo-controlled, double-blind, randomized trial of cyclosporine therapy in active chronic Crohn's disease. *N Engl J Med.* 1989;321:845–850.

21. Stange EF, Modigliani R, Pena AS, Wood AJ, Feutren G, Smith PR. European trial of cyclosporine in chronic active Crohn's disease: a 12-month study. The European Study Group. *Gastroenterology* 1995;109:774–782.
22. Feagan BG, McDonald JW, Rochon J, et al. Low-dose cyclosporine for the treatment of Crohn's disease. The Canadian Crohn's Relapse Prevention Trial Investigators. *N Engl J Med.* 1994;330:1846–1851.
23. Lochs H, Mayer M, Fleig WE, et al. Prophylaxis of postoperative relapse in Crohn's disease with mesalamine: European Cooperative Crohn's Disease Study VI. *Gastroenterology* 2000;118:264–273.
24. Korelitz B, Hanauer S, Rutgeerts P, et al. Postoperative prophylaxis with 6-MP, 5-ASA or placebo in Crohn's disease: A 2 year multicenter trial. *Gastroenterology* 1998;114:A1011.
25. Eaden J, Abrams K, Ekbom A, Jackson E, Mayberry J. Colorectal cancer prevention in ulcerative colitis: a case-control study. *Aliment Pharmacol Ther.* 2000;14:145–153.
26. Brandt LJ, Bernstein LH, Boley SJ, Frank MS. Metronidazole therapy for perineal Crohn's disease: a follow-up study. *Gastroenterology* 1982;83:383–387.
27. Sutherland L, Singleton J, Sessions J, et al. Double blind, placebo controlled trial of metronidazole in Crohn's disease. *Gut* 1991;32:1071–1075.
28. Prantera C, Zannoni F, Scribano ML, et al. An antibiotic regimen for the treatment of active Crohn's disease: a randomized, controlled clinical trial of metronidazole plus ciprofloxacin. *Am J Gastroenterol.* 1996;91:328–332.
29. Rutgeerts P, Hiele M, Geboes K, et al. Controlled trial of metronidazole treatment for prevention of Crohn's recurrence after ileal resection. *Gastroenterology* 1995;108:1617–1621.
30. Rutgeerts P, Van Assche G, D'Haens G, et al. Ornidazol for prophylaxis of postoperative Crohn's disease: final results of a double blind placebo controlled trial. *Gastroenterology* 2002;122:A-135.
31. Sanderson JD, Moss MT, Tizard ML, Hermon-Taylor J. Mycobacterium paratuberculosis DNA in Crohn's disease tissue. *Gut* 1992;33:890–896.
32. Gui GP, Thomas PR, Tizard ML, Lake J, Sanderson JD, Hermon-Taylor J. Two-year-outcomes analysis of Crohn's disease treated with rifabutin and macrolide antibiotics. *J Antimicrob Chemother.* 1997;39:393–400.
33. Thomas GA, Swift GL, Green JT, et al. Controlled trial of antituberculous chemotherapy in Crohn's disease: a five year follow up study. *Gut* 1998;42:497–500.
34. Stokkers PC, Camoglio L, van Deventer SJ. Tumor necrosis factor (TNF) in inflammatory bowel disease: gene polymorphisms, animal models, and potential for anti-TNF therapy. *J Inflamm.* 1995–1996;47:97–103.
35. Cominelli F. Tumor necrosis factor modulation: from bench to bedside. *Inflamm Bowel Dis.* 2000;6:S21–S22.
36. Targan SR, Hanauer SB, van Deventer SJ, et al. A short-term study of chimeric monoclonal antibody cA2 to tumor necrosis factor alpha for Crohn's disease. Crohn's Disease cA2 Study Group. *N Engl J Med.* 1997;337:1029–1035.
37. Best WR, Becktel JM, Singleton JW, Kern F Jr. Development of a Crohn's disease activity index. National Cooperative Crohn's Disease Study. *Gastroenterology* 1976;70:439–444.
38. Rutgeerts P, D'Haens G, Targan S, et al. Efficacy and safety of retreatment with anti-tumor necrosis factor antibody (infliximab) to maintain remission in Crohn's disease. *Gastroenterology* 1999;117:761–769.

39. Hanauer SB, Feagan BG, Lichtenstein GR, et al, for the ACCENT I Study Group. Maintenance infliximab for Crohn's disease: the ACCENT I randomised trial. *Lancet* 2002;359:1541–1549.
40. Present DH, Rutgeerts P, Targan S, et al. Infliximab for the treatment of fistulas in patients with Crohn's disease. *N Engl J Med.* 1999;340:1398–1405.
41. D'haens G, Van Deventer S, Van Hogezand R, et al. Endoscopic and histological healing with infliximab anti-tumor necrosis factor antibodies in Crohn's disease: A European multicenter trial. *Gastroenterology* 1999;116:1029–1034.
42. Sandborn WJ, Targan SR. Biologic therapy of inflammatory bowel disease. *Gastroenterology* 2002;122:1592–1608.
43. Farrell R, Alsahli M, Falchuk K, Peppercorn M, Michetti P. Human antichimeric antibody levels correlate with lack of efficacy and infusion reactions following infliximab therapy. *Gastroenterology* 2001;120:A-69.
44. Norman M, Baert F, D'Haens G, et al. HACA formation after infliximab (Remicade) treatment in Crohn's disease is clearly associated with infusion reactions. *Gastroenterology* 2001;120:A261.
45. Farrell R, Alsahli M, Falchuk K, Peppercorn M, Michetti P. A randomised, double-blind placebo-controlled trial of intravenous hydrocrtisone in reducing human anti-chimeric antibody formation following infliximab therapy. *Gastroenterology* 2001;120:A618–619.
46. Hanauer S, Rutgeerts P, Targan S, et al. Delayed hypersensitivity to infliximab (Remicade) re-infusion after a 2–4 year interval without treatment. *Gastrenterology.* 1999;116:A731.
47. Vermeire S, Norman M, Van Assche G, et al. Infliximab (Remicade) treatment in Crohn's disease and antinuclear antibody (ANA) formation. *Gastroenterology* 2001;120:A-69.
48. Gardam MA, Keystone EC, Menzies R, et al. Anti-tumour necrosis factor agents and tuberculosis risk: mechanisms of action and clinical management. *Lancet Infect Dis.* 2003;3:148–155.
49. Salmon-Ceron D. Recommendations for the prevention and management of tuberculosis in patients taking infliximab. *Ann Med Interne (Paris).* 2002; 153:429–431.
50. Brown SL, Greene MH, Gershon SK, Edwards ET, Braun MM. Tumor necrosis factor antagonist therapy and lymphoma development: twenty-six cases reported to the Food and Drug Administration. *Arthritis Rheum.* 2002; 46:3151–3158.
51. Stack WA, Mann SD, Roy AJ, et al. Randomised controlled trial of CDP571 antibody to tumour necrosis factor-alpha in Crohn's disease. *Lancet* 1997; 349:521–524.
52. Sandborn WJ, Feagan BG, Hanauer SB, et al. An engineered human antibody to TNF (CDP571) for active Crohn's disease: a randomized double-blind placebo-controlled trial. *Gastroenterology* 2001;120:1330–1338.
53. Feagan BG, Sandborn WJ, Baker J, et al. A randomized, double-blind, placebo-controlled, multi-center trial of the engineered human antibody to TNF (CDP571) for steroid sparing and maintenance of remission in patients with steroid-dependent Crohn's disease. *Gastroenterology* 2000;118: A655.
54. D'Haens G, Swijsen C, Noman M, et al. Etanercept in the treatment of active refractory Crohn's disease: a single-center pilot trial. *Am J Gastroenterol.* 2001; 96:2564–2568.

55. Sandborn WJ, Hanauer SB, Katz S, et al. Etanercept for active Crohn's disease: a randomized, double-blind, placebo-controlled trial. *Gastroenterology* 2001; 121:1088–1094.
56. Rutgeerts P, Lemmens L, Van Assche G, Noman M, Borghini-Fuhrer I, Goedkoop R. Treatment of active Crohn's disease with onercept (recombinant human soluble p55 tumour necrosis factor receptor): results of a randomized, open-label, pilot study. *Aliment Pharmacol Ther.* 2003;17:185–192.
57. Papadakis KA, Targan SR. Tumor necrosis factor: biology and therapeutic inhibitors. *Gastroenterology* 2000;119:1148–1157.
58. Facchini S, Candusso M, Martelossi S, Liubich M, Panfili E, Ventura A. Efficacy of long-term treatment with thalidomide in children and young adults with Crohn disease: preliminary results. *J Pediatr Gastroenterol Nutr.* 2001; 32:178–181.
59. Vasiliauskas EA, Kam LY, Abreu-Martin MT, et al. An open-label pilot study of low-dose thalidomide in chronically active, steroid-dependent Crohn's disease. *Gastroenterology* 1999;117:1278–1287.
60. Ehrenpreis ED, Kane SV, Cohen LB, Cohen RD, Hanauer SB. Thalidomide therapy for patients with refractory Crohn's disease: an open-label trial. *Gastroenterology* 1999;117:1271–1277.
61. Lee JC, Kumar S, Griswold DE, Underwood DC, Votta BJ, Adams JL. Inhibition of p38 MAP kinase as a therapeutic strategy. *Immunopharmacology* 2000;47:185–201.
62. Hommes D, van den Blink B, Plasse T, et al. Inhibition of stress-activated MAP kinases induces clinical improvement in moderate to severe Crohn's disease. *Gastroenterology* 2002;122:7–14.
63. van Deventer SJ, Elson CO, Fedorak RN. Multiple doses of intravenous interleukin 10 in steroid-refractory Crohn's disease. Crohn's Disease Study Group. *Gastroenterology* 1997;113:383–389.
64. Schreiber S, Fedorak RN, Nielsen OH, et al. Safety and efficacy of recombinant human interleukin 10 in chronic active Crohn's disease. Crohn's Disease IL-10 Cooperative Study Group. *Gastroenterology* 2000;119:1461–1472.
65. Fedorak RN, Gangl A, Elson CO, et al. Recombinant human interleukin 10 in the treatment of patients with mild to moderately active Crohn's disease. The Interleukin 10 Inflammatory Bowel Disease Cooperative Study Group. *Gastroenterology* 2000;119:1473–1482.
66. Steidler L, Hans W, Schotte L, et al. Treatment of murine colitis by Lactococcus lactis secreting interleukin-10. *Science* 2000;289:1352–1355.
67. Neurath MF, Fuss I, Kelsall BL, Stuber E, Strober W. Antibodies to interleukin 12 abrogate established experimental colitis in mice. *J Exp Med.* 1995;182: 1281–1290.
68. Duchmann R, Schmitt E, Knolle P, Meyer zum Buschenfelde KH, Neurath M. Tolerance towards resident intestinal flora in mice is abrogated in experimental colitis and restored by treatment with interleukin-10 or antibodies to interleukin-12. *Eur J Immunol.* 1996;26:934–938.
69. Fuss IJ, Marth T, Neurath MF, Pearlstein GR, Jain A, Strober W. Anti-interleukin 12 treatment regulates apoptosis of Th1 T cells in experimental colitis in mice. *Gastroenterology* 1999;117:1078–1088.
70. Debinski H, Forbes A, Kamm MA. Low dose interferon gamma for refractory Crohn's disease. *Ital J Gastroenterol Hepatol.* 1997;29:403–406.

71. Siegmund B, Fantuzzi G, Rieder F, et al. Neutralization of interleukin-18 reduces severity in murine colitis and intestinal IFN-gamma and TNF-alpha production. *Am J Physiol Regul Integr Comp Physiol.* 2001;281:R1264–R1267.
72. Van Assche G, Dalle I, Noman M, et al. A pilot study on the use of the humanized anti-interleukin-2 receptor antibody daclizumab in active ulcerative colitis. *Am J Gastroenterol.* 2003;98:369–376.
73. Yacyshyn BR, Bowen-Yacyshyn MB, Jewell L, et al. A placebo-controlled trial of ICAM-1 antisense oligonucleotide in the treatment of Crohn's disease. *Gastroenterology* 1998;114:1133–1142.
74. Schreiber S, Nikolaus S, Malchow H, et al. Absence of efficacy of subcutaneous antisense ICAM-1 treatment of chronic active Crohn's disease. *Gastroenterology* 2001;120:1339–1346.
75. Yacyshyn BR, Chey WY, Goff J, et al. Double blind, placebo controlled trial of the remission inducing and steroid sparing properties of an ICAM-1 antisense oligodeoxynucleotide, alicaforsen (ISIS 2302), in active steroid dependent Crohn's disease. *Gut* 2002;51:30–36.
76. Yacyshyn BR, Barish C, Goff J, et al. Dose ranging pharmacokinetic trial of high-dose alicaforsen (intercellular adhesion molecule-1 antisense oligodeoxynucleotide) (ISIS 2302) in active Crohn's disease. *Aliment Pharmacol Ther.* 2002;16:1761–1770.
77. Ghosh S, Goldin E, Gordon FH, et al. Natalizumab for active Crohn's disease. *N Engl J Med.* 2003;348:24–32.
78. Gordon FH, Lai CW, Hamilton MI, et al. A randomized placebo-controlled trial of a humanized monoclonal antibody to alpha4 integrin in active Crohn's disease. *Gastroenterology* 2001;121:268–274.
79. Gordon FH, Hamilton MI, Donoghue S, et al. A pilot study of treatment of active ulcerative colitis with natalizumab, a humanized monoclonal antibody to alpha-4 integrin. *Aliment Pharmacol Ther.* 2002;16:699–705.
80. Hesterberg PE, Winsor-Hines D, Briskin MJ, et al. Rapid resolution of chronic colitis in the cotton-top tamarin with an antibody to a gut-homing integrin alpha 4 beta 7. *Gastroenterology* 1996;111:1373–1380.
81. Feagan B, McDonald J, Greenberg G, et al. An ascending dose trial of humanized A4B7 antibody in ulcerative colitis (UC). *Gastroenterology* 2000;118:A874.
82. James SP. Remission of Crohn's disease after human immunodeficiency virus infection. *Gastroenterology* 1988;95:1667–1669.
83. Emmrich J, Seyfarth M, Fleig WE, et al. Treatment of inflammatory bowel disease with anti-CD4 monoclonal antibody. *Lancet* 1991;338:570–571.
84. Canva-Delcambre V, Jacquot S, Robinet E, et al. Treatment of severe Crohn's disease with anti-CD4 monoclonal antibody. *Aliment Pharmacol Ther.* 1996;10:721–727.
85. Vaughan D, Drumm B. Treatment of fistulas with granulocyte colony-stimulating factor in a patient with Crohn's disease. *N Engl J Med.* 1999;340:239–240.
86. Korzenik J, Dieckgraefe B. Immunostimulation in Crohn's disease: results of a pilot study of G-CSF (R-Methug-CSF) in mucosal and fistulizing Crohn's disease. *Gastroenterology* 2000;118:A874.
87. Korzenik J, Dieckgraefe B. Immunostimulation in Crohn's disease: safety and efficacy of rhuGM-CSF for the treatment of active Crohn's disease. *Gastroenterology* 2001;120:A277–A287.

88. Kuijpers AL, van de Kerkhof PC. Risk-benefit assessment of methotrexate in the treatment of severe psoriasis. *Am J Clin Dermatol.* 2000;1:27–39.
89. Suarez-Almazor ME, Belseck E, Shea B, Wells G, Tugwell P. Methotrexate for rheumatoid arthritis. *Cochrane Database Syst Rev.* 2000;2:CD000957.
90. Kozarek RA, Patterson DJ, Gelfand MD, Botoman VA, Ball TJ, Wilske KR. Methotrexate induces clinical and histologic remission in patients with refractory inflammatory bowel disease. *Ann Intern Med.* 1989;110:353–356.
91. Feagan BG, Rochon J, Fedorak RN, et al. Methotrexate for the treatment of Crohn's disease. The North American Crohn's Study Group Investigators. *N Engl J Med.* 1995;332:292–297.
92. Feagan BG, Fedorak RN, Irvine EJ, et al. A comparison of methotrexate with placebo for the maintenance of remission in Crohn's disease. North American Crohn's Study Group Investigators. *N Engl J Med.* 2000;342:1627–1632.
93. Arora S, Katkov W, Cooley J, et al. Methotrexate in Crohn's disease: results of a randomized, double-blind, placebo-controlled trial. *Hepatogastroenterology* 1999;46:1724–1729.
94. Egan LJ, Sandborn WJ, Tremaine WJ, et al. A randomized dose-response and pharmacokinetic study of methotrexate for refractory inflammatory Crohn's disease and ulcerative colitis. *Aliment Pharmacol Ther.* 1999;13: 1597–1604.
95. Oren R, Moshkowitz M, Odes S, et al. Methotrexate in chronic active Crohn's disease: a double-blind, randomised, Israeli multicenter trial. *Am J Gastroenterol.* 1997;92:2203–2209.
96. Lemann M, Chamiot-Prieur C, Mesnard B, et al. Methotrexate for the treatment of refractory Crohn's disease. *Aliment Pharmacol Ther.* 1996;10: 309–314.
97. Mack DR, Young R, Kaufman SS, Ramey L, Vanderhoof JA. Methotrexate in patients with Crohn's disease after 6-mercaptopurine. J Pediatr. 132: 830–835.
98. Te HS, Schiano TD, Kuan SF, Hanauer SB, Conjeevaram HS, Baker AL. Hepatic effects of long-term methotrexate use in the treatment of inflammatory bowel disease. *Am J Gastroenterol.* 2000;95:3150–3156.
99. Moshkowitz M, Oren R, Tishler M, et al. The absorption of low-dose methotrexate in patients with inflammatory bowel disease. *Aliment Pharmacol Ther.* 1997;11:569–573.
100. Kanof ME, Lake AM, Bayless TM. Decreased height velocity in children and adolescents before the diagnosis of Crohn's disease. *Gastroenterology* 1988;95: 1523–1527.
101. Markowitz J, Grancher K, Rosa J, Aiges H, Daum F. Growth failure in pediatric inflammatory bowel disease. *J Pediatr Gastroenterol Nutr.* 1993;16: 373–380.
102. Katschinski B, Logan RF, Edmond M, Langman MJ. Smoking and sugar intake are separate but interactive risk factors in Crohn's disease. *Gut* 1988;29: 1202–1206.
103. Riordan AM, Ruxton CH, Hunter JO. A review of associations between Crohn's disease and consumption of sugars. *Eur J Clin Nutr.* 1998;52:229–238.
104. Ostro MJ, Greenberg GR, Jeejeebhoy KN. Total parenteral nutrition and complete bowel rest in the management of Crohn's disease. *J Parenter Enteral Nutr.* 1985;9:280–287.

105. Seo M, Okada M, Yao T, Furukawa H, Matake H. The role of total parenteral nutrition in the management of patients with acute attacks of inflammatory bowel disease. *J Clin Gastroenterol.* 1999;29:270–275.
106. Kobayashi K, Katsumata T, Yokoyama K, Takahashi H, Igarashi M, Saigenji K. [A randomized controlled study of total parenteral nutrition and enteral nutrition by elemental and polymeric diet as primary therapy in active phase of Crohn's disease]. *Nippon Shokakibyo Gakkai Zasshi* 1998;95:1212–1221.
107. Teahon K, Pearson M, Levi AJ, Bjarnason I. Elemental diet in the management of Crohn's disease during pregnancy. *Gut* 1991;32:1079–1081.
108. Teahon K, Smethurst P, Pearson M, Levi AJ, Bjarnason I. The effect of elemental diet on intestinal permeability and inflammation in Crohn's disease. *Gastroenterology* 1991;101:84–89.
109. O'Morain C, Segal AW, Levi AJ. Elemental diets in treatment of acute Crohn's disease. *Br Med J.* 1980;281:1173–1175.
110. Harries AD, Jones LA, Danis V, et al. Controlled trial of supplemented oral nutrition in Crohn's disease. *Lancet* 1983;1:887–890.
111. O'Morain C, Segal AW, Levi AJ. Elemental diet as primary treatment of acute Crohn's disease: a controlled trial. *Br Med J (Clin Res Ed).* 1984; 288:1859–1862.
112. Lochs H, Steinhardt HJ, Klaus-Wentz B, et al. Comparison of enteral nutrition and drug treatment in active Crohn's disease. Results of the European Cooperative Crohn's Disease Study. IV. *Gastroenterology* 1991;101:881–888.
113. Griffiths AM, Ohlsson A, Sherman PM, Sutherland LR. Meta-analysis of enteral nutrition as a primary treatment of active Crohn's disease. *Gastroenterology* 1995;108:1056–1056.
114. Teahon K, Bjarnason I, Pearson M, Levi AJ. Ten years' experience with an elemental diet in the management of Crohn's disease. *Gut* 1990;31:1133–1137.
115. Teahon K, Pearson M, Levi AJ, Bjarnason I. Practical aspects of enteral nutrition in the management of Crohn's disease. *J Parenter Enteral Nutr.* 1995;19:365–368.
116. Heuschkel RB, Menache CC, Megerian JT, Baird AE. Enteral nutrition and corticosteroids in the treatment of acute Crohn's disease in children. *J Pediatr Gastroenterol Nutr.* 2000;31:8–15.
117. Verma S, Brown S, Kirkwood B, Giaffer MH. Polymeric versus elemental diet as primary treatment in active Crohn's disease: a randomized, double-blind trial. *Am J Gastroenterol.* 2000;95:735–739.
118. Leiper K, Woolner J, Mullan MM, et al. A randomised controlled trial of high versus low long chain triglyceride whole protein feed in active Crohn's disease. *Gut* 2001;49:790–794.
119. Gassull MA, Fernandez-Banares F, Cabre E, et al. Fat composition may be a clue to explain the primary therapeutic effect of enteral nutrition in Crohn's disease: results of a double blind randomised multicentre European trial. *Gut* 2002;51:164–168.
120. Sakurai T, Matsui T, Yao T, et al. Short-term efficacy of enteral nutrition in the treatment of active Crohn's disease: a randomized, controlled trial comparing nutrient formulas. *J Parenter Enteral Nutr.* 2002;26:98–103.
121. Tsujikawa T, Satoh J, Uda K, et al. Clinical importance of n-3 fatty acid-rich diet and nutritional education for the maintenance of remission in Crohn's disease. *J Gastroenterol.* 2000;35:99–104.

122. Belluzzi A, Brignola C, Campieri M, Pera A, Boschi S, Miglioli M. Effect of an enteric-coated fish-oil preparation on relapses in Crohn's disease. *N Engl J Med.* 1996;334:1557–1560.
123. Gionchetti P, Rizzello F, Venturi A, et al. Oral bacteriotherapy as maintenance treatment in patients with chronic pouchitis: a double-blind, placebo-controlled trial. *Gastroenterology* 2000;119:305–309.
124. Borruel N, Carol M, Casellas F, et al. Increased mucosal tumour necrosis factor alpha production in Crohn's disease can be downregulated ex vivo by probiotic bacteria. *Gut* 2002;51:659–664.
125. Gupta P, Andrew H, Kirschner BS, Guandalini S. Is lactobacillus GG helpful in children with Crohn's disease? Results of a preliminary, open-label study. *J Pediatr Gastroenterol Nutr.* 2000;31:453–457.
126. Prantera C, Scribano ML, Falasco G, Andreoli A, Luzi C. Ineffectiveness of probiotics in preventing recurrence after curative resection for Crohn's disease: a randomised controlled trial with Lactobacillus GG. *Gut* 2002;51:405–409.
127. Lomer MC, Harvey RS, Evans SM, Thompson RP, Powell JJ. Efficacy and tolerability of a low microparticle diet in a double blind, randomized, pilot study in Crohn's disease. *Eur J Gastroenterol Hepatol.* 2001;13:101–106.

5 The Management of Perianal Crohn's Disease

Arthur Allan and Philip E. Bearn

1. Introduction

"In patients with Crohn's disease, perianal problems are common . . . but when planning treatment for such lesions it must be against the background of a strong tendency for spontaneous resolution and the risk of incontinence by surgical intervention" [1]. This view was expressed 20 years ago, based on a series of patients studied at the Birmingham General Hospital and peer-review journals from 1964–1980. The intervening years have brought with them a more selective approach based on more sophisticated imaging and new medical and surgical therapies.

2. The Manifestations of Perianal Crohn's Disease

Patients with perianal Crohn's disease (PACD) develop a variety of lesions: anal skin tags and fissures, abscess and fistula, and anal strictures. In the long term, malignant change may supervene. Ironically, Crohn, Ginzburg, and Oppenheimer initially reported that "none of the perianal fistulas, condylomas or peri-rectal abscesses that characterise the complications of true colitis" were present in the patients in their first description of "regional ileitis" [2].

Perianal Crohn's disease is a common manifestation of Crohn's disease. In 5% of patients it will be the only manifestation but it will be found in at least one third of patients with Crohn's disease elsewhere. If asymptomatic disease or tags are included, the frequency is higher [3–5].

Perianal Crohn's disease in the absence of coexistent disease is more difficult to recognize and although the multiplicity of perianal lesions, eccentricity of fissures, and the presence of rectal disease is helpful, this may only be obvious after a positive biopsy [3,6]. Perianal Crohn's disease should be differentiated from the perianal dermatitis (excoriation, superficial abrasion, and maceration) associated with chronic diarrhoea [7].

3. The Natural History of PACD

A few centres have recorded the natural history of PACD in Crohn's disease and many patients have an indolent course without surgery. In Birmingham, 109 patients with perianal fissure or fistula in ano were identified and followed up. Ten patients had undergone proctectomy but only 5 for clinical reasons specifically related to PACD. After allowing for exclusions, including 24 patients who were asymptomatic and declined examination, 61 patients first examined in 1968 were available for examination 10 years later. Almost 30% of those with fissure had no fissure on review. Fifty percent with persistent fissures progressed to anal canal stenosis or induration but without breach of the mucosa in the majority of cases. Less than a third of 7 patients without fissure initially developed anal stenosis or induration. In 21 patients with fistula in ano, 8 had no detectable fistula at 10 years. Seven others underwent surgery but only 1 patient had residual disease 10 years later [8–9].

In a subsequent review of medical treatment and limited surgical intervention, laying open a low fistula achieved healing in only 1 out of 12 patients and 6 patients had impaired continence [1]. The realisation that aggressive surgery and its complications could have a more devastating effect on the patient than the Crohn's disease has traditionally led to a conservative approach—encapsulated by the expression that "faecal incontinence is the result of aggressive surgeons, and not progressive disease" [10]. In recent years, this stance has given ground to a greater use of surgical techniques.

4. The Classification of PACD

Where there is a classification of a disease, there is the potential to compare treatment and outcomes. For PACD, the simplest, proposed by Fielding, recognised abscess formation, sinus and fistula, anal tags, and anal fissure [8].

In Birmingham. a further classification defined skin lesions (ulcers, abscesses, and skin tags), anal canal lesions (fissure, ulcer, and stenosis), and fistula that were subdivided in to low (anal canal to skin), high (rectum to skin), or rectovaginal [11].

The most widely adopted classification is the Hughes' classification, based on the surgical pathology and clinical findings in 150 patients with clinically significant PACD over a 20-year period [12]. This classification defines primary (considered part of CD) and secondary lesions (arising from mechanical and/or infective complications). Basic primary midline and the less common lateral fissures may lead to low or intersphincteric fistulas. These fissures correspond to superficial ulcers elsewhere in the intestine of Crohn's patients. The penetrating ulcers (corresponding to the intestinal lesion that leads to intraabdominal abscess and fistulation) arise at or above the dentate line. They lead to high, complex fistula. In some cases a collar-stud fistula through the levator plate may lead to a supralevator abscess. Horseshoeing of this particular variant leads to extrarectal stricture while more superficial intraluminal strictures result from superficial ulceration.

5. Initial Assessment of Perianal Disease

A good classification will enable the clinician to assess the stage and severity of PACD. Symptoms may be surprisingly minor, so before embarking on medical or surgical therapy it is well to check how any PACD affects day-to-day activity. A full physical examination should be carried out. The nutritional status of the patient should be noted. Patients receive an anorectal and vaginal examination and scars of previous sepsis or surgery noted. Proctoscopy and sigmoidoscopy are essential, the latter to exclude proctitis. A rectal biopsy should be taken. Because PACD rarely presents as the solitary focus of Crohn's disease, careful assessment for disease elsewhere by conventional radiology or endoscopy should be undertaken. Routine haematological and biochemical tests, including inflammatory markers, should be part of the assessment of disease activity. In the emergency situation or where there is chronic sepsis or previous surgery, a full assessment of PACD may only be possible under a general anesthetic and even then may be difficult without specialised radiology.

5.1. The Use of Magnetic Resonance Imaging (MRI) and Endo–Anal Ultrasound (EAUS)

The recognition, classification, and treatment of PACD, and, in particular, perianal fistula and abscess, depends on an understanding of the underlying anatomy. Endo–anal ultrasound (EAUS) and magnetic resonance imaging (MRI) are both helpful in defining the extent and direction of fistula and abscess [13].

Endo–anal ultrasound is now more readily available because anorectal physiology units are requirements for a full colorectal service. Scanners may give linear or 360-degree scans but currently the latter is more commonly used in anorectal physiology facilities. The results of EAUS are operator dependent. Studies may identify previously undetectable pathology and, of course, there may be a false-positive rate as is recognised in early studies investigating anal sphincter damage. The interpretation of the anatomy in PACD is made more difficult by scarring from recurrent sepsis or previous surgery. It is our practice to scan at the time of potential surgical intervention. Assessment in the presence of anal stenosis may be impossible and anal mucosal distortion may make acoustic contact difficult. The use of hydrogen peroxide may make interpretation of scans easier and increase detection of fistula. The role of three dimensional EAUS in PACD is yet to be established.

In one study of 41 patients with PACD, radial EAUS augmented by 3% H_2O_2, defined 4 types of fistula. Twenty-two percent were low fistulas (single track subsphincteric, intersphincteric, and transphincteric fistulas) and 78% were high fistulas (suprasphincteric and extrasphincteric), ramified fistulas, or anovaginal fistulas [14]. A much higher incidence of low fistulas has been reported in another study but this may be explained by selection bias of patients for surgery, treatment, and complexity of disease [15].

Magnetic resonance imaging is helpful in assessing deep pelvic sepsis and as an adjunct to EAUS [15]. Two recent studies have investigated the place of EAUS and MRI. Thirty-two patients were studied to determine the accuracy of EAUS (radial and linear) and MRI (body coil and pelvic phased array coil) and EUA (with methylene blue). The accuracy of all 3 was >85%. but this was increased to 100% when any 2 tests were combined. Magnetic resonance imaging tended to miss short or superficial tracks where EAUS was superior [16]. In another study where the gold standard was the operative findings at EUA, EAUS using a linear probe gave an accuracy of 82% compared with 50% with MRI [17].

In summary, pelvic MRI, EAUS, and EUA are all reasonably accurate ways of classifying PACD, defining the anatomy of the pelvic floor, and differentiating superficial from deep sepsis. It seems sensible to use two modalities to optimise results but accuracy of interpretation still depends on local expertise.

6. Treatment of PACD

The aim of both medical and surgical treatment of PACD is the resolution of sepsis, closure of fistula, and symptomatic improvement. This should be achieved with preservation of continence, avoidance of a stoma, and return to normal activity. Indications for urgent local surgery include pain from an abscess and obstructed defaecation with anal stenosis.

6.1. Management of Perianal Abscess

It is rare to see a Crohn's abscess as the first manifestation of PACD. Patients will often have had previous perianal surgery or be on systemic treatment, such as infliximab, for PACD or CD elsewhere. Presenting features include a painful swelling, painful defaecation, and incontinence for stool. That the site of sepsis may be recurrent has been well recognised. A typical experience has been reported from Tubingen, in a prospective series of 126 patients with PACD, 61 of whom developed a perianal abscess. In all there were 110 episodes of sepsis with 145 anatomically distinct sites over a mean follow up of 32 months. Approximately one half of patients developed recurrent sepsis and immunosuppressive agents had no effect on prevention of recurrence. In only 3 patients was abscess the first manifestation of CD. The site of sepsis was subcutaneous in 33%, intersphincteric in 21%, ischiorectal in 43%, and supralevator in 12% [18].

Although the treatment of a superficial abscess is by incision and drainage, it is more complex with deeper abscesses. Where CD has been previously diagnosed, all patients should be warned that surgery is often followed by the development of fistula. Indeed, a postoperative fistula may be the first clue to a diagnosis of PACD. It is therefore better for a more senior surgeon to drain perianal sepsis in this situation and at the same time carry out a careful EUA, sigmoidoscopy, and rectal biopsy. A superficial abscess cavity may need to be packed and any fistula tract treated by seton. Rarely, a low fistula can be opened but this should be in the absence of rectal disease. Recurrence rates of sepsis may be lower if a seton is placed after partial sphincterotomy [19]. Deeper cavities (supralevator and ischiorectal) can be drained with a 10 to 14 F mushroom catheter. Such a catheter may prevent early recurrence and facilitate identification of any internal opening and secondary placement of a seton [6,18,20]. Supralevator abscess without communication with the perianal skin, rectum, or ischiorectal space can be drained transrectally by mushroom catheter. Some patients may need defunctioning if sepsis is severe and these patients have less recurrence of sepsis [18].

Healing rates following abscess surgery vary between 33% to 83% and depend on the type of abscess. Study comparisons are limited because of the absence of data including anatomic type of abscess, frequency of rectal disease, and follow up data. Patients with supralevator abscesses are in the long term at risk of proctectomy [4,18,21–23].

6.2. *Management of Anal Fissures and Skin Tags*

Most patients with isolated oedematous skin tags will avoid surgery if PACD has been diagnosed because of the risk of chronic fissure and because they are normally asymptomatic. In contrast, anal fissures, the commonest manifestation of PACD with an incidence of 5% to 43%, are symptomatic in up to 85% of patients [24,25].

Acute fissures differ from chronic fissure by the absence of a sentinel tag, hypertrophied anal papilla, scar tissue at the edge of the fissure, or any associated fistula. Chronic fissure may be associated with anal stenosis. Acute and chronic fissures may have similar symptoms. Forty-nine out of 56 patients (20 acute, 36 chronic fissure) did have symptoms: pain (70%), bleeding (55%), discharge (9%), and pruritus (4%) [25].

Treatment of fissure is initially medical and includes topical ointments, metronidazole, prednisolone, and sulfasalasine. Early uncontrolled studies suggested healing rates of up to 81%, but 50% is more realistic. Acute and painless fissures are more likely to heal. When fissures fail to respond to medical or surgical treatment there is often progression to more complex PACD, but this is not necessarily associated with active rectal disease [8,24,25].

Local surgical treatment of fissure in ano is little reported. Anal dilatation has been reported to be helpful but has fallen out of general favor for fear of faecal incontinence reported in one study [1,24,26]. Sphincterotomy with and without fissurectomy may lead to healing. In the Lahey study, lateral internal sphincterotomy and/or fissurectomy led to healing in 7 out of 8 patients with isolated PACD [25]. Two other studies report similar data [27,28]. Careful use of sphincterotomy may be appropriate in patients who fail medical treatment.

6.3. The Treatment of Crohn's Perianal Fistula

Anal fistulas are common manifestations of CD with an incidence ranging between 11% and 28% [28]. Both low and high fistulas will be associated with recurrent episodes of sepsis, but high fistulas are more likely to be associated with other manifestations of PACD such as anal stenosis.

The object of surgical treatment of an anal fistula in cryptoglandular disease is to eradicate it without disturbing anal continence. In PACD it is control of symptoms without disturbing anal continence, rather than eradication of disease. Patients with extensive and unsightly perianal fistulas may be more troubled by CD at other sites where attention is better directed. Many patients will have had previous fistulas. It is important to establish the course and level of the fistula tract but this will not be easy in a scarred, inflamed, and indurated perineum even with EAUS and MRI. When comparing the outcome of various treatments reported in the literature, different proportions of high and low fistula, evolution of medical and surgical therapies, imaging, and recruitment of patients with active CD elsewhere create difficulties. Generally the higher and more complex the fistula, the worse the outcome of aggressive surgery. Faecal incontinence occurs for several reasons, including simple division of healthy sphincter muscle, division of a scarred but continent sphincter, especially when challenged by diarrhoea, and, finally, unmasking of previously unrecognised pudendal neuropathy. Overlap sphincter repair can be carried out after iatrogenic injury, but in a study of 6 patients it was suggested that a covering stoma improved healing [30].

The following surgical procedures have been undertaken in fistula associated with PACD: fistulotomy, seton placement, fistulectomy, advancement flaps, stoma formation, and proctectomy.

6.3.1. Low Fistulas

Outcome results of surgery for low fistula in PACD compare favorably with non-Crohn's disease, with primary healing occurring in 78%–100%

[4,23,26,31–36]. Longer term follow up is less optimistic with healing down to 40% [22,37,38]; five studies are helpful although they contain high and low fistula. Makowiec prospectively studied 90 patients over a median follow up period of 22 months. EAUS and MRI were available. Seventy-seven percent had undergone previous surgery for PACD. Sixty-one percent had rectal disease. Active treatment included both surgery and medical treatment. Sepsis was initially controlled by mushroom catheter or simple incision. Active fistulas were then treated by seton until inactive (when purulent discharge or local pain disappeared). Healing was defined as closure of the fistula for 4 weeks. Fourteen patients underwent faecal diversion before or during the trial period. There were 12 ischiorectal or suprasphincteric fistulae, 50 trans-sphincteric fistulae, and 28 subcutaneous or intersphincteric fistulas. Seventy-one had active perianal fistulas/abscesses and all became inactivated between 2 and 81 weeks. Recurrence rates were 48% at 1 year and 59% at 2 years. Healing was seen in 51 fistulas at 2 years but 44% reoccurred within a further 18 months. Faecal diversion and rectal sparing improved outcome. The lower the fistula, the better the outcome. No patient became incontinent as a result of treatment in the non-defunctioned group [15].

Williams reported the Mayo Clinic series of 33 patients with low fistulas treated by conventional fistulotomy. There were 17 subcutaneous, 19 intersphincteric, and 5 low transphincteric fistulas in this group. Of these, 30% had rectal disease. Within 6 months 93% healed but there was worsening of incontinence in 7 patients. By contrast, 22 patients with a high fistula (16 high transphincteric, 5 suprasphincteric, and 1 extrasphincteric) were treated by laying open the superficial component and then introducing a noncutting seton in to the residual tract. In this group only 3 fistulas healed and 7 remained asymptomatic. Eight patients ultimately underwent proctocolectomy for PACD or associated colonic disease and of these, 7 patients underwent the procedure within 2 years [33].

As mentioned above, curettage and partial internal sphincterotomy led to healing in 11 out of 15 patients with fistula and recurrent abscess and no case of incontinence was reported [19].

Finally in the series of 35 patients with low and high fistula treated at the Oschner Clinic, there were 29 low fistulas and 6 high fistulas. Fistulotomy was performed in 19 patients, 8 patients underwent a partial fistulotomy and seton insertion, 5 patients underwent faecal diversion and then fistulotomy, and 3 patients went straight to proctectomy. Thirty out of 32 patients with sphincter preservation had complete healing. Seven patients who healed required more than one procedure. A further patient required a proctectomy and another developed an asymptomatic fistula. Successful outcome correlated with absence of rectal disease and quiescent disease elsewhere [34].

Hellers reported poor long-term results. In a study with much longer follow up, spontaneous fistula healing was reported in 47% of 184 patients over a median follow up of 9.4 years. The recurrence rate was 35% by 2 years and the proctectomy rate over the study period reached 40%. Fistulas that remained healed were characterised by rectal sparing in all but 4% [37].

Another surgical option is to core the fistula tract and close the internal opening. In a series of 81 patients, 17 fistulas reoccurred and again rectal disease increased the chance of this happening [39].

6.3.2. High Fistulas

6.3.2.1. Setons

Setons are the mainstay of the initial and sometimes long-term treatment of high fistula. A correctly inserted seton marks the level in the anal canal of the internal opening of a fistula and by stimulating fibrosis and settling sepsis can make fistulotomy a safe second procedure. Nylon, silk, and silastic vascular slings have all been used.

Loose drainage setons are used in patients with the more complex high fistulas encountered in PACD and especially when the fistula involves more than one third of the sphincter. A long-term loose seton can drain the perianal sepsis, prevent recurrence, and is well accepted by patient and therefore by the clinician. Loose setons are placed at EUA preferably with EAUS imaging to pick up secondary tracts. Patients should understand that the seton is not a cure and indeed repeat insertion may be necessary. Although, many patients with severe PACD will eventually undergo proctectomy as the disease progresses, this technique may put off the moment [35,40].

In a review of patients with high fistula treated at the Mayo Clinic, Williams reported a series of 23 patients treated by seton. Patients were complex: 18 patients had had previous abscess, 2 had anal strictures, and only 3 had not undergone perianal surgery at all.

Details of medical treatment were not reported. A good result was observed in 11 (48%) of 23 patients. The seton was removed from 3 out of 11 patients with the fistula tract remaining closed during the follow-up period (18–36m). In the remaining 8 successes, the tract remained quiescent for between 6 months and 5 years but of these, 2 eventually underwent proctocolectomy for colitis. Nine patients developed recurrent abscess between 6 months and 3.5 years after initial treatment but importantly in all of these the seton had been removed or fallen out. In 3 patients the seton failed and proctectomy was performed without further treatment. Five patients developed minor incontinence (of flatus or episodic loose stool) and 3 reported a mucus discharge. The conclusion was that in high Crohn's fistula, setons preserved sphincter function but recurrence was common on removal of the seton [40].

Tight cutting setons migrate through internal and external sphincter muscle fibers, drawing the fistula tract with it and leaving fibrous tissue to re-establish the sphincter. In the absence of Crohn's disease, the technique can be applied when one third or less of the sphincter is involved. Unfortunately that judgement is difficult and where recorded, cutting setons can lead to faecal incontinence in over one third of patients [41,42].

A selective approach is necessary. In a series of 27 patients with high complex fistula in ano, 4 patients with Crohn's disease were treated with a modified cutting seton in whom the internal sphincter was preserved. The authors reported that all fistulas healed but in patients with PACD, 3 subsequently underwent proctectomy for severe recurrent perianal disease and proctitis [43].

An interesting therapeutic innovation has been laser ablation, but because this has only been reported in combination with a laparoscopic ileostomy and seton insertion [44], the laser may be best employed by colorectal surgeons as a pointer at meetings!

6.4. *Defunctioning*

The faecal stream plays a significant role in the pathogenesis of Crohn's disease [45]. A defunctioning procedure can induce remission of Crohn's colitis or PACD, at least in the short term. This may be appropriate for patients who are too debilitated to undergo major surgery such as proctocolectomy or segmental resection or for those in whom medical treatment has not been given a fair chance. Newer medical therapies for Crohn's colitis have reduced the need for such procedures, but before this there was healthy debate as to the short- and long-term benefits of temporary diversion. At the very least diversion may still provide relief from the discomfort of perianal pain from local sepsis after drainage.

In a series from Oxford, 29 patients with severe perianal disease underwent a defunctioning ileostomy. In all, 16 out of 19 fistulas improved and 5 healed in the face of active rectal or intestinal disease [46]. In another study, sepsis and discomfort were improved in 22 out of 23 patients by a loop ileostomy [47]. Diversion in Crohn's colitis is less satisfactory [48].

In Oxford, between 1970 and 1997, an average of 2.8 diversionary procedures were performed annually for Crohn's colitis or PACD (out of a total 70–80 operations performed annually for Crohn's disease), 18 out of 73 patients with PACD underwent diversion and all had a combination of complex fistulas and perianal sepsis. There were 6 anovaginal or rectovaginal fistulas, 1 rectovesical fistula, and 1 anal stenosis. No patient had isolated PACD. Early remission was achieved in 15 patients (83%). Stoma closure, however, was only achieved in 4 out of 15 and only 2 of these had good function and no subsequent relapse; 6 out of 11 underwent proctocolectomy. The conclusion from this study is that because only 2 of 18 avoided a permanent stoma, patients will go in to remission but at the cost of a permanent stoma or eventual proctocolectomy [49]. Defunctioning the colon and rectum may obscure the development of active colitis made worse by anal stenosis [50].

Are there any factors that might predict complete remission in PACD? The Birmingham group examined the records of 31 patients who underwent faecal diversion between 1970 and 1997 for PACD. The group was similar to those in Oxford: severe perianal sepsis (13), deep anal ulcer (3), complex anorectal fistula (9), and rectovaginal fistula (6). Eighteen patients had undergone either seton or abscess drainage. No rectovaginal fistula had been subject to surgery. Twenty-five (81%) went in to early remission and 6 (19%) failed to respond. Early responders (17/25) failed at a median of 81 months. Eventually 22 patients underwent proctectomy at median 20 months. One patient required repeated drainage of perianal sepsis. Only 3 (10%) patients (2 perianal abscess and 1 anorectal fistula) have been able to have the stoma reversed. All 6 patients with rectovaginal fistula underwent proctectomy after failing to go in to complete remission. Age, gender, disease duration, steroid use, smoking, coexisting Crohn's disease, blood indices, and CD activity index affected outcome [51].

6.5. The Influence of Proximal Resection and Disease Activity on Healing of PACD

In the largest series of 826 patients followed from 1955 to 1974, 23% had either high or low fistula. After definitive surgery for small-bowel or ileocolic disease, 60% healed. Patients with colonic CD did not heal. Of fistulas, 47% healed spontaneously after resection of active proximal disease although in 35% of cases fistulas recurred in 2.5 years. However, in the 65 patients with rectal CD and anal fistula, 58 patients still underwent proctocolectomy. At this time, however, medical therapy was less advanced [37].

Is there any evidence that medical or surgical treatment that leads to reduction in disease activity benefits PACD? Reports are equivocal [26,29,32,38]. In one series of 35 patients, 3 patients underwent early proctectomy. Out of the remaining 32, 30 demonstrated healing even though 6 had high fistulas. Healing was less likely in the presence of active intestinal disease particularly rectal involvement [34,52,53]. Other studies were less certain that rectal disease was so important [35,54]. Surgery may also reduce arthralgia [55].

6.6. Advancement Flaps in Anorectal PACD

In the absence of proctitis, high fistulas (trans-sphincteric, anovaginal) have been treated by a variety of advancement flaps (endoanal, cutaneous, endorectal, and sleeve) with excision of the fistula tract [52,53,56–58]. Extensive, circumferential ulceration, perianal stricture, and inflammation in the anal canal up to anorectal ring preclude this operation as much on technical grounds as on the absence of a functioning anal canal [59]. Even in centers of excellence the technique is not extensively performed so it is surprising that the technique is much quoted for anorectal fistulas [58,60]. Failure often leads to proctectomy as it reflects aggressive Crohn's disease.

In a small series of 5 patients with PACD, 3 patients with low anal fistulas were healed by the so-called house flap [61].

In the sleeve technique, a cylinder of diseased anal canal is resected and the healthy low rectum is mobilised to form a full-thickness sleeve flap that is then anastomozed to the dentate line. Thirteen patients with rectovaginal or rectovaginal and perianal fistulas underwent the procedure. All but 2 patients were on some form of immunosuppression. Six were defunctioned. A 60% healing rate over 36-month median follow up was seen, although 2 patients required a transrectal advancement flap for persistent sinus [59].

Advancement techniques for purely trans-sphincteric perianal fistulas in CD have been associated with healing rates from 33% to 100% in small series [23,52,62]. In the largest study (20 patients), a 75% healing rate was reported at 2 years with healing less likely in patients with Crohn's colitis. This compares favourably with healing rates of 30% to 40% after seton from the same group [15,57].

In summary, this is a complex technique, little carried out for trans-sphinteric fistulas but with potential in the absence of proctitis.

6.7. *The Treatment of Vaginal Fistula in PACD*

Rectovaginal fistulas may occur in 10% of women with Crohn's disease and an intact distal colon [63]. Unpleasant though this symptom may be, treating coexistent Crohn's disease elsewhere in the gastrointestinal tract may be more of a priority. Medical treatment may alleviate symptoms but rarely results in complete or sustained healing of this type of fistula. As with perianal fistula, the aim of surgery is to alleviate symptoms and, by defining the anatomy, consider the possibility of repair and eradication of the tract. Surgery may improve symptoms by controlling sepsis by simple drainage and placement of a loose seton. In some patients, it may be reasonable to attempt secondary repair procedures. Where repair of a rectovaginal fistula is undertaken, the level of the internal vaginal opening guides surgery. Repairs that do not divide the sphincter should not compromise continence. A diversionary procedure to prevent perineal contamination may improve healing. In all cases, failure of treatment with recurrent fistulation points to aggressive CD and likely rectal involvement. In this situation, proctectomy may be optimum treatment, eradicating symptoms of rectal disease, faecal incontinence, and vaginal discharge. Morbidity from delay in healing of the perineum should not be ignored.

Rectovaginal fistulas are classified as follows: high (involves the vault), medium (involves the vaginal wall above the level of the sphincter), and low (directly involve the anal sphincter). High vault fistulas are managed transabdominally and will not be discussed further.

Repair of Crohn's rectovaginal fistulas are carried out using a transvaginal and transrectal approach. Anovaginal fistulas recur more frequently after local repair than other trans-sphincteric procedures [52]. In severe PACD, the approach utilised is an endoanal or endorectal advancement flap for localised low or high disease and a circumferential sleeve advancement flap for circumferential disease, both in the absence of active proctitis [52,59]. Alternatively, a vaginal approach can be taken [64].

Twelve patients underwent rectal advancement flap repair for trans-sphincteric anovaginal fistula using the technique described by Lewis and Bartolo [62]. Healing at 1 year was 54% but had dropped to 28% by 2 years. This was much worse than the 72% healing for the trans-sphinteric perianal group also reported by this group [57].

The Bristol group reported a series of 10 patients, none of whom had undergone previous fistula surgery, but they were less rigid in their surgical approach. Symptoms had been present for a mean of 4.8 years before definitive repair. Sepsis was controlled by seton drainage and defunctioning in 8 patients. This was a mixed group (5 low trans-sphincteric; 3 high trans-sphincteric; 2 supra-sphincteric). Six patients underwent transanal advancement flap, 1 a low fistulotomy, 2 transperineal, and 1 transvaginal repair. Two patients underwent 2 repairs and 1 patient 3 repairs. Eight out of 10 fistulas remained healed with preservation of a functioning anus in follow up between 6 and 66 months [65].

In a series of 14 patients treated by endoanal advancement flap, there was healing in 10 patients but in mean follow up to 39 months the overall rate dropped to 50% [66].

The transanal approach has also been reported by the Cleveland clinic. In this series of 48 women, 9 patients with severe anorectal and/or colonic CD, however, immediately underwent proctocolectomy.

Curvilinear advancement flaps (CARF) were carried out in patients with mild or minimal anorectal disease. Thirteen out of 24 patients healed primarily rising to 16 out 24 after additional repairs. Five out of 6 with a covering stoma had a successful stoma closure.

If the fistula was long or high or associated with an anal ulcer, a linear advancement flap was chosen (LARF). In this vertical repair, the fistula is excised and the rectal wall and mucosa closed but the vaginal defect left open. Three out of 6 fistulas were healed. Two patients underwent a CARF and one remained healed.

An advancement sleeve flap (ASF) is indicated in women with minimal or mild rectal disease associated with severe anal ulceration. In this technique, a circumferential mucosectomy is performed, exposing the internal sphincter. The rectum is advanced after carrying out an Altemeier-type dissection, and after the fistula tract has been cored out and sutured, the cuff of normal rectum is sutured to the level of the internal sphincter. Again the vaginal side of the fistula tract is left open. In this small group of 5 patients, 3 were defunctioned. Three patients healed after the primary procedure, 1 healed after a second ASF, and 1 underwent a total proctocolectomy and ileostomy [67].

In a study from Mt. Sinai Hospital, 13 patients with rectovaginal fistulas associated with colitis were repaired transvaginally. All patients had received metronidazole and immunosuppressant therapy before surgery. All but 1 fistula measured less than 1 cm and 3 patients had anorectal fistula as well. In this technique, a vaginal flap was raised; the rectal fistula was closed and firstly covered by approximated levator ani and then by the advanced vaginal flap. Postoperatively patients remained on medical treatment that was steroid sparing in all but 1 case. The results were excellent with fistulas eradicated in 12 out of 13 patients followed up between 9 and 68 months and in 13 out of 14 in a follow-up study [64,68].

In summary, vaginal fistula associated with PACD are difficult to treat and flap repair carried out transanally can achieve 60%, but in larger studies this drops to 28% [52,57]. The results of the transvaginal repair appear to be more encouraging [68].

6.8. Anorectal Stricture

Crohn's disease is characterised by stricture formation so it is hardly surprising that strictures can develop in the anal canal, anorectum, and rectum. Distortion of the anatomy by PACD and stricture length may make it difficult to categorize the site of origin [12]. There will usually be coexistent proctitis or sepsis. Presenting features are usually of the underlying sepsis or proctitis (perineal pain, tenesmus, mucus PR, or bloody diarrhoea) rather than obstruction or constipation. The diagnosis is may be made at EUA for other manifestations of PACD such as fistula, fissure, or skin tag.

Quiescent strictures require no treatment in themselves but medical therapy may help symptoms of proctitis. Local medication may be impossible to deliver rectally, in which case stricture dilatation (digital, balloon, or Hegar) may be helpful but is associated with local sepsis. Care should be taken to prove the stricture to be benign and to exclude and treat an associated fistula if there is recurrent sepsis. Many patients with anorectal stricture will come to proctectomy.

The Birmingham group reported a series of 44 patients with rectal (22), anal (15), and anorectal (11) strictures. Patients almost always had proctitis (98%) and severe PACD (93%). Six patients underwent immediate proctocolectomy. Conversely, 5 needed no treatment at all. Thirty-three patients underwent dilatation of the stricture. Fourteen patients required more invasive surgery including defunctioning (2) and proctocolectomy (13). In the remaining 19 patients, healing was delayed in 9 and failed to occur in 3 patients. Fourteen, however, became symptom free and 2 required repeated dilatations [69].

In summary, anal strictures should be managed conservatively once the diagnosis is established because surgery is associated with complications and the outlook is poor.

6.9. Proctocolectomy in PACD

Proctocolectomy with ileostomy is indicated for severe unremitting PACD, proctitis, and malignancy. All patients need to be warned that delayed or failure of perineal healing as well as recurrent Crohn's disease are recognised complications. This is not confined to this disease as a persistent perineal sinus occurred in 14% of patients with carcinoma, 31% with ulcerative colitis, and 36% with CD in one series [70].

In a series from Birmingham, perineal healing was defined as early within 12 weeks, delayed between 12 and 6 months, and as a persistent sinus if the wound remained unhealed for over 6 months. A persistent sinus was present in 33 out of 145 (23%) patients.

The unhealed perineum may be a source of pain and discharge and in women involvement of the posterior wall of the vagina may prevent sexual activity. Patients may be left with a large granulating cavity or a simple sinus. For a simple sinus, simple curettage is rarely successful and radical excision of the sinus with closure has achieved variable results. Studies report healing rates from just under 30% to 100% [71,72].

6.10. PACD, Sexual Function, and the Mode of Delivery

Women with CD have significantly more sexual problems than controls. Many are sexually inactive because of dyspareunia, abdominal pain, diarrhoea, and fear of faecal incontinence during intercourse [73].

Mode of delivery did not appear to exacerbate inactive PACD although patients are more likely to undergo delivery by Caesarean section [74]. Active PACD is an indication for Caesarean section [75].

6.11. Malignant Change and PACD

Crohn's disease is associated with malignant change with reports citing anything from 4- to 20-fold increase in relative risk. The risk is related to early onset of disease and prolonged duration [76]. The risk of development of carcinoma within Crohn's anorectal fistula, rectovaginal fistula, and stricture and defunctioned rectum are well described. Both adenocarcinoma and squamous-cell carcinoma may occur. Pain and bleeding may be features. Malignant transformation has been reported to be associated with anal tags [77].

Malignancy has been reported in 2 patients: one with a defunctioned rectal stump and the other in the perineum 13 years postproctocolectomy but with the intervening chronic sepsis of enterocutaneous fistula [11]. Stricture formation may be significant with 10 (6.8%) malignancies in 175 colonic strictures in 980 patients with Crohn's ileocolitis or colitis. The relative risk of developing cancer was 10-fold in patients with strictures. It is recommended that all Crohn's strictures should be brushed for cytology and biopsied. This is applicable to anorectal strictures [78].

In a series from New York, there were 7 patients with carcinoma (3 adenocarcinomas; 4 squamous-cell carcinomas) arising in anorectal fistulas in a series of more than 1000 patients with anorectal CD treated between 1983 and 1997. All patients had suffered from CD for 8 years or more. In 4 patients the delay in diagnosis was substantial [79].

This data suggests that PACD should be biopsied on a regular basis especially after 10 years. Biopsy will often need to be undertaken under general anaesthetic. A defunctioned rectum should be regarded as temporary and proctectomy carried out in the medium term.

Dysplastic tissue should be re-biopsied on a regular basis but patients counseled for early definitive surgery. Any fistula that does not respond to conventional therapy or that occurs distal to a stricture site must arouse suspicion and be brushed for cytology and biopsied for histological confirmation.

7. The Medical Management of PACD

Outcomes of medical management are more difficult to establish because fistula mapping is rarely reported. Some, but not all, will use a Perianal Disease Activity Index that records the presence or absence of discharge, pain, or restriction of everyday activities, restriction of sexual activity, the type of perianal disease, and the degree of induration.

7.1. Metronidazole and Ciprofloxacin

The mode of action of metronidazole in Crohn's disease may be anti-inflammatory and immunosuppressive. Reducing antigenic stimulation by anaerobic bacteria such as bacteriodes may be significant [80]. Metronidazole decreases perianal odor and discharge. In an early nonrandomised study by Bernstein, there was an early response in 21 out of 21 patients with complete healing in 10 out of 18 patients who continued on therapy [76]. Jacobovits and Schuster reported the results of 8 patients with a variety of perineal fistula whom had received medical therapy and surgery. After treatment of an average of 6.6 weeks, the number of fistulae decreased 20-fold and 50% of the fistulous tracts closed completely. All patients experienced side effects and 5 out of 8 stopped treatment because of them. All patients noticed improvement in Crohn's symptoms during 6 months follow up off treatment [81]. Metronidazole use long term is limited by toxicity and side effects. There is no randomised trial looking specifically at PACD and metronidazole.

Ciprofloxacin may be used in patients unable to tolerate metronidazole. In a small series, ciprofloxacin improved well being and subjective symptoms in 8 patients, but all patients relapsed off treatment [82]. A 12-week course of both ciprofloxacin and metronidazole led to healing of fistulas in 3 and improvement in 9 out of 14 patients but again symptoms returned on cessation of treatment [83].

7.2. *Azathioprine and 6-Mercaptopurine (6-MP)*

The antimetabolite agents azathioprine and 6-MP are purine analogues that interfere with nucleic-acid metabolism and cell proliferation and have immunosuppressive properties. Azathioprine is rapidly converted in to 6-MP in vivo. The use of these drugs is limited by a slow onset of action, requiring up to 3 months to reach clinical efficiency tolerable in long-standing PACD disease. In a meta-analysis of 9 trials, fistula responses were reported in 5 studies. Out of 41 patients, 22 (54%) responded compared with 6 out of 29 (21%) patients receiving placebo. Most patients came from one study from Mount Sinai Hospital and the authors expressed caution in interpretation of this result because two other less detailed studies had demonstrated no significant benefit in healing [84].

There have been encouraging reports using cyclosporin in PACD [85].

7.3. *Infliximab*

Infliximab is a genetically constructed IgG1 murine–human chimeric monoclonal antibody that binds both the soluble subunit and the membrane-bound precursor of tumour necrosis factor α. TNF-α is thought to have a key role in the initiation and propagation of Crohn's disease. It is the first drug that may act with substantial efficacy and a durable response.

In a prospective, randomised, double-blind placebo-controlled multicentre trial, 94 adults with perianal or abdominal wall fistula of 3 months duration were treated with infliximab infusions. Crohn's strictures and abscess were excluded. Patients could be on concomitant therapy, excluding cyclosporin-A. The primary end- point was defined as a reduction in the number of fistula sites by greater or more than 50%. Infliximab was given at weeks 0, 2 and 6. A seton, if present, was removed at 2 weeks. Patients were assessed on weeks 10, 14, 18, 26, and 34. There was a significant reduction in the number of draining fistulas after 2 or 3 treatments. The effect of treatment was rapid (about 2 weeks) and with a median duration of 3 months. The primary end-point was achieved in 68 or 56% (depending on dosage) versus 26% in the placebo group. A complete response occurred in 46% compared with 13 %. Perianal sepsis developed in 11%. Closure of all fistulas was seen overall in 46% versus 13%. Within the study period however fistulas reappeared in more than 50% of cases. This suggests that the fistulous tract persists despite closure of the internal openings. Interestingly, benefit was independent of concomitant steroids, 6-MP, or antibiotics [86]. This has been confirmed in another study by endoanal ultrasound [87].

A similar experience was reported from the Mayo Clinic. The first 100 patients treated included 39 patients with a total of 74 fistulas (50 perianal; 15 rectovaginal or pouch–vaginal; 6 enterocutaneous; 3 peristomal). Each patient received between 1 and 3 doses of infliximab over 8 weeks as induction therapy. Eighteen (46.2%) patients had fistulas that healed and 9 (23.1%) patients had fistulas that improved. Two patients (5%) developed abscesses during treatment. Six patients had had treatment with seton and 3 drainage of abscess at the time of treatment. This prophylactic surgery, as well as antibiotic therapy, reduced the abscess rate in this study. Infusion-related reactions were seen in 19 patients, of which 2 involved hypotensive episodes. Interestingly 18 out of 19 were on concomitant immune modifier treatment [88]. In another study, 23 (69%) of 33 patients with fistulous disease demonstrated a response with a mean duration of response of 10.9 weeks and 78% maintained this response at 18 weeks [89].

The place of infliximab in PACD and CD generally is still to be decided. The high cost of infliximab at £1350 per infusion (dose: 5 mg/kg) has prevented widespread clinical experience and confidence that comes with a new treatment adoption. Perhaps this will come from its parallel use in rheumatoid diseases. Current NICE recommendations are to be reviewed in 2005. Current recommendations direct infliximab should not be used for CD with any type of fistula unless the patient has severe active CD, treatment with immunomodulators and corticosteroids have not worked (or have caused intolerable side effects), and in patients whom surgery would not be the right treatment because of patient condition (NICE April 2002). Repeat infusions of infliximab could be used as a long-term maintenance treatment or as bridge therapy while azathiaprine/6-MP takes affect. In PACD, however, infliximab may be a useful adjunct to surgery by reducing inflammation around the fistula so optimising corrective surgery.

In the future, gastroenterologists and colorectal surgeons will continue to discuss the place of each modality on an individual bases. Perhaps medical advances will make Crohn's surgery generally less common. For the moment the optimal timing, frequency, and duration of infliximab treatment, long-term toxicity, best concomitant therapy, prevention of complications, and cost effectiveness will only be established if it is used in clinical practice [90].

References

1. Allan A, Keighley MRB. Management of perianal Crohn's disease. *World J Surg.* 1988;12:198–202.

2. Crohn BB, Ginzburg L, Oppenheimer GD. Regional ileitis: a pathologic and clinical entity. *J Am Med Assoc.* 1932;99:1323–1328.
3. Alexander-Williams J, Buchmann P. Perianal Crohn's disease. *World J Surg.* 1980;4:203–208.
4. Frizelle FA, Santoro GA, Pemberton JH. The management of perianal Crohn's disease. *Int J Colorect Dis.* 1996;11:227–237.
5. Lapidus A, Bernell O, Hellers G, Lofberg R. Clinical course of colorectal Crohn's disease: a 35-year follow-up study of 507 patients. *Gastroenerology* 1998;114:1151–1160.
6. McClane SJ, Rombeau JL. Anorectal Crohn's disease. *Surg Clin North Am.* 2001;81:169–183.
7. Pescatori M, Interisano MD, Basso L, et al. Management of perianal Crohn's Disease: results of a multicenter study in Italy. *Dis Colon Rectum.* 1995;8: 121–124.
8. Fielding JH. Perianal lesions in Crohn's disease. *J R Coll Surg Edin.* 1972:17: 32–37.
9. Buchmann P, Keighley MRB, Allan RN, Thompson H, Alexander-Williams J. Natural history of perianal Crohn's disease. Ten year follow up: a plea for conservatism. *Am J Surg.* 1980;140:642–644.
10. Alexander-Williams J. Fistula-in-ano: management of Crohn's fistula. *Dis Colon Rectum.* 1976;19:518–529.
11. Buchmann P, Alexander-Williams J. Classification of perianal Crohn's disease. *Clin Gastroenterol.* 1980;9:323–331.
12. Hughes LE. Clinical classification of perianal Crohn's disease. *Dis Colon Rectum.* 1992;35:928–932.
13. Bayer I, Gordon PH. Selected management of fistula in ano in Crohn's disease. *Dis Colon Rectum.* 1994;37:760–765.
14. Sloots CEJ, Felt-Bersma RJF, Poen AC, Cuesta MA, Meuwissen SGM. Assessment and classification of fistula-in-ano in patients with Crohn's disease by hydrogen peroxide enhanced transanal ultrasound. *Int J Colorectal Dis.* 2001; 16:292–297.
15. Makowiec F, Jehle EC, Starlinger M. Clinical course of perianal fistulas in Crohn's disease. *Gut* 1995;37:696–701.
16. Schwartz DA, Wiersema MJ, Dudiak KM, et al. A comparison of endoscopic ultrasound, magnetic resonance imaging, and exam under anesthesia for evaluation of Crohn's perianal fistulas. *Gastroenterology* 2001;121:1064–1072.
17. Orsoni P, Barthet M, Portier F, Panuel M, Desjeux A, Grimaud AC. Prospective comparison of endosonography, magnetic resonance imaging and surgical findings in anorectal fistula and abscesses complicating Crohn's disease. *Br J Surg.* 1998;86:360–364.
18. Makowiec F, Jehle EC, Becker H-D, Starlinger M. Perianal abscess in Crohn's disease. *Dis Colon Rectum.* 1997;40:443–450.
19. Sohn N, Korelitz BI, Weinstein MA. Anorectal Crohn's disease: definitive surgery for fistulas and recurrent abscesses. *Am J Surg.* 1980;139:394–397.
20. Pritchard TJ, Schoetz DJ, Roberts PL, Murray JJ, Coller JA, Veidenheimer MC. Perirectal abscess in Crohn's disease: drainage and outcome. *Dis Colon Rectum.* 1990;33:933–937.
21. Williamson PR, Hellinger MD, Larah SW, Ferrara A. Twenty year review of the surgical management of perianal Crohn's disease. *Dis Colon Rectum.* 1995;38: 389–392.

22. Keighley MRB, Allan RN. Current status and influence of operation on perianal Crohn's disease. *Int J Colorectal Dis.* 1986;1:104–107.
23. Fry RD, Shemesh EI, Kodner IJ, Timmcke A. Techniquest and results in the management of anal and perianal Crohn's disease. *Surg Gynaecol Obstet.* 1989; 168:42–48.
24. Sweeney JL, Ritchie JK, Nicholls RJ. Anal fissure in Crohn's disease. *Br J Surg.* 1988;75:56–57.
25. Fleshner PR, Schoetz DJ Jr, Roberts PL, et al. Anal fissure in Crohn's disease: a plea for aggressive management. *Dis Colon Rectum.* 1995;38:1137–1143.
26. Hobbis JH, Schofield PF. Management of perianal Crohn's disease. *J Roy Soc Med.* 1982;75:414–417.
27. Sohn N, Korelitz BI. Local operative treatment of anorectal Crohn's disease. *J Clin Gastroenterol.* 1982;4:395–399.
28. Wolkomir AF, Luchtefeld MA. Surgery for symptomatic hemorrhoids and anal fissures in Crohn's disease. *Dis Colon Rectum.* 1993;36:545–547.
29. Halme L, Sanio AP. Factors related to frequency, type, and outcome of anal fistulas in Crohn's disease. *Dis Colon Rectum.* 1995;38:55–59.
30. Scott A, Hawley PR, Phillips RKS. Results of external sphincter repair in Crohn's disease. *Br J Surg.* 1989;76:959–960.
31. Marks CG, Ritchie JK, Lockhart-Mummery HE. Anal fistulas in Crohn's disease. *Br J Surg.* 1981;68:525–527.
32. Nordgren S, Fasth S, Hulten L. Anal fistulas in Crohn's disease: incidence and outcome of surgical treatment. *Int J Colorectal Dis.* 1992;7:214–218.
33. Williams JG, Rothenberger DA, Nemer FD, et al. Fistula-in-ano in Crohn's disease: results of aggressive surgical treatment. *Dis Colon Rectum.* 1991;34: 378–384.
34. Morrison JG, Gathright JB Jr, Ray JE, Ferrari BT, Hicks TC, Timmcke AE. Surgical management of anorectal fistulas in Crohn's disease. *Dis Colon Rectum.* 1989;32:492–496.
35. Van Dongen LM, Lubbers E-J. Perianal fistulas in patients with Crohn's disease. *Arch Surg.* 1986;121:1187–1190.
36. Fuhrmann G, Larch SW. Experience with perirectal fistulas in patients with Crohn's disease. *Dis Colon Rectum.* 1989;32:847–848.
37. Hellers G, Bergstrand O, Ewerth S, Holmstrom B. Occurrence and outcome after primary treatment of anal fistulae in Crohn's disease. *Gut* 1980;21:525–527.
38. Levien DH, Surrell J, Mazier WP. Surgical treatment of anorectal fistula in patients with Crohn's disease. *Surg Gynaecol Obstet.* 1989;169:133–136.
39. Athanasiadis S, Girona J. New methods of treatment of perianal fistulas in Crohn's disease. Long term results in 81 patients. *Langenbecks Arch Chir.* 1983; 360:119–132.
40. Williams JG, MacLeod CA, Rothenberger DA, et al. Seton treatment of high anal fistulae. *Br J Surg.* 1991; 78:1159–1161.
41. Van Tets WF, Kuijpers JH. Seton treatment of perianal fistula with high anal or rectal opening. *Br J Surg.* 1995;82:895–897.
42. Garcia-Aguilar J, Belmonte C, Wong DW, Goldberg SM, Madoff RD. Cutting seton versus two-stage seton fistulotomy in the surgical management of high anal fistula. *Br J Surg.* 1988; 85:243–245.
43. McCourtney JS, Finlay IG. Cutting seton without preliminary internal sphincterotomy in management of complex high fisula-in-ano. *Dis Colon Rectum.* 1996;39:55–58.

44. Bodzin JH. Laser ablation of complex perianal fisulas preserves continence and is a rectum-sparing alternative in Crohn's disease patients. *Am Surg.* 1998;64: 627–632.
45. Janowitz HD, Creon EC, Sachar DB. The role of the fecal stream in Crohn's disease: an historical and analytical review. *Inflamm Bowel Dis.* 1998;4:29–39.
46. Harper PH, Kettlewell MG, Lee EC. The effect of split ileostomy on perianal Crohn's disease. *Br J Surg.* 1982;69:608–610.
47. Zelas P, Jagelman DG. Loop ileostomy in the management of Crohn's colitis in the debilitated patient. *Ann Surg.* 1980;191:164–168.
48. Burman JH, Thompson H, Cooke WT, Williams J. The effect of diversion of intestinal contents on the progress of Crohn's disease of the large bowel. *Gut* 1971;12:11–15.
49. Edwards CM, George BD, Jewell DP, et al. Role of a defunctioning stoma in the management of large bowel Crohn's disease. *Br J Surg.* 2000;87:1063–1066.
50. Williamson MER, Hughes LE. Bowel diversion should be used with caution in stenosing anal Crohn's disease. *Gut* 1994;35:1139–1140.
51. Yamamoto T, Allan RN, Keighley MR. Effect of faecal diversion alone on perianal CD. *World J Surg.* 2000;24:1258–1263.
52. Jones IT, Fazio VW, Jagelman DG. The use of trans anal rectal advancement flap in the management of fisulas involving the anorectum. *Dis Colon Rectum.* 1987; 30:919–923.
53. Kodner IJ, Mazor A, Shemesh EI, et al. Endorectal advancement flap repair of rectovaginal an dother complicated anorectal fistulas. *Surgery* 1993;114:682–690.
54. Bergstrand O, Ewerth S, Hellers G, Holmstrom B, Ullman J, Wallberg P. Outcome following treatment of anal fistulae in Crohn's disease. *Acta Chir Scand.* 1980; (suppl 500):43–44.
55. Heuman R, Bolin T, Sjodahl R, Tagesson C. The incidence and course of perianal complications and arthralgia after intestinal resection with restoration of continuity for Crohn's disease. *Br J Surg.* 1981;68:528–530.
56. Robertson WG, Mangione JS. Cutaneous advancement flap closure: alternative method for treatment of complicated anal fistulas. *Dis Colon Rectum.* 1998;41: 884–887.
57. Makowiec F, Jehle EC, Becker HD, Starlinger M. Clinical course after transanal advancement flap repair of perianal fistula in patients with Crohn's disease. *Br J Surg.* 1995;82:603–606.
58. Rothenberger DA, Christenson CE, Balcos EG. Endorectal advancement flap for the treatment of simple rectovaginal fistula. *Dis Colon Rectum.* 1982;25: 297–300.
59. Marchesa P, Hull TL, Fazio VW. Advancement sleeve flaps for treatment of severe perianal Crohn's disease. *Br J Surg.* 1998;85:1695–1698.
60. Scott HJ, Northover JMA. Evaluation of surgery for perianal Crohn's fistulas. *Dis Colon Rectum.* 1996;39:1039–1043.
61. Christensen MA, Ptisch RM, Cali RL, Blatchford GJ, Thorson AG. "House" advancement pedicle flap for anal stenosis. *Dis Colon Rectum.* 1992;35:201–203.
62. Lewis P, Bartolo DCC. Treatment of trans-sphincteric fistulae by full thickness anorectal advancement flaps. *Br J Surg.* 1990;77:1187–1189.
63. Radcliffe AG, Ritchie JK, Hawley PR, Lennard-Jones JE, Northover JMA. Anovaginal and rectovaginal fistulas in Crohn's disease. *Dis Colon Rectum.* 1988;31:94–99.

64. Bauer JJ, Sher ME, Jaffin H, Present D, Gelerent I. Transvaginal approach for repair of rectovaginal fistulae complicating Crohn's disease. *Ann Surg.* 1991;213: 151–158.
65. O'Leary DP, Milroy CE, Durdey P. Definitive repair of anovaginal fistula in Crohn's disease. *Ann R Coll Surg Engl.* 1998;80:250–252.
66. Hyman N. Endoanal advancement flap repair for complex anorectal fistulas. *Am J Surg.* 1999;178:337–340.
67. Hull TL, Fazio VW. Surgical approaches to low anovaginal fistula in Crohn's disease. *Am J Surg.* 1997;173:95–98.
68. Sher ME, Bauer JJ, Gelernt I. Surgical repair of rectovaginal fistulas in patients with Crohn's disease: transvaginal approach. *Dis Colon Rectum.* 1991;34: 641–648.
69. Linares L, Moreira LF, Andrews H, Allan RN, Alexander-Williams J, Keighley MRB. Natural history and treatment of anorectal strictures complicating Crohn's disease. *Br J Surg.* 1988;75:653–655.
70. Baudot P, Keighley MR, Alexander-Williams J. Perineal wound healing after proctectomy for carcinoma and inflammatory disease. *Br J Surg.* 1980;67: 275–276.
71. Ferrari BT, DenBesten L. The prevention and treatment of the persistent perineal sinus. *World J Surg.* 1980;4:167–172.
72. Yamamoto T, Bain IM, Allan RN, Keighley MRB. Persistent perineal sinus after proctocolectomy for Crohn's disease. *Dis Colon Rectum.* 1999;42:96–101.
73. Moody G, Probert CSJ, Srivastava EM, Rhodes J, Mayberry JF. Sexual dysfunction amongst women with Crohn's disease: a hidden problem. *Digestion* 1992;52:179–183.
74. Rogers RG, Katz VL. Course of Crohn's disease during pregnancy and its effect on pregnancy outcome: a retrospective review. *Am J Perinatol.* 1995;12:262–264.
75. Ilnyckyj A, Blanchard JF, Rawsthorne P, Bernstein CN. Perianal Crohn's disease and pregnancy: role of the mode of discovery. *Am J Gastroenterol.* 1999;94: 3274–3278.
76. Bernstein D, Rogers A. Malignancy in Crohn's disease. *Am J Gastroenterol.* 1996;91:434–440.
77. Somerville KW, Langman MJS, Da Cruz DJ, Balfour TW, Sully L. Malignant transformation of anal skin tags in Crohn's disease. *Gut* 1884;25:1124–1125.
78. Yamazaki Y, Ribiero MB, Sachar DB et al. Malignant colorectal strictures in Crohn's disease. *Am J Gastroenterol.* 1991;86:882–885.
79. Ky A, Sohn N, Weinstein MA, Korelitz BI. Carcinoma arising in anorectal fistulas of Crohn's disease. *Dis Colon Rectum.* 1998;41:992–996.
80. Stein RB, Lichtenstein GR. Medical therapy for Crohn's disease: the state of the art. *Surg Clin North Am.* 2001;81:71–101.
81. Jakobovits J, Schuster MM. Metronidazole therapy for Crohn's disease and associated fistulae. *Am J Gastroenterol.* 1984;79:533–541.
82. Turunen U, Farkkila M, Seppala K. Long-term treatment of perianal or fistulous Crohn's disease with Ciprofloxacin. *Scand J Gastroenterol.* 1989;24:144.
83. Solomon M, McCleod R, O'Connor B, et al. Combination of ciprofloxacin and Metronidazole in severe perianal Crohn's disease. *Can J Gastroenterol.* 1993;7: 571–573.
84. Pearson DC, May GR, Fick GH, Sutherland LR. Azathioprine and 6-Mercaptopurine in Crohn disease. *Ann Intern Med.* 1995;122:132–142.

85. Present DH, Lichtiger S. Efficacy of Cuclosporine in treatment of fistula of Crohn's disease. *Dig Dis Sci.* 1994;39:374–380.
86. Present DH, Rutgeerts P, Targan S, et al. Infliximab for the treatment of fistulas in patients with crohn's disease. *N Engl J Med.* 1999;340:1398–1405.
87. Van Bodegraven AA, Sloots EJ, Felt-Bersma RJF, Meuwissen SGM. Endosonographic evidence of persistence of Crohn's disease—associated fistulas after infliximab tretement, irrespective of clinical response. *Dis Colon Rectum.* 2002; 45:39–46.
88. Ricart E, Panaccione R, Loftus EV, Tremaine WJ, Sandborn WJ. Successful management of Crohn's disease of the ileoanal pouch with infliximab. *Gastroenterology* 1999;117:429–432.
89. Farrell RJ, Shah SA, Lodhavia PJ, et al. Clinical experience with infliximab therapy in 100 patients with Crohn's disease. *Am J Gastroenterol.* 2000;95: 3490–3497.
90. Ricart E, Sandborn WJ. Infliximab for the treatment of fistulas in patients with Crohn's disease—comment. *Gastroenterology* 1999;117:1247–1251.

6
Investigation and Management of Malignant Anal-Canal Tumours

Najjia N. Mahmoud and Robert D. Madoff

1. Introduction

Tumours of the anal margin and canal are a rare but histologically diverse group of neoplasms. In the United States, anal-canal carcinoma accounts for 1.5% of digestive system cancers, with an estimated 3400 new cases diagnosed each year [1]. Despite its infrequency, insights into anal-cancer biology over the past 30 years have radically altered its management. In the past, chronic conditions such as haemorrhoids, fistulas, and fissures were thought to cause anal cancer. This belief has been replaced with the knowledge that human papilloma viruses and chronic immunosuppression play critical roles. Thirty years ago, abdominoperineal resection was the standard treatment for patients with anal cancer. Today, chemoradiation has redefined therapy, allowing many patients to retain gastrointestinal continuity with lower morbidity. This chapter overviews the causes, diagnosis, and treatment of anal-canal carcinoma in the context of the rapid changes in this field in the past 30 years.

2. Anatomic Features

Traditionally, the anus is divided into the mucosa-lined anal canal and the more distal epidermis-covered anal margin. Confusion in the literature over precise anatomic localisation of tumours has resulted from reporting errors and differences of opinion among clinicians and researchers. These inconsistencies have made comparisons of studies difficult and may confound outcomes. The World Health Organization (WHO) recently defined the anal canal and margin in histologic and anatomic terms, in keeping with the American Joint Committee on Cancer (AJCC)/International Union Against Cancer (UICC) staging system; it is this definition that most clinicians and researchers have now agreed on [2]. By this definition, the anal canal extends from the rectum to the perianal skin and is lined by the mucosa overlying the internal sphincter. Importantly, this definition includes the anal transition zone (ATZ) epithelium and the non–hair-bearing and non–sweat-gland bearing squamous mucosa extending distally to its junction with skin. Anal margin refers to the junction of the skin and the squamous mucosa of the anal canal. Anal-margin tumours are, for this reason, staged according to the system used for skin cancers.

Histologically, the mucosa of the anal canal is divided into three zones. The upper zone is located above the ATZ and comprises colorectal-type mucosa. The ATZ extends variably above and below the dentate line for about 1–2 centimeters vertically, in fingerlike projections that vary in length both between subjects and within the same individual [3]. Fenger, in a classic study of the anatomy and histology of the anal canal, defined the extent of the ATZ and its relationship to the dentate line with alcian blue—a stain that renders mucin-rich columnar epithelium dark blue, mucin-poor transitional epithelium light blue, and squamous epithelium colorless. According to Fenger, the dentate line ranged from 5 to 19 mm above the lower end of the anal canal. The ATZ was generally located above the dentate line, but in a number of canals, the borders of this zone extended 3 to 6 mm below it [4].

Tumours arising distal to the dentate line are usually keratinising squamous-cell carcinomas, whereas those arising in the ATZ and above are typically nonkeratinising. Because of the complex gross and histologic anatomy of this region, classification of anal neoplasms has been a source of confusion and inconsistency. Most pathologists use the World Health Organization (WHO) classification. According to the WHO classification, anal canal lesions consist of squamous-cell (cloacogenic) variants, including keratinising, nonkeratinising, and basaloid tumours [2]. Anal-canal lesions may also include adenocarcinoma, and other more rare lesions such as carcinoid, anal lymphoma, and melanoma. Anal-margin tumours include squamous-cell carcinoma, giant condyloma (verrucous carcinoma), basal-cell carcinoma, and variants of anal intraepithelial neoplasia sometimes termed Bowen's disease. Paget's disease refers to adenocarcinoma-in-situ. For more detailed discussion of these subtypes, see the Histology section.

The dentate line provides an anatomic reference point for lymphatic drainage of the anal canal and margin. Above the dentate line, drainage is primarily via the superior rectal lymphatics to the inferior mesenteric nodes and laterally along the middle and inferior rectal vessels [5,6]. Lesions distal to the line drain to the inguinal and femoral lymphatics (Figure 6.1). Tumours in the ATZ may follow both lymphatic routes. Patients with unexplained inguinal lymphadenopathy should undergo a careful examination of the anal canal.

3. Presentation and Physical Findings

By far, the most common presenting symptom of anal cancer is rectal bleeding, which occurs in 45% of patients. Another 30% have pain or the sensation of a rectal mass, whereas 20% have no symptoms at all [7,8]. Initially,

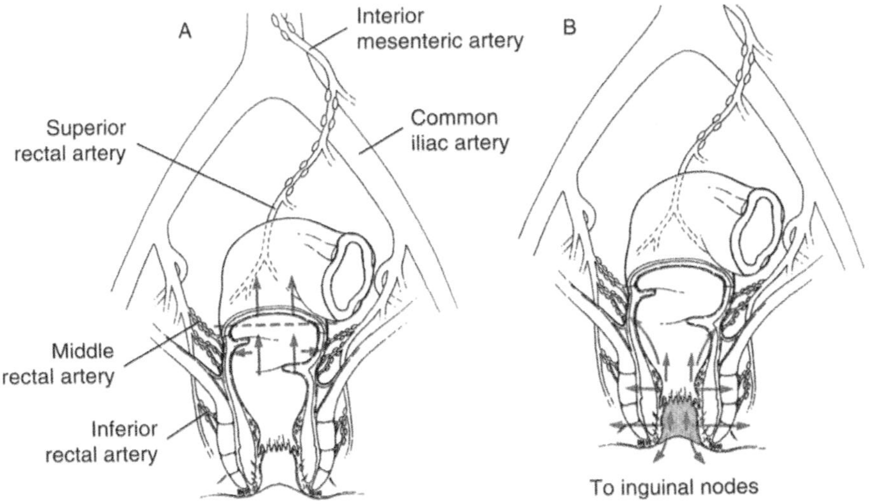

FIGURE 6.1. Lymphatic drainage routes of the rectum and anus. (Reprinted with permission from Gordon PH, Nivatvongs S, eds. *Principles and Practice of Surgery of the Colon, Rectum, and Anus*. St. Louis, MO: Quality Medical Publishing, Inc, 1992:30.)

many patients may have symptoms of persistent bleeding and itching. In one series, more than 50% of the cases documented were diagnosed more than 2 years after the onset of symptoms [9]. Prompt diagnosis and treatment of anal-canal and -margin cancers can be difficult. Stearns and Quan reported that one third of such cancers in their series were initially misdiagnosed as benign inflammatory disease [10]. More advanced cases involving the anal sphincter can cause tenesmus and incontinence. A common problem arises when haemorrhoid specimens sent for routine histopathology are found to contain areas of cellular atypia, high- or low-grade intraepithelial neoplasia, or invasive cancer; in such individuals, treatment and follow up are controversial.

4. Risk Factors

In the past, the commonly held notion was that benign anorectal conditions, such as haemorrhoids, fissures, and fistulas, predispose to the development of squamous-cell carcinoma (SCC). The cause or common mechanism was presumed to be prolonged exposure of the anal-canal epithelium and margin to chronic inflammatory conditions. Similarly, patients with inflammatory bowel disease were believed, on this basis, to be at increased risk, particularly when anal fistulas were present. In 1994, Frisch examined this issue in a large population and did not find a causal relationship between benign anorectal conditions and anal cancer, up to 13 years after resolution of the benign condition [11]. In a similar large population study, Frisch identified 9602 Danish patients with a diagnosis of either Crohn's disease or ulcerative colitis (mean follow up, 10 years). Only 2 patients developed anal squamous-cell carcinoma in this time, both of whom had had Crohn's disease or ulcerative colitis more than 15 years. Frisch concluded that although long-term sufferers of irritable bowel disorders may be at slightly increased risk of anal SCC, short- and mid-term risk is not significantly different from that of the general population [12].

4.1. Lessons from Cervical Cancer

In contrast, striking evidence links human papilloma virus (HPV) infection with the development of anal SCC and anal intraepithelial neoplasia (AIN). HPV is a double-stranded DNA tumour virus with a predilection for mucoepithelial tissues. More than 100 types of HPV have been identified overall, but only 30 types have been found in conjunction with either anal SCC or AIN. Furthermore, HPV 6 and 11 are nononcogenic—they are associated with lesions such as low-grade anal squamous intraepithelial lesions (LSIL) and condyloma acuminatum. Oncogenic or high-risk types 16 and 18 are associated with invasive anogenital cancers and lesions with the potential to progress to invasive cancer, such as high-grade squamous intraepithelial lesions (HSIL) [13].

In the general population, the incidence of anal cancer has been observed to have a female predilection, occurring in women at almost twice the rate as men. However, for more than 60 years, an increased risk of anal cancer in homosexual men has been noted [14]. The identification of a high-risk population with numerous sexual partners and other venereal diseases made an infectious agent seem likely. This likelihood is strengthened by recent studies demonstrating an increase in anal-canal cancer in heterosexual men and in women with numerous partners of the opposite sex; both these subgroups have a heavy burden of venereal disease. Current estimates show that the risk of anal cancer in American homosexual men practicing anal-receptive sex may be even higher than the risk of cervical cancer in American women [15]. The incidence of cervical cancer in the United States is now about 8 per 100,000. The incidence of anal cancer, in both men and women in the general population, is about one tenth that figure. The estimated incidence in men with a history of receptive anal intercourse is about 35 per 100,000—a figure on par with the incidence of cervical cancer in women before screening programs were instituted [13]. In the United States, according to the Surveillance, Epidemiology, and End Results (SEER) program, the relative risk of developing anal cancer is 4.6 in women who had a prior diagnosis of cervical cancer [16].

Interest in the viral pathogenesis of anal intraepithelial lesions and invasive anal cancer began with the investigation of the HIV epidemic. Most current studies focus on data collected before the advent of highly active anti-retroviral therapy (HAART) in HIV-positive homosexual men. Again, cervical cancer provides an excellent model for the study of anal cancer. Both types occupy anogenital mucoepithelium in an epithelial transformation zone, both are frequently associated with HPV, and both are recognized to have a noninvasive dysplastic precursor lesion. Most of the hypotheses about the natural history and pathogenesis of anal cancer are directly extrapolated from the well-documented example of cervical cancer. Prospective data on the biological ramifications of HPV infection and on the HSIL and LSIL precursor lesions in the HIV-positive as well as HIV-negative subpopulations are just now being gathered. No published studies to date have documented the progression of HSIL to anal cancer; however, it seems likely that—with time and adequate follow up, in light of the cervical cancer literature—this connection can be established. Obviously, investigation is hampered by low case numbers in the non-HIV subpopulation and by short follow-up times among study patients in the HIV-positive population (because of the morbidity of their underlying disease). It is not known how HAART will affect the natural history of HSIL and LSIL. Similarly, it is unclear how close follow-up with concomitant clinical intervention might change outcome data [13,17–19].

4.2. *HIV Infection*

Emerging data from ongoing studies show that 93% of HIV-positive homosexual men and 61% of HIV-negative homosexual men have HPV DNA as detected by PCR sampling. HPV 16 was the most prevalent viral serotype, but 73% of HIV-positive men had multiple types compared with 23% of HIV-negative men [20]. In one recent study, the relative risk of developing ASIL increased with decreasing CD4 counts. Other investigators, following a San Francisco cohort of homosexual men, found that 49% of the 277 HIV-positive men and 17% of the 221 HIV-negative men developed HSIL over a 4-year period [13]. Risk factors for progression to HSIL include infection with multiple HPV types, high-level infection with oncogenic HPV types, and chronic anal infection. A limited number of small studies have documented the effects of HAART on the natural history of anal-canal cancer. Evidence from these studies suggests that those patients progressing to anal cancer had lower CD4 counts [13,17,21,22]. In these same studies, those patients with high CD4 counts had the highest rate of HSIL regression to LSIL. Clearly, it is still too early to make definitive statements regarding the impact of HAART on the natural history and progression of ASIL to invasive cancer; however, trends suggest that patients on chronic immunosuppression and HAART nonresponders may have a greater risk of developing invasive precursors. Longer follow up is needed to establish this definitively.

4.3. Smoking

Several case-control studies have demonstrated that smoking increases the risk of anal cancer by a factor of 2 to 5, independently of sexual practices [16,23]. The antiestrogenic effect of smoking is speculated to potentiate the neoplastic effects of oncogenic HPV serotypes [24]. Conversely, lung cancer is more than twice as frequent in those with anal cancer as in the general population.

4.4. Chronic Immunosuppression

An increased risk of persistent HPV infection is correlated with an increased likelihood of anal cancer. Patients on long-term corticosteroid immunosuppression do not have an increased risk of anal-canal cancer, but they do harbor persistent HPV infection [29].

5. Diagnosis

The diagnosis of anal-margin and -canal tumours can be delayed when mistaken for benign conditions. Malignancy must be considered when treatment for anal dermatitis fails, or when pruritus ani proves refractory to medical therapy. Obvious firm masses and bleeding, friable, ulcerated lesions require prompt biopsy. A thorough physical examination includes specific attention to the anogenital region and the inguinal lymph nodes. Computed tomography (CT) of the abdomen and pelvis and a chest X-ray are the standard extent-of-disease evaluation of anal cancer. Other imaging studies that may help determine depth of invasion include magnetic resonance imaging (MRI) and endoanal ultrasound (EAUS). There is currently no specific EAUS protocol for the diagnosis or posttreatment follow up of patients. However, at our institution, we use this technique for all newly diagnosed anal-canal cancers to quantify the size of the lesion, to determine the extent of sphincter involvement, and to detect the presence of regional lymph nodes (although the significance of the latter finding remains uncertain). EAUS is also used in the follow up of treated patients to detect early recurrences (Figure 6.2) [25,26].

The role of total colonic evaluation for patients diagnosed with anal-canal carcinoma has been debated. Current evidence seems to support the view that squamous-cell carcinoma variants do not represent an increased risk for synchronous colonic adenomas or adenocarcinomas [27]. However, full colonoscopic evaluation remains a part of many clinicians' practice. Many patients evaluated for anal-cancer require colonic screening for routine preventive reasons.

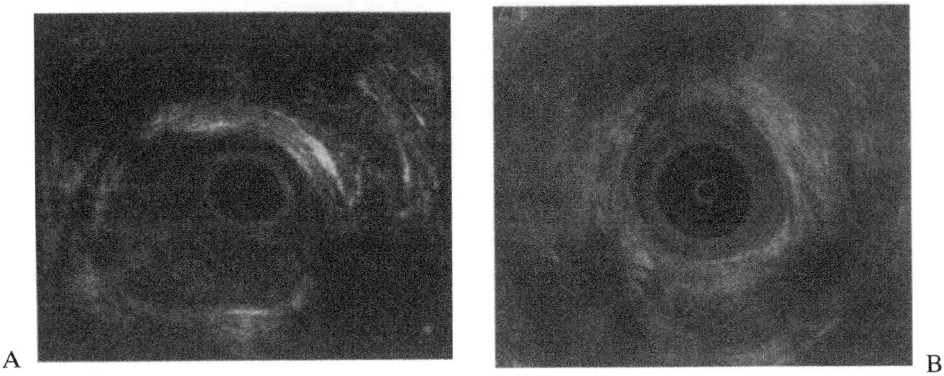

FIGURE 6.2. (A) Pre-chemoradiation therapy. (B) Eighteen months post-chemoradiation therapy. (Ultrasound images courtesy Dr. Julio Garcia-Aguilar.)

6. Classification and Terminology

6.1. Location

Anal-canal tumours are defined by their location and histologic grade. The most commonly accepted anatomic description of the anal canal has been put forth by the WHO and agreed on by the AJCC/UICC. The canal extends from the rectum to the perianal skin and is lined by the mucous membrane overlying the internal sphincter (Figure 6.3). Therefore, the anal

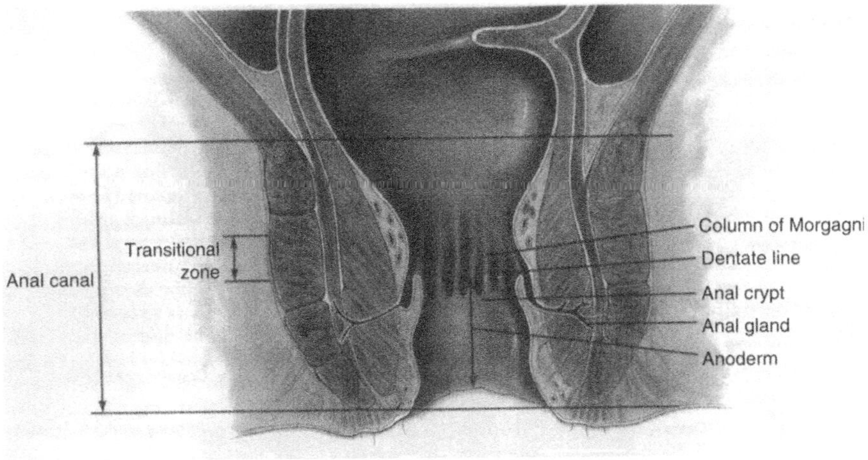

FIGURE 6.3. The anal canal, ATZ, and anal margin. (Reprinted with permission from Gordon PH, Nivatvongs S, eds. *Principles and Practice of Surgery of the Colon, Rectum, and Anus*. St. Louis, MO: Quality Medical Publishing, Inc, 1992:12.)

canal encompasses the ATZ epithelium and the non–hair-bearing and non–sweat-gland-bearing squamous mucosa extending distally to its junction with skin. Anal margin refers to the junction of the skin and the squamous mucosa of the anal canal. Anal-margin tumours are, for this reason, staged according to the TNM system used for skin cancers.

6.2. Histology

Before the WHO classification proposed by Jass and Sobin in 1989, anal-canal tumour location and histologic information was highly variable and confusing [28]. Terminology was nonstandard and even now makes meaningful retrospective meta-analysis of the literature quite difficult. Although the majority of anal-canal tumours are variants of squamous-cell carcinoma, the anal canal and margin contain numerous examples of mixed histologic cell types that have spawned various histologic designations. For example, although the WHO classification designates all anal-canal squamous-cell variants as cloacogenic, other systems regard only those variants with basaloid features (that is, containing small palisading cells that histologically resemble basal-cell carcinoma) as cloacogenic. Other variants are designated mucoepidermoid, referring to the histologic admixture of squamous cells and mucus-producing cells. In the anal canal, about 50% of squamous-cell tumours show a degree of keratinisation; in the anal margin, about 80%. All of these cell types are thought to arise from the transitional epithelial tissue that constitutes the dentate line [6]. Fortunately, neither treatment nor prognosis seems to depend on these rather arbitrary designations (Table 6.1).

7. Treatment

7.1. Background

Nearly 80% of anal-canal tumours are either SCC or histologic variants of SCC such as epidermoid, transitional cell, or basaloid [29]. All of these variants arise in the anal transition zone. As mentioned before, variable terminology has led to confusion in the literature; however, there is no difference in treatment or outcome among these tumours [2]. Another 10% of anal-canal tumours are adenocarcinomas; the remaining 10% are mainly melanomas, carcinoids, and leiomyosarcomas.

The treatment of anal-canal carcinoma has a dynamic recent history, having undergone major changes within the past 3 decades. Before 1974, the standard of care was either wide local excision (for tumours judged to be superficial), or abdominoperineal resection (APR) (for tumours invading the external sphincter). Outcomes were poor, with overall survival rate after APR ranging from 30% to 70% depending on tumour grade, stage,

Table 6.1. WHO classification of carcinoma of the anus.

Histologic Classification

Anal Canal

Malignant epithelial tumours
- Squamous-cell (cloacogenic) carcinoma
- Large-cell keratinising
- Large-cell nonkeratinising (transitional)
- Basaloid

Adenocarcinoma
- Rectal type
- Of anal gland
- Within anorectal fistula

Small-cell carcinoma (designated as histologic grade 3)

Undifferentiated (designated as histologic grade 4)

Anal Margin

Malignant epithelial tumours
- Squamous-cell carcinoma
- Giant condyloma (verrucous carcinoma)*
- Basal-cell carcinoma*
- Others
- Bowen's disease (squamous intraepithelial neoplasia)*
- Paget's disease (adeno intraepithelial neoplasia)

*These types are not usually graded, although Bowen's disease corresponds to high-grade squamous intraepithelial lesions (HSIL) and squamous carcinoma-in-situ (CIS).

Histologic Grade

Histologic grade for anal squamous-cell cancers are listed. In tumours with mixed grades, the most poorly differentiated is recorded.

Grade X	Grade cannot be assessed
Grade 1	Well differentiated
Grade 2	Moderately differentiated
Grade 3	Poorly differentiated
Grade 4	Undifferentiated

Regional Lymph Nodes

In the TNM system, regional lymph nodes in anal-canal or -margin cancer consist of the perirectal, mesorectal, internal iliac (hypogastric), and superficial and deep inguinal nodes. All other nodal groups are regarded as metastatic disease and given an M designation.

TNM Staging

TNM staging (AJCC/UICC designations) for anal-canal carcinoma is shown below. Anal-margin tumours are staged according to skin cancer classifications, and melanomas are grouped separately as well. T refers to primary tumour size and local extension. N designates locoregional nodal involvement, and M implies distant spread.

Primary Tumour (T)

TX	Primary tumour cannot be assessed
T0	No evidence of primary tumour
Tis	Carcinoma in situ
T1	Tumour <2 cm in greatest dimension
T2	Tumour >2 cm but not >5 cm in greatest dimension
T3	Tumour >5 cm in greatest dimension
T4	Tumour of any size invades adjacent organ(s), e.g., vagina, urethra, bladder (involvement of muscle alone is not classified as T4)

Table 6.1. *Continued*

The TNM system allows for the classification of nonsurgically treated tumours whether by chemoradiation, chemotherapy, radiation alone, or polypectomy. The R designates residual disease.

RX Presence of residual tumour cannot be assessed
R0 No residual tumour
R1 Microscopic residual tumour
R2 Macroscopic residual tumour

Regional Lymph Nodes (N)
NX Regional lymph nodes cannot be assessed
N0 No regional lymph node metastasis
N1 Metastasis in perirectal lymph nodes
N2 Metastasis in unilateral internal iliac and/or inguinal lymph nodes
N3 Metastasis in perirectal and inguinal lymph nodes and/or bilateral internal iliac and/or inguinal lymph nodes

Distant Metastasis (M)
MX Presence of distant metastasis cannot be assessed
M0 No distant metastasis
M1 Distant metastasis

Stage Groupings

Stage 0	Tis	N0	M0
Stage I	T1	N0	M0
Stage II	T2	N0	M0
	T3	N0	M0
Stage IIIA	T1	N1	M0
	T2	N1	M0
	T3	N1	M0
	T4	N0	M0
Stage IIIB	T4	N1	M0
	Any T	N2	M0
	Any T	N3	M0
Stage IV	Any T	Any N	M1

and size [30–32]. In a series from Singh et al. at Roswell Park Memorial Institute, the local recurrence rate after wide resection or APR was 25% to 35% for all stages; for tumours invading through the submucosa, 100% [8]. Perineal or pelvic recurrence occurs in 50% to 70% of patients undergoing APR; only 10% die of distant disseminated disease [9].

7.2. Local Excision

Although chemotherapy and radiation result in higher disease-free survival rates, local excision still has a role in anal-canal carcinoma. Local resection with curative intent should be restricted to small (less than 1 cm), well-differentiated tumours confined to the submucosa. A retrospective analysis of local excision and survival rates at the University of Minnesota revealed a direct correlation between survival and tumour size. For tumours greater than 2.5 cm, 5-year survival rates were 60% [29]. For those that were less than 1 cm, survival rates were much higher. Corman and Haggitt reported a similar experience: all tumours confined to the submucosa were cured by local excision or APR; those that extended beyond the submucosa eventually recurred [33]. Longo recorded a 62% failure rate in stage I–III tumours that were treated solely by local excision: all stage II and III tumours recurred [34]. Tumour accessibility, full-thickness excision, and 1-cm margins seem imperative for local resection.

7.3. Preoperative Chemotherapy and Radiation

The treatment of anal-canal carcinoma has changed radically with the advent of chemoradiation protocols in the late 1970s. In 1974, Norman Nigro, working at Wayne State University School of Medicine, defined a treatment protocol involving the administration of 5-FU, mitomycin-C, and preoperative radiation to shrink the tumours. The radiation (30 Gy total) was given in 15 sessions over a 3-week period. The 5-FU was administered at a dose of 1000 mg/m2/d for 4 days, starting on the first day of radiation therapy, as a continuous infusion; it was then repeated on days 29 through 32. Mitomycin-C (15 mg/m2) was administered as a single dose on day 1 of treatment [35]. Although the pretreatment tumour size averaged 5 cm, pathologic examination yielded residual tumour in only 7 of the 45 patients studied. All 7 patients with residual tumour died of disseminated disease [35]. Follow up was under 5 years for many of the patients, but their 89% disease-free survival rate fueled intense interest in preoperative chemoradiation and spawned a number of studies with similar multimodality regimens. Some of these studies used radiation, alone or with other therapies, followed by surgical excision to assess pathologic response.

A number of radiation delivery techniques have been described in the literature. The 2-field anterior–posterior (AP–PA) technique and the 3-field posterior–anterior technique are most commonly used. Typically, a dose of 1.8 Gy/d 5 times per week results in a standard total dose of 45 Gy in 5 weeks. If N1 disease is detected, the fields can be flared to include the inguinal nodes [4,7]. Enker at Memorial Sloan-Kettering Hospital reported that 59% of patients treated with both chemotherapy and radiation were downstaged to pT0 [36]. All of these patients had undergone APR or wide local excision after radiation treatment.

Most multimodality studies since Nigro's 1974 publication have used 5-FU and mitomycin-C as the chemotherapeutic agents. However, several have made dose and infusion modifications, and nearly all have varied the radiation dose upward. Maximal doses have been in the range of 50 Gy. Because of such variability among similar therapies, meta-analysis is difficult. However, direct comparison between studies is useful (Table 6.2).

TABLE 6.2. Results of combined chemoradiation.

Author, Year	Patients (n)	Type of Chemotherapy	Dose (Gy)	Complete Regression (%)	Follow Up (m)
Cummings et al., 1984	16	5-FU MTC	50	94	48–84
Cummings et al., 1984	14	5-FU MTC	25 + 25	100	30–48
Sischy, 1985	33	5-FU MTC	55–65	91	12–108
Cummings, 1987	18	5-FU MTC	24 + 24	89	6–30
Meeker et al., 1986	19	5-FU MTC	30	87	30 (median)
Flam et al., 1987	30	5-FU MTC	41–50	87	9–76
Nigro, 1987	104	5-FU MTC	30	93	24–132

Table modified from Gordon PH, Nivatvongs S, eds. *Principles and Practice of Surgery of the Colon, Rectum, and Anus*. St. Louis, MO: Quality Medical Publishing, Inc, 1992:412.

In 1996, the United Kingdom Coordinating Committee on Cancer Research (UKCCCR) published the largest prospective randomised study of chemotherapy and radiation versus radiation alone. The trial enrolled 585 patients, assigning them to either combined therapy or radiation alone, and then assessed them at 6 weeks. Poor responders were then offered APR and good responders were given a boost of radiotherapy and reassessed. Those patients receiving radiation alone had a local failure rate of 59%, whereas those on combined therapy had a 36% local failure rate (mean follow up, 42 months) [37]. The early morbidity of combined therapy was higher than with radiation alone; in fact, 2 patients died of sepsis. However, the late morbidity rate was the same. With combined therapy, the local failure rate was halved, as was the number of patients requiring salvage surgery. In all, of 174 patients on combined therapy (with a boost of radiotherapy), 29 required salvage APR; of 188 on radiation alone, 72 required salvage APR. Although the local failure rate for radiation alone was higher, overall survival between the groups was the same [37].

Also in 1996, Flam et al. further explored the role of 5-FU and mitomycin-C as radiation-sensitising agents in a phase III prospective randomised RTOG/ECOG trial [38]. A total of 310 patients were randomised to receive either radiation with 5-FU or radiation with both 5-FU and mitomycin-C. Flam concluded that, although the addition of mitomycin-C produced slightly greater toxicity, at 4 years the disease-free survival was higher (73% vs 51%, P = .0003). However, as in the UKCCCR trial, improved overall survival rates could not be demonstrated [38].

In 1997, the third large randomised trial comparing combined therapy with radiation alone for of anal-canal carcinoma was reported by the European Organisation for Research and Treatment of Cancer (EORTC); this phase III trial involved 110 patients [39]. The addition of chemotherapy (5-FU and mitomycin-C) resulted in a complete response rate of 54% with radiation alone and 80% with combined therapy. The actuarial 5-year locoregional control rate improved by 18%; colostomy-free survival, by 32%. As in the UKCCCR study, however, no definite overall survival advantage could be demonstrated. Most patients whose cancer recurred did not respond to local excision, yet the authors observed an advantage to adding chemotherapy to radiation in larger tumours: the event-free survival rate was lower, with similar toxicities [39] (Table 6.3).

7.4. *Inguinal Lymphadenectomy*

Before the advent of chemoradiation, radical inguinal lymphadenectomy was advocated as a useful adjunct to primary resection. Recent evidence reveals an extremely high morbidity associated with it, with little apparent benefit in preventing local or distant recurrence [7,10,33]. Current recommendations focus on the use of therapeutic inguinal lymphadenectomy to reduce the complications and discomfort of rapidly growing groin tumours. The inguinal area is frequently included in the radiation portal when delivering adjuvant therapy; however, this technique is not complication-free. Fibrosis and inflammation can result in debilitating lymphedema that can be permanent, thus requiring the judicious use of fitted graded-compression garments, leg elevation, or both.

8. Recurrent Disease and Surgical Salvage

Anal-canal carcinoma metastasises rarely (in less than 10% of patients) and late. The most common sites of distant spread are the liver and lungs. Patients with recurrence tend to die of locoregional complications, including ureteral obstruction, perineal sepsis and necrosis, bowel obstruction, and venous thrombosis. The goal of early detection of perineal posttreatment recurrences is to prevent lymphatic disease spread. In a retrospective analysis of salvage therapy for recurrent disease after chemoradiation, Allal et

TABLE 6.3. Five-year local recurrence rates and disease-free survival rates in prospective studies.

Author, Year	Patients (n)	Radiation Dose (rads)	Median Follow Up (m)	5-year Local Recurrence Rate (%)	5-year, Disease-free Survival Rate (%)
UKCCCR, 1996[a]	290	45	42	59	60
UKCCCR, 1996	295	45	42	36	39
EORTC, 1997[a]	52	45	42	46	n/a
EORTC, 1997	51	45	42	20	n/a
Flam et al., 1996[a] (5-FU)	145	45–50.4	36	34	51[b]
Flam et al., 1996[a] (5-FU + MMC)	146	45–50.4	36	16	73[b]

[a]Combined chemotherapy with radiation administered. Flam et al. prospectively compared radiation with 5-FU vs 5-FU+mitomycin C (MMC).
[b]4-year actuarial disease-free survival rates.

al. found that patients who underwent APR had a 53% actuarial 5-year survival rate; those who didn't receive additional treatment, 28% [40]. Pocard's data from St. Antoine University Hospital examined salvage APR in 21 patients who had either residual disease after sphincter conservation or recurrence [41]. The actuarial 5-year survival rate was 30%. Factors resulting in failure were lymphadenopathy, positive margins, and distant disease. Recent studies documenting experience with salvage APR after sphincter-sparing treatment are recorded below (Table 6.4).

Contraindications for salvage surgery include medical debilitation, known distant metastases, invasion of the pelvic sidewalls, and obvious inguinal lymphadenopathy. The preoperative assessment should include a chest X-ray and an MRI or CT scan. Imaging of the abdomen and pelvis should include fine cuts (2–3 mm) through the pelvis, to help visualize proximity to unresectable structures (such as the iliac arteries or the sciatic nerve). A multidisciplinary approach is appropriate when local invasion of resectable structures occurs (such as the urinary bladder, cervix, vagina, or sacrum below the S2 level). The team should include a urologist, neurosurgeon, orthopedic surgeon, and perhaps a plastic surgeon. Recurrences close to the pelvic sidewall may be indistinguishable intraoperatively from fibrosis and scarring from prior radiation or surgery. An intraoperative frozen section may be useful if after-loading brachytherapy catheters, iodine seeds, or intraoperative radiation therapy (boost of 1740 Gy) will be used. The role and long-term outcomes of brachytherapy as an adjunct for salvage surgery has not yet been validated.

The complications of salvage pelvic surgery are often difficult, for both the patient and the surgeon. Perineal wound dehiscence and necrosis can have debilitating consequences. Tissue coverage in previously radiated fields provides a way to improve wound healing; many consider it essential in postexenteration reconstruction. Pedicle flaps are routinely taken from the gluteus, gracilis, or rectus abdominus muscles.

TABLE 6.4. Abdominoperineal resection (APR) after failure of radiation (with or without chemotherapy) for anal cancer.

Author	Year	No. of APRs	Median Follow Up (m)	Alive (%)	5-year Survival Rate (%)
Zelnick et al.	1992	9	20	<10	—
Tanum	1993	9	36	67	—
Lasser	1993	14	36	50	—
Ellenhorn et al.	1994	38	47	—	44
Longo et al.	1994	11	25	18	—
Hill et al.	1996	11	25	18	—
Pocard et al.	1997	21	40	48	33

Table modified from Pocard M, Tiret E, Nugent K, Dehni N, Parc R. Results of salvage abdominoperineal resection for anal cancer after radiotherapy. *Dis Colon Rectum.* 1998; 41:1488–1493.

9. Chemoradiation Salvage After Local Resection

Long-term follow-up data is lacking regarding radiation or chemoradiation salvage after local excision. Patients who undergo primary excision for anal-canal carcinoma do so for a number of reasons, including polypectomy, haemorrhoidectomy, excisional biopsy, as well as local excision with intent-to-cure. It is unclear at this point whether further treatment for completely excised, early-stage lesions is appropriate. Nonetheless, patients with positive margins, or with tumours harbouring vascular or lymphatic invasion with poorly differentiated characteristics, are candidates for further therapy. A retrospective analysis from Memorial Sloan-Kettering Hospital in 1999 involved 14 patients who underwent postoperative chemoradiation (either 30 or 45–50 Gy) [42]. Actuarial 5-year local control rates were 93%, with no differences in outcome with the higher versus lower doses [42].

Longo published the largest single retrospective analysis of outcomes in 1994 documenting his experience with chemoradiation after local excision. The overall local control rate at 5 years was 79% in 109 patients (median dose, 42 Gy). Stratification of the data by stage revealed a 90% local control rate for stage I; 54%, stage II; and 100%, stage III [34]. Current studies suggest that incompletely excised tumours, those with poor histologic characteristics, and those that are stage II and above are candidates for chemoradiation after excision. As with primary therapy, chemotherapy (principally infusional 5-FU with mitomycin-C) seems to promote effective local control at lower radiation doses [29,31,34,42].

10. Evaluation After Treatment

Close follow up is considered imperative, but the modalities and frequency are matters of debate. After multimodality therapy, it is not known exactly what time period is required before maximal tumour regression occurs. After that time, any disease detected is residual and salvage therapy is warranted. Most surgeons require follow up every 2 to 3 months. Tumours regress rather slowly after treatment, so 2 to 3 months probably represents a logical initial time period [44]. Biopsy of any residual mass may reveal nonviable cancer cells and fibrosis. Because local failure is the rule in 80% of cases that recur, some surgeons advocate interval biopsy every 3 months, but there is no consensus on the duration of this practice. An alternative strategy involves the use of ERUS inspection and physical examination. At the University of Minnesota, the current protocol is ERUS inspection every 4 months for 3 years, then every 6 months for 2 years. Suspicious tissue or lymph nodes can then be biopsied under ultrasound guidance. The presence of inguinal lymphadenopathy after excision and multimodality therapy may represent a normal response to ongoing inflammation. However, persistent or new adenopathy must be biopsied to rule out lymphatic spread.

11. Screening, Evaluation, Treatment, and Follow-Up of ASIL

Retrospective analysis of outcome for patients undergoing wide local excision of HSIL has reinforced the shortcomings of this technique. Total excision is difficult and recurrence frequent. Brown found that nearly one half of 19 such patients had an incomplete excision with positive margins, and that 12 of them had biopsy-proven recurrent HSIL within 1 year. No patient developed invasive cancer, but 5 had complications (ranging from anal stenosis to faecal incontinence postoperatively) [46]. Even so, when surveyed, most colorectal surgeons opt for wide local excision for patients with small lesions (<3 cm); 87% also use wide local excision for larger lesions. However, 74% treat patients with microscopic disease conservatively, at widely varying follow-up intervals, but without further surgery; most patients in that category have an incidental finding of HSIL in a haemorrhoidectomy specimen [17,47].

Prior to wide local excision, most surgeons advocate some sort of anal mapping to delineate extent of disease, for example, serial punch biopsies (with 2- to 4-mm corneal punch biopsy forceps at 1-cm intervals circumferentially). The use of 5% acetic acid solution with high-resolution anoscopy is also common. The vinegar solution causes dysplastic mucosa and skin to blanch. Biopsies are then taken from this area [17].

Wide local excision presents reconstruction issues in an area that is difficult to heal. Small defects can be primarily closed or left open to granulate and then secondarily close. Large defects merit advancement flap or skin graft closure. Other techniques described to eradicate HSIL include ablative therapies (such as cautery fulguration, CO2 laser ablation, photodynamic therapy, and argon-beam destruction). None of these techniques yield a pathologic specimen, and none have been studied prospectively. Some retrospective series with very small patient numbers have indicated that photodynamic therapy, in particular, may be promising, offering ablation without severe morbidity. However, prospective trials must first be done prior to recommending these treatments as primary therapy for HSIL [17,48,49].

Medical treatments for HSIL have not been well-validated or prospectively studied. Oral and topical retinoids, immune modifiers such as imiquimod and intralesional interferon, and 5-FU cream have not proven effective, although clinical trials are ongoing [13].

Palefsky's group at the University of California, San Francisco, has the most experience with the evaluation, treatment, and follow up of a large high-risk population with ASIL, consisting of both HIV-positive and HIV-negative men. Palefsky advocates a cost-effective prevention program in high-risk populations that is very similar to cervical-cancer–screening strategies. A complete history is taken, with specific questions asked con-

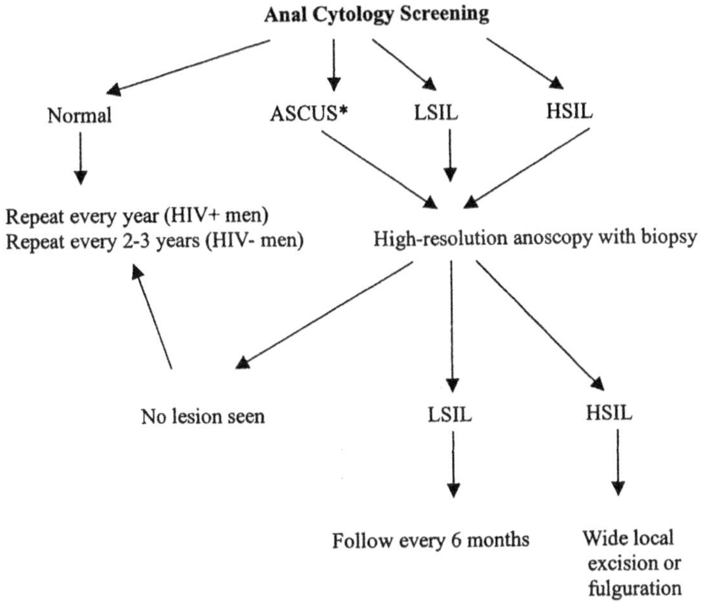

FIGURE 6.4. Protocol for screening for anal squamous intraepithelial lesions in HIV+ and HIV- homosexual men. *ASCUS is "atypical squamous cells of indeterminate significance." (Reprinted with permission from Palefsky JM. Anal squamous intraepithelial lesions in human immunodeficiency virus-positive men and women. *Semin Oncol.* 2000;27: 476.)

cerning anal discharge, pain, or bleeding. An anal Pap smear with high-resolution anoscopy is performed, followed by a digital rectal exam and inguinal lymph node palpation. Further treatment is based on Pap smear findings (Figure 6.4) [13,50].

Unfortunately, optimal follow-up for other, lower-risk groups (such as heterosexual men and women with anal condyloma) are not defined. Prospective studies in these groups are much more difficult, the numbers of affected individuals are fewer, and medical follow up is less likely. Even so, a number of possibly high-risk subgroups, including women diagnosed with cervical dysplasia and prostitutes, may benefit from this algorithm as well.

References

1. Spratt JS. Cancer of the anus. *J Surgical Oncol.* 2000;74:173–174.
2. Rickert RR, Compton CC. Protocol for the examination of specimens from patients with carcinomas of the anus and anal canal: a basis for checklists. Cancer Committee of the College of American Pathologists. *Arch Pathol Lab Med.* 2000;124:21–25.

3. Thompson-Fawcett MW, Mortensen NJ McC. Anal transitional zone and columnar cuff in restorative proctocolectomy. *Br J Surg.* 1996;83:1047–1055.
4. Fenger C. The anal transitional zone. *Acta Pathol Microbiol Scand.* 1979;87: 379–386.
5. Shun Wong C, Tsao MS, Sharma V, Chapman WB, Pintilie M, Cummings BJ. Prognostic role of p53 protein expression in epidermoid carcinoma of the anal canal. *Int J Radiat Oncol Biol Phys.* 1999;45:309–314.
6. Gordon PH, Nivatvongs S, eds. *Principles and Practice of Surgery of the Colon, Rectum, and Anus.* St. Louis, MO: Quality Medical Publishing, Inc, 1992:412.
7. Beahrs OH, Wilson SM. Carcinoma of the anus. *Ann Surg.* 1976;184:422–428.
8. Singh R, Nime F, Mittleman A. Malignant epithelial tumors of the anal canal. *Cancer* 1981;48:411–415.
9. Greenall MJ, Quan SHQ, Stearns MW, Urmacher C, DeCosse JJ. Epidermoid cancer of the anal margin. Pathologic features, treatment, and clinical results. *Am J Surg.* 1985;149:95–101.
10. Stearns MW Jr, Quan SHQ. Epidermoid carcinoma of the anorectum. *Surg Gynecol Obstet.* 1970;131:953–957.
11. Frisch M, Olsen JH, Bautz A, Melbye M. Benign anal lesions and the risk of anal cancer. *N Engl J Med.* 1994;331:300–307.
12. Frisch M, Johansen C. Anal carcinoma in inflammatory bowel disease. *Br J Cancer.* 2000;83:89–90.
13. Palefsky JM. Anal squamous intraepithelial lesions in human immunodeficiency virus-positive men and women. *Semin Oncol.* 2000;27:471–479.
14. Daling JR, Weiss NS, Hislop TG, et al. Sexual practices, sexually transmitted disease, and the incidence of anal cancer. *N Engl J Med.* 1987;317:973–977.
15. Palefsky J, Holly EA, Hogeboom CJ, et al. Virologic, immunologic, and clinical parameters in the incidence and progression of anal squamous intraepithelial lesions in HIV-positive and HIV-negative homosexual men. *J Acquir Immune Defic Syndr.* 1998;17:314–319.
16. Ryan DP, Compton CC, Mayer RJ. Carcinoma of the anal canal. *N Engl J Med.* 2000;342:792–800.
17. Cleary RK, Schaldenbrand JD, Fowler JJ, Schuler JM, Lampman RM. Perianal Bowen's disease and anal intraepithelial neoplasia: Review of the literature. *Dis Colon Rectum.* 1999;42:945–951.
18. Goedert JJ. The epidemiology of acquired immunodeficiency syndrome malignancies. *Semin Oncol.* 2000;27:390–401.
19. Melbye M, Frisch M. The role of human papillomaviruses in anogenital cancers. *Semin Cancer Biol.* 1998;8:307–313.
20. Brown DR, Schroeder JM, Bryan JT, Stoler MH, Fife KH. Detection of multiple human papillomavirus types in condylomata acuminata lesions from otherwise healthy and immunosuppressed patients. *J Clin Microbiol.* 1999; 37:3316–3322.
21. Scholefield JH. Anal intraepithelial neoplasia. *Br J Surg.* 1999;86:1363–1364.
22. Moscicki A-B, Hills NK, Shiboski S, et al. Risk factors for abnormal anal cytology in young heterosexual women. *Cancer Epidemiol Biomarkers Prev.* 1999;8:173–178.
23. Stephenson J. Health agencies update: anal cancer screening. *JAMA.* 2000; 283:3060.

24. Frisch M, Glimelius B, Wohlfahrt J, Adami H-O, Melbye M. Tobacco smoking as a risk factor in anal carcinoma: an antiestrogenic mechanism? *J Natl Cancer Inst.* 1999;91:708–715.
25. Magdeburg B, Fried M, Meyenberger C. Endoscopic ultrasonography in the diagnosis, staging and follow-up of anal carcinomas. *Endoscopy* 1999;31: 359–364.
26. Maier AG, Kreuzer SH, Herbst F, et al. Transrectal sonography of anal sphincter infiltration in lower rectal carcinoma. *Am J Roentgenol.* 2000;175: 735–739.
27. Wasvary HJ, Barkel DC, Klein SN. Is total colonic evaluation for anal cancer necessary? *Am Surg.* 2000;66:592–594.
28. Jass JR, Sobin LH. *Histologic Typing of IntestinalTtumours: World Health Organization.* 2nd ed. New York, NY: Springer-Verlag; 1989:41–47.
29. Klas JV, Rothenberger DA, Wong WD, Madoff RD. Malignant tumors of the anal canal: the spectrum of disease, treatment, and outcomes. *Cancer* 1999;85: 1686–1693.
30. Staib L, Gottwald T, Lehnert T, et al. Sphincter-saving treatment in epidermoid anal cancer: cooperative analysis of 142 patients in five German university surgical centers. *Int J Colorectal Dis.* 2000;15:282–290.
31. Rich TA. Infusional chemoradiation of rectal and anal cancer. *Oncology* 1999; 13:131–134.
32. Cummings BJ. The role of radiation therapy with 5-fluorouracil in anal canal cancer. *Semin Radiat Oncol.* 1997;7:306–312.
33. Corman ML, Haggitt RC. Carcinoma of the anal canal. *Surg Gynecol Obstet.* 1977;145:674.
34. Longo WE, Vernova AM, Wad TP. Recurrent squamous cell carcinoma of the anal canal: predicators of initial treatment failure and results of salvage therapy. *Ann Surg.* 1994;220:40–49.
35. Nigro ND, Vaitkevicuis VK, Considine B. Combined therapy for cancer of the anal canal: a preliminary report. *Dis Colon Rectum.* 1974;17:354–356.
36. Enker WE, Heilwell M, Janov AJ. Improved survival in epidermoid carcinoma of the anus in association with preoperative multidisciplinary therapy. *Arch Surg.* 1986;121:1386.
37. UKCCR Anal Cancer Trial Working Party. Epidermoid anal cancer: results from the UKCCCR randomized trial of radiotherapy alone versus radiotherapy, 5-fluourouracil, and mitomycin. *Lancet* 1996;348:1049–1054.
38. Flam M, John M, Pajak TF, et al. Role of mitomycin in combinaton with fluorouracil and radiotherapy, and of salvage chemoradiation in the definitive nonsurgical treatment of epidermoid carcinoma of the anal canal: results of a phase III randomized intergroup study. *J Clin Oncol.* 1996;14:2527–2539.
39. Bartelink H, Roelofsen F, Eschwege F, et al. Concomitant radiotherapy and chemotherapy is superior to radiotherapy alone in the treatment of locally advanced anal cancer: results of a phase III randomized trial of the European Organization for Research and Treatment of Cancer Radiotherapy and Gastrointestinal Cooperative Groups. *J Clin Oncol.* 1997;15:2040–2049.
40. Allal AS, Obradovic M, Laurencet F, et al. Treatment of anal carcinoma in the elderly: feasibility and outcome of radical radiotherapy with or without concomitant chemotherapy. *Cancer* 1999;85:26–31.

41. Pocard M, Tiret E, Nugent K, Dehni N, Parc R. Results of salvage abdominoperineal resection for anal cancer after radiotherapy. *Dis Colon Rectum.* 1998;41:1488–1493.
42. Hu K, Minsky BD, Cohen AM, et al. 30 Gy may be an adequate dose in patients with anal cancer treated with excisional biopsy followed by combined-modality therapy. *J Surg Oncol.* 1999;70:71–77.
43. Tyring S. Immune response modification: imiquimod. *Aust J Dermatol.* 1998; 39:S11–S13.
44. Cummings BJ, Keane TJ, O'Sullivan B, et al. Epidermoid anal cancer: treatment by radiation alone or by radiation and 5-fluorouracil with and without mitomycin-C. *Int J Radiat Oncol Biol Phys.* 1993;21:1115–1125.
45. Volberding P. Looking behind: time for anal cancer screening. *Am J Med.* 2000; 108:674–675.
46. Brown SR, Skinner P, Tidy J, Smith JH, Sharp F, Hosie KB. Outcome after surgical resection for high-grade anal intraepithelial neoplasia (Bowen's disease). *Br J Surg.* 1999;86:1063–1066.
47. Cleary RK, Schaldenbrand JD, Fowler JJ, Schuler JM, Lampman RM. Treatment options for perianal Bowen's disease: survey of American Society of Colon and Rectal Surgeons members. *Am Surg.* 2000;68:686–688.
48. Morton CA, Whitehurst C, McColl JH, Moore JV, MacKie RM. Photodynamic therapy for large or multiple patches of Bowen disease and basal cell carcinoma. *Arch Dermatol.* 2001;137:319–324.
49. Runfola MA, Weber TK, Rodriguez-Bigas MA, Dougherty TJ, Petrelli NJ. Photodynamic therapy for residual neoplasms of the perianal skin. *Dis Colon Rectum.* 2000;43:499–502.
50. Goldie SJ, Kuntz KM, Weinstien MC, Freedberg KA, Welton ML, Palefsky JM. The clinical effectiveness and cost-effectiveness of screening for anal squamous intraepithelial lesions in homosexual and bisexual HIV-positive men. *JAMA.* 1999;281:1822–1829.

7
Difficult Intraoperative Problems in Pelvic Surgery

Finlay J.M. Curran and Nigel A. Scott

1. Introduction

Colorectal surgery in the pelvis is directed at removing a neoplastic or inflammatory process from the confines of the pelvic cavity and/or reconstructing intestinal continuity to the anal canal. Both types of pathological processes, unrestrained by anatomical planes, can involve adjacent pelvic viscera, the pelvic nerves, the musculature of the pelvic floor, pelvic vessels, and the bony pelvis in an unpredictable fashion. Intraoperative problems and dilemmas in the pelvis are posed by the complexity of the structures that are involved by the pathology compounded by the narrow confines and restricted access of the true pelvis. In addition, the restoration of rectal and genitourinary function along with wound reconstruction presents a wide range of technical intraoperative challenges [1].

The best approach to difficult intraoperative pelvic problems in colorectal surgery is anticipation of the problem and its planned management to optimise patient outcomes. Preoperative planning involves meticulous imaging and detailed patient discussion, assembly of an experienced multiprofessional team, and appropriate operating room and preoperative resources.

2. Preoperative Planning

For the colorectal surgeon, difficulties in the pelvis are compounded by unexpected tumour or inflammatory involvement of vascular structures, genitourinary structures, and pelvic musculoskeletal components. Loss of tissue planes due to previous pelvic surgery and/or radiotherapy exacerbates these surgical difficulties (Figure 7.1). Anticipation of anatomical problems is based on a comprehensive preoperative imaging strategy might include the processes in Table 7.1.

Having delineated the extent of the pelvic pathology and established the feasibility of excision, detailed involvement of the patient and relatives in

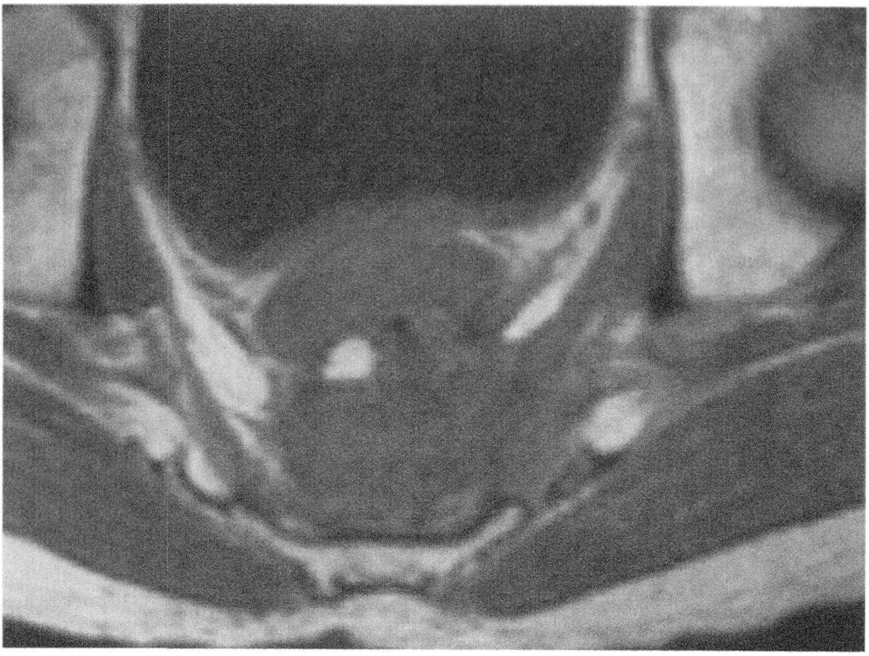

FIGURE 7.1. Magnetic resonance imaging of a rectal-cancer recurrence.

the operative strategy is essential. Excisional pelvic surgery has a range of potentially devastating mental and physical consequences for the patient. Addressing these concerns preoperatively considerably simplifies the management of problems encountered intraoperatively (Table 7.2).

The final aspect of preparedness for complex pelvic surgery and associated intraoperative problems is the identification of the resources and per-

TABLE 7.1. Preoperative imaging strategy.

Inflammatory Process	Neoplastic Process
Physical, including pelvic examination under anaesthetic	Physical, including pelvic examination under anaesthetic
Lower gastrointestinal endoscopy	Lower gastrointestinal endoscopy
Cystoscopy	Cystoscopy
Computed tomography of the pelvis	Computed tomography of the pelvis
Magnetic resonance imaging of the pelvis	Magnetic resonance imaging of the pelvis
Gastrointestinal contrast series	Transrectal ultrasound
Intravenous pyelogram	Staging computed tomography chest and abdomen
Excretion renogram	Positron emission tomography scan
	Intravenous pyelogram
	Excretion renogram

TABLE 7.2. Potential mental and physical consequences of excisional pelvic surgery for the patient.

Loss of anorectal function and stoma formation
Loss of bladder function and stoma formation
Loss of sexual function
Postoperative morbidity including nonhealing perineum
Postoperative mortality
Adjuvant morbidity
Risk of noncurative procedure

sonnel required for the planned procedure and anticipated intraoperative problems. Multidisciplinary team operating is a skill that is developed by frequent practice. Consultants that commonly operate together develop intraoperative patterns of working that are difficult to emulate in ad hoc surgical teams summoned to the operating room on an urgent unplanned basis. Although not all are applicable to the majority of cases, access to the resources listed in Table 7.3 should be considered in the planning of a complex colorectal pelvic case.

It is mandatory that a complex colorectal procedure be conducted with the correct personnel and within the correct environment. Senior theater nurses with an extensive colorectal experience are essential for difficult pelvic surgery to both anticipate problems and manage the technical requirements of a multidisciplinary surgical team. Junior surgical trainees are not suitable sole assistants for complex pelvic surgery. Senior trainees, colorectal specialist surgical assistants, and/or joint consultant operating are more appropriate.

Exposure of the pelvic operative field can present a problem. While the pelvis of a thin female allows easy, direct visualisation of the procedure, the obese male pelvis is a much more difficult environment to operate within. The majority of colorectal pelvic surgery is conducted in the Lloyd Davis position (Figure 7.2). Careful attention has to be paid to the positioning of the lower limbs to avoid compression of the lateral popliteal nerve and

TABLE 7.3. Identification of the resources and personnel that should be considered in the planning of a complex colorectal pelvic case.

Consultant Surgical Personnel	Operating Room Resource	Perioperative Care
Colorectal surgeon	Three-session day	MPT discussion
Urologist	Three scrub teams	Stoma care
Gynaecologist	Two consultant anaesthetists	Preoperative clinic
Neurosurgeon (spinal)	Image intensifier, epidural placement	Bowel preparation
Plastic surgeon	Repositioning (Lloyd Davies, prone, supine)	Blood bank on site
Vascular surgeon		HDU bed provision
	Cell Saver® access	ITU bed provision

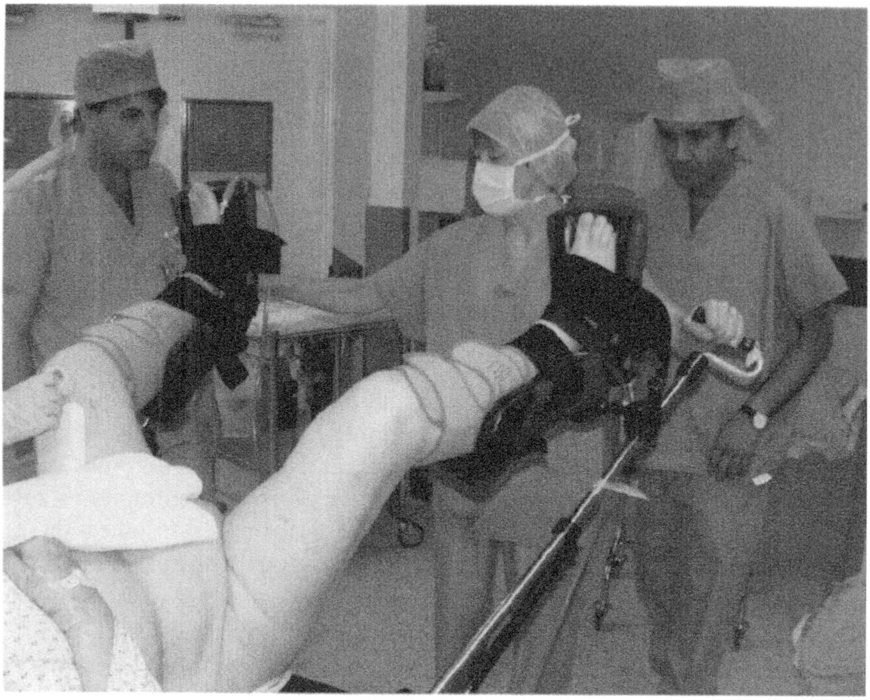

A

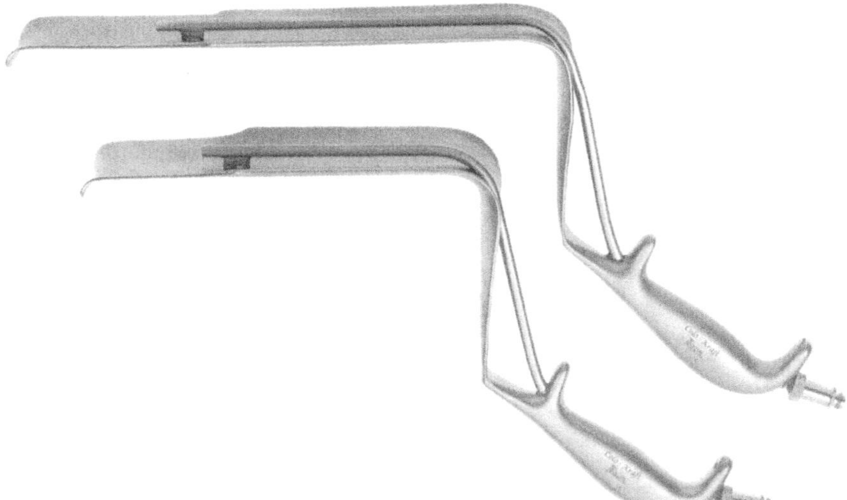

B

FIGURE 7.2. (A) Overall view: Lloyd Davis position with head down. (B) St. Mark's retractors.

lower-leg compartment syndrome. For removal of the anal canal, the coccyx must be advanced beyond the edge of the operating table. When a mucosectomy or intersphincteric dissection is contemplated, it is helpful to retract the buttocks of an obese patient with adhesive tape. A posterior approach to the sacrum necessitates intraoperative repositioning of the patient into the prone jackknife position.

The dissection techniques used for a malignant process differ fundamentally from those used for an inflammatory mass. An inflammatory process is pinched off adjacent to the involved structures in the expectation that removal of the inflammatory focus will be followed by resolution of the inflammation. By contrast, a malignant process must never be transgressed by the dissection—malignancy must be removed intact within a block of normal structures for local cure to be effected. The pelvis is cleared of small bowel loops by positioning the patient head down. Early in the process of defining a malignant pelvic mass, loops of small bowel adherent to the mass should be divided across with a 55-mm stapling gun. Similarly, the sigmoid should be divided from the rectum and all the abdominal viscera packed away from the pelvis into the upper abdomen.

Access and retraction is greatly assisted by using a mechanical retractor such as the Omnitract. Two short blades are used to retract the abdominal wall laterally and the large fence retractor placed over packs keeps the small bowel out of the pelvis. Finally, the lipped retractors can be used to retract the bladder or the vagina and uterus anteriorly away from the rectum. Standard theater lighting can be adequate for illuminating the generality of the operative field, but detailed dissection on the pelvic floor requires lighting directed into the pelvis. Headlamps offer a consistently high standard of pelvic illumination. An alternative is a lighted retractor, which is useful for dissection deep onto the pelvic floor.

Difficult intraoperative pelvic problems consist of (a) vascular or urogenital collateral damage, (b) specific excisional problems, and (c) pelvic visceral and soft tissue reconstruction.

3. Collateral Damage

3.1. *Intraoperative Pelvic Haemorrhage*

Colorectal pelvic surgery can be complicated by difficult intraoperative haemorrhage. Haemorrhage during surgery in the pelvis can be a life-threatening event and usually arises from either the presacral venous plexus or from branches of the internal iliac vessels on the pelvic sidewall.

3.1.1. Presacral Venous Haemorrhage

There are two separate systems of veins in the presacral space and each is a potential source of bleeding [2]. The presacral venous plexus forms one system and this communicates with the internal sacral venous drainage by a series of basivertebral veins. The adventitia of the valveless basivertebral veins is continuous with the sacral periosteum as the vein enters the sacral foramen. The damaged the veins can retract into the sacral foramina and form a second potential source of major presacral bleeding.

Presacral bleeding in the majority of cases is due to performing the dissection of the mesorectum posterior to the rectum in the wrong plane [3]. The correct plane for mesorectal excision is through loose areolar tissue, which is almost completely avascular. If this plane is not defined correctly by sharp dissection, the surgeon can begin to remove the presacral fascia, particularly if conducting a blunt dissection behind the rectum with the hand or a swab on a stick. Such a blunt stripping disrupts the hypogastric plexus and exposes the lumbosacral disc, the sacral periosteum, and the very thin-walled veins of the presacral plexus. Continued blunt stripping of the presacral fascia tears these veins and initiates torrential venous bleeding.

Haemorrhage from the presacral plexus will not improve by placing the patient in a steep Trendelenburg position, as this increases the pressure within the basivertebral veins, facilitating further bleeding. The best initial manoeuvre is to stop operating and use the pressure of a pack accurately placed over the bleeding point to stem the blood loss. Keep the pressure applied with your hand to ensure that you have control while you consider your options. Do not waste time and circulating blood volume by sucking at a bleeding field that you cannot define due to the torrential loss of blood. Do not take the pack in and out frequently to be greeted by severe blood loss—be prepared to sustain the pressure with the help of an assistant for 30 minutes or so.

While gaining control of the bleeding by pressure, inform the anaesthetist that you have a significant problem with pelvic bleeding. Give the anaesthetist time to consider the following while you maintain haemorrhage control by pressure: (a) immediate blood and/or fluid infusion if clinically appropriate, (b) arranging for cross-matched units to be brought to theatre, (c) arranging for further cross-match units, or (d) arranging for a Cell Saver® (Haemonetics), if available.

You should also consider the personnel, equipment, and manoeuvres you may need to employ to stop the presacral bleeding. Do you have a suitable assistant to help you visualise the bleed and deal with it? If not, consider sending for more experienced help, including a fellow consultant, at this stage. Is the lighting adequate? Would a lighted retractor or a headlight improve the view? Do you need two suckers to clear the operative field for a good view when the packs are removed?

What technique might arrest the haemorrhage?

- Pressure alone with haemostatic Surgicel (Johnson & Johnson)
- Diathermy with spray on
- Argon beam plasma coagulation

- Suture
- Thumbtack with Surgicel
- Leave the pelvis packed postoperatively

Talk these options over with your assistants and the scrub staff and assemble all the options in the theater while you continue to maintain control with pressure on the haemorrhage site. Do not be tempted to begin to move the pack and visualise the bleeding point until all the anaesthetic preparations for torrential bleeding and all your requirements for personnel and equipment are assembled in the operating room.

3.1.2. Surgical Control of Presacral Haemorrhage

After 30 minutes of direct pressure on the haemorrhage site, with suitable experienced assistance, suction, and lighting in place, the pack is removed. It is not uncommon at this stage for pressure alone to be responsible for a considerable reduction in the ferocity of the blood loss. If this is the case, the application of haemostatic Surgicel with further pressure may arrest the bleeding entirely and allow mesorectal excision, in the right plane, to continue.

Continued significant presacral bleeding requires intervention, and brief direct visualisation of the bleeding point using brief suction before reapplying the packs allows a decision to be made about the best option. Is there a length of visible vein on the sacrum that can be sutured or does the blood loss emerge straight from a torn vein in the bony sacrum?

Diathermy is usually quite useless for presacral venous bleeding, often making the situation worse by disrupting the delicate venous plexus further. Argon beam plasma coagulation offers the theoretical advantage of noncontact coagulation, preventing inadvertent removal of the eschar, but is unlikely to be effective against the full force of a torrential bleed.

A visible length of disrupted vein (i.e., bleeding from a vein in the presacral plexus) allows an attempt at suture ligation using a 3-0 prolene vascular suture. Suturing into the pelvis onto the sacral periosteum requires experienced assistance to help pick up the needle without tearing the sacral vein further. Under-running the vessel and tying the suture requires great care and delicacy to prevent further venous damage. However, with care and good assistance and exposure, haemorrhage from an exposed length of presacral vein can be controlled by suture ligation.

Direct torrential haemorrhage from a venous source in the sacrum (i.e., bleeding from a basivertebral vein), if not controlled by pressure, cannot be controlled by diathermy or suture ligation. Occlusion of the venous os by a metallic thumbtack offers a means of controlling such bleeding. Although various sterilised metallic tacks have been reported, titanium thumbtacks are now commercially available [2,4–8]. The thumbtack is inserted directly over the bleeding into the sacral bone to stop the haemorrhage from the basivertebral vein in the sacral foramen. The thumbtack may also be inserted through a sheet of the synthetic coagulant Surgicel to produce greater tamponade in addition to the procoagulant properties of the Surgicel. In the elderly osteoporotic pelvis, the tack can be easily inserted by direct digital pressure. By contrast, the sacrum of a young man can be so dense that the occlusive tack requires considerably more force to place it into the bone.

3.1.3. Surgical Control of Iliac Venous Bleeding

Dissection within the mesorectal plane does not involve any branches of the iliac vessels. Iliac-vein injury is the result of dissection that accidentally or deliberately strays out of this plane to deal with disease that involves the pelvic sidewall. Injury to the common and/or external iliac veins is uncommon but potentially devastating. Careful control and exposure of the venous laceration is required before direct repair with a single ended 4–0 vascular prolene suture is attempted. Early involvement of a vascular surgeon is essential if this injury is not rapidly brought under control.

More commonly, dissection taken out to the pelvic sidewalls disrupts branches of the internal iliac arteries and or internal iliac veins. Careful and knowledgeable dissection identifies and controls vascular pedicles with ligaclips before division. Suture ligation of arterial bleeding points is relatively straightforward. Venous branches are more difficult, producing poorly localised torrential venous loss. Direct pressure for several minutes allows anaesthetic preparations and surgical assembly of personnel and options. Venous loss is reduced by a period of pressure and the venous injury visualised and controlled by suture ligation. Haemostasis in the operative field should be re-established before the dissection is continued, but in some circumstances rapid removal of the pathology is required to gain access to a bleeding point within the confines of the true pelvis.

3.1.4. Postoperative Pelvic Packing

If direct means of pelvic haemostasis are not successful, postoperative packing of the pelvis may be required [9,10]. Application of haemostatic gauze to the haemorrhaging point is maintained by the pressure of several lengths of 6-inch ribbon gauze. The gauze may be used dry and the packs are left in place for 48 to 72 hours while coagulation studies and the patient's haemoglobin are normalised. Care should be exercised when removing the packs. Pulling adherent gauze from the sacral fascia may cause further bleeding. This can be prevented by placing the gauze in an intestinal bag prior to packing.

The patient should be returned to the operating room for removal of the pack with the personnel and equipment available for a full laparotomy if pelvic haemorrhage resumes on removal of the pack.

Leaving the ends of the gauze packs emerging from the lower end of the laparotomy wound allows removal in some instances without laparotomy.

Alternatively pack removal is carried out via a formal laparotomy when pelvic haemostasis can be checked under direct vision as the packs are removed.

3.2. Urogenital Collateral Damage

Surgery in the pelvis for colorectal cancer or inflammatory bowel disease including diverticular disease places the ureters at risk of injury—division and/or suture occlusion. In reoperative pelvic surgery, these risks are increased by the ureters being pulled in towards the rectum.

3.2.1. Strategies for Protecting the Ureters

The possibility of ureteric injury is a concern in all pelvic colorectal surgery. The incidence of ureteric injury during mobilisation or excision of the rectum is reported as being up to 6% [11–14]. Protection is best afforded by early and direct visualisation of both the left and the right ureter. The surgeon must maintain a rigid policy of not dividing any vascular pedicle, especially the inferior mesenteric pedicle, without checking the position of each ureter. Simple identification can be augmented by gently slinging each ureter with a rubber sling, as this reduces the time spent on re-establishing the position of each ureter prior to continuing with the dissection. Reoperative pelvic surgery in which normal tissue planes have been violated and surgery for inflammatory bowel disease, especially a diverticular mass or a Crohn's mass, can make ureteric identification difficult. If a ureter is pulled on to an inflammatory mass it can be gently separated from the mass by blunt finger dissection. The index finger is placed between the ureter and the inflammatory mass with the nail towards the ureter and the pulp of the fingertip towards the mass. The index finger is then pushed down between the ureter and the inflammatory process to separate the ureter away and laterally from the mass.

Ureteric stents can be of great help if ureteric identification is anticipated to be difficult. Standard 4F stents placed at the beginning of the case allow for the ureters to be easily identified by palpation in the majority of cases. However, hard atheromatous plaques in the iliac vessels can make identification of the course of the stented ureter difficult by palpation alone. The use of illuminated ureteric stents adds another dimension to ensuring ureteric safety in complex cases by giving a direct visual guide to ureteric position throughout the dissection (Figure 7.3).

3.2.2. Colorectal Cancer Involvement of the Urogenital Tract

Cure of a colorectal cancer that involves the urological tract mandates en bloc resection of the involved structures. Trial dissections that cross tumour planes condemn the patient to pelvic recurrence. It is imperative that before

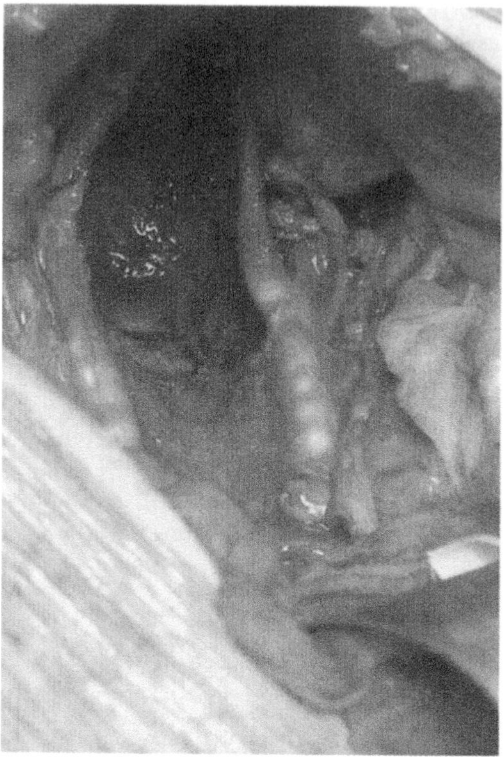

FIGURE 7.3. Illuminated stents.

proceeding with this type of surgery that the following conditions are satisfied:

- Preoperative imaging excludes distant metastases so local cure is possible by radical excision.
- Consideration is given to adjuvant radical (50 Gy) preoperative radiotherapy (with or without chemotherapy).
- Relative bilateral renal function is established by isotope renogram.
- Joint review of the case with a consultant urologist is conducted.
- Preoperative counselling of the patient and family as to possible outcomes, including impotence and ileal conduit.

Cancer invasion of the dome of the bladder can usually be handled by entering the dome of the bladder away from the tumour (telling the anaesthetist that urine output via the catheter will temporarily cease) and visualising both ureteric orifices to be clear of the planned resection. A disc of bladder to include the invasion and a good circumferential margin is then excised and the bladder repaired in 2 layers of vicryl. A urethral or suprapubic catheter is then left in place for 10 days. If this excision threatens to considerably reduce bladder volume then an urologist should be involved in this simple excision to consider bladder augmentation with a length of small bowel.

Cancer invasion of a ureter has to be handled by en bloc resection with good margins of normal tissue around the tumour. In these circumstances considerable ureteric length can be lost and reconstruction options that the urologist might consider include reimplantation with Psoas hitch, uretero–ureteric anastomosis to the normal ureter on the other side, Boari flap and reimplantation, or interposition of a length of small bowel.

Locally advanced, low rectal cancers can directly invade the prostate gland and/or seminal vesicles. Cystoscopy, digital examination under anaesthesia, and magnetic resonance imaging are all useful in preoperative assessment of this possibility. If surgical cure is the therapeutic intention, total pelvic clearance is required with an end sigmoid colostomy and an ileal (or sigmoid) conduit. A possible alternative strategy to bladder excision if only the prostate is involved is radical prostatectomy with vesico–urethral reconstruction in the hands of an experienced urologist. Urinary continence is likely to be impaired and prostatectomy will be likely be associated with impotence.

Uterine involvement by a colorectal cancer being resected for cure requires en bloc resection of the involved uterus and relevant adenexal structures. This can be a modest partial excision of the uterus or a subtotal hysterectomy with careful attention to the protection of the ureters. A low rectal cancer that involves the lower vagina can be excised en bloc with the posterior vaginal wall, with or without vaginal reconstruction. Involvement of the vaginal fornices and the distal uterus requires a radical hysterectomy with division of the uterine arteries and release of the ureters away from the cervix and vaginal fornix.

4. Specific Excisional Problems

4.1. Benign Proctectomy

Proctectomy for inflammatory bowel disease can be carried out as part of proctocolectomy or as a separate procedure some time following subtotal colectomy and ileostomy. Intraoperative considerations and difficulties include dissection of the rectal stump, ureteric protection, and autonomic nerve protection.

4.1.1. Dissection of the Rectal Stump

After subtotal colectomy and ileostomy for inflammatory bowel disease, the rectal stump is managed in two different ways. Either a long rectal stump is left with a mucus fistula on the abdominal wall or closure just behind the midline wound. Alternatively, the dissection is taken low into the pelvis and the stump stapled off at or below the peritoneal reflection. When reoperating to remove the rectal stump subsequently, it is much preferable to encounter a long rectum with undisturbed tissue planes in the pelvis. Rectal-stump identification in these circumstances is easy and the pelvic dissection, including identification of the ureters, is straightforward.

By contrast, low division of the rectal stump immediately presents problems of rectal identification as reperitonealisation of the pelvis can obliterate any evidence of the stump as viewed by the abdominal operator (Figure 7.4). This difficulty can be overcome by running a blue 2-0 prolene suture

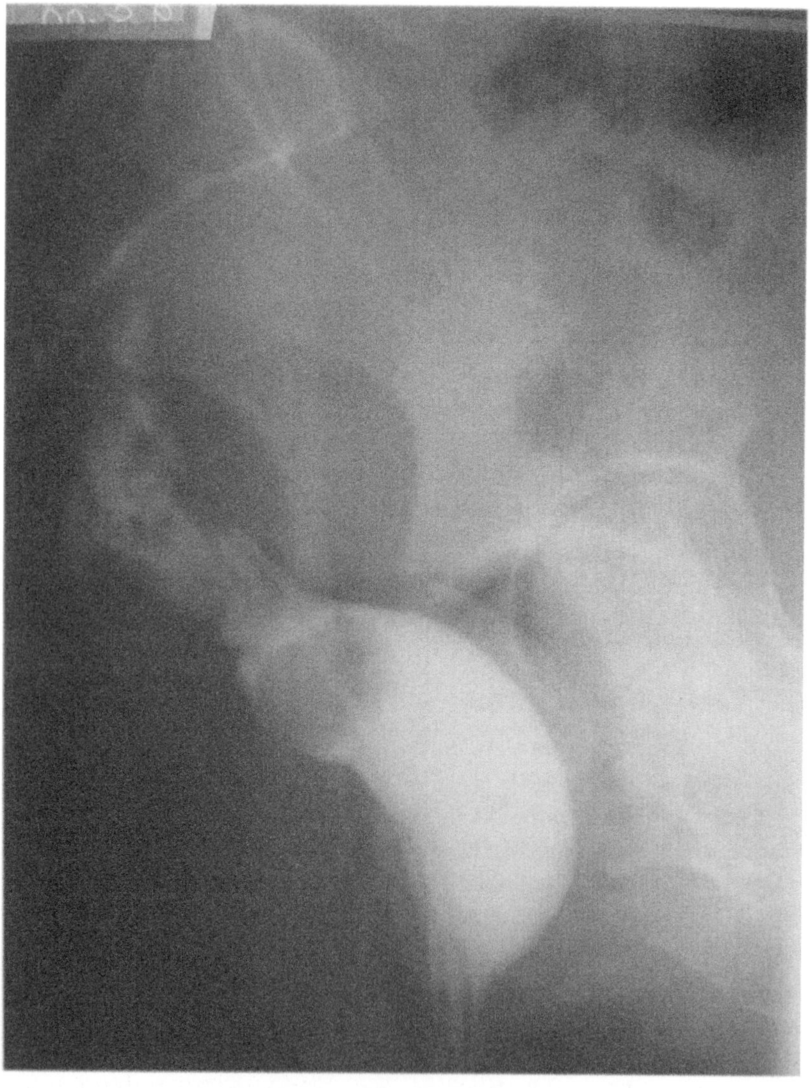

FIGURE 7.4. Proctogram of a small stump.

over the staple line and leaving the ends of the suture 10–15-cm long. At the subsequent proctectomy, the long prolene suture ends, marking the rectal stump, are easily identified. Alternatively, rigid sigmoidoscopy with palpation of the sigmoidoscope enables stump identification and allows the abdominal operator to direct dissection.

Typically, if the rectal stump is inflamed the mesorectum is thickened and edematous. Crohn's ulceration and/or rectal-stump apical abscess formation can produce an extremely dense fibrous reaction. After establishing the position and protection of the ureters, a very dense fibrotic response around the rectal stump is best handled by knife dissection or diathermy.

4.1.2. Autonomic Injury

Proctectomy for inflammatory bowel disease and other benign conditions should have an extremely low incidence [15] of autonomic nerve injury. Preoperatively, patient discussion should include questions defining preoperative erectile and bladder function. A conventional mesorectal excision can be practised above the peritoneal reflection with identification and protection of the hypogastric plexus and nerves at the sacral promontory and out to the pelvic sidewalls. However, below the peritoneal reflection dissection should be taken onto the rectal muscular wall and the mesorectum left intact.

In contrast to dissection in the mesorectal plane, close rectal dissection can be extremely bloody. Numerous small vessels (1–3 mm) passing from mesorectum into the rectal muscular wall have to be divided. This dissection may be performed by either diathermy or sharp dissection followed by diathermy to the bleeding points. However, the lateral thermal effects of diathermy, particularly at the pelvic floor, also pose a risk to autonomic nerve integrity. The harmonic scalpel [16,17] seals and divides small vessels using ultrasonic vibration with minimal lateral thermal effect. The short handpiece is ideal for open pelvic dissection with traction being placed on the rectum and the mesorectum to identify small vessels running to the rectal wall. The blades of the scalpel are placed across the vessel and slow coagulation with division is carried. Gradual progress along the rectal wall allows a bloodless close rectal dissection with a reduced risk of pelvic parasympathetic injury.

4.2. The Pouch of Douglas Mass

The colorectal surgeon must be involved in the surgery of the malignant ovarian pelvic mass [18] if the rectum or colon is involved and radical removal of the mass is appropriate for the patient (Figure 7.5). Preoperative planning must include bowel preparation and discussion of stomas. The ovarian malignant pelvic mass can initially appear unresectable due to extensive peritoneal involvement. Mobilisation should be commenced

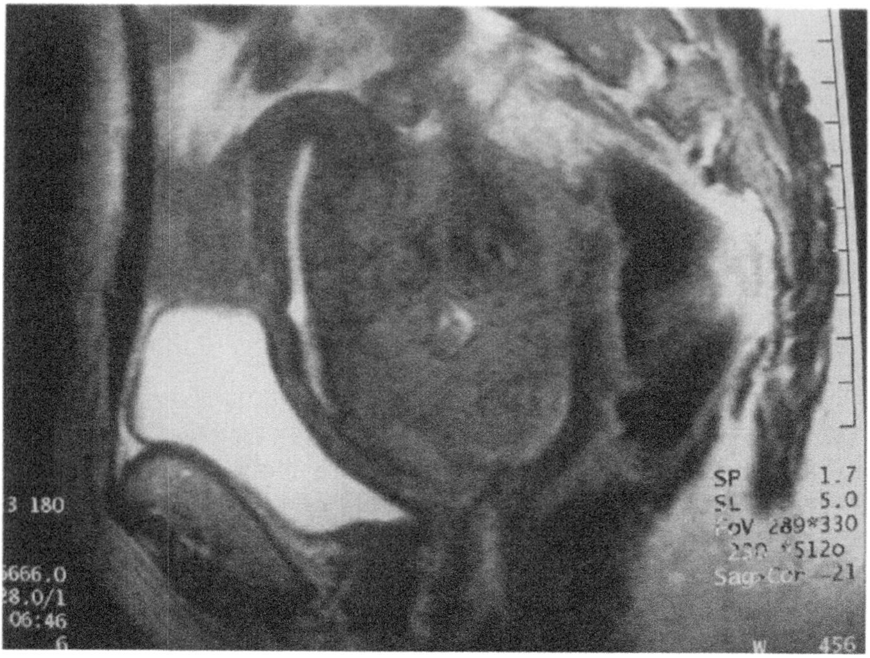

FIGURE 7.5. Magnetic resonance imaging of a POD mass.

behind the rectum in the normal mesorectal plane and extended laterally so the rectum is freed up from the pelvis in continuity with the pelvic mass. The round ligaments and the ovarian pedicles are divided, as is the peritoneum over the bladder to enter the plane between the vagina and the bladder. Division of the uterine arteries allows the ureters to be swept away from the vaginal fornices. Having exposed the anterior vaginal wall, the anterior aspect of the vagina is divided below the cervix and the lumen of the vagina entered. Sharp division is then continued through the posterior vaginal wall to expose the normal rectum below the pouch of Douglas tumour mass. The exposed rectum is then cross stapled and divided. The tumour mass is removed in continuity with the rectum, the uterus, and the proximal vagina. A cross-stapled anastomosis is then fashioned between the colon and the rectum with a proximal loop ileostomy.

4.3. Sacral Excision

The successful management of a neoplastic process involving the sacrum is best secured by preoperative diagnosis, assessment, and planning. Recurrent rectal cancer [19], along with presacral chordomas and teratomas, constitute the majority of cases that require en-bloc sacral excision. The visceral component of the excision may encompass the rectum alone or may be combined with total pelvic exenteration. An anterior approach with the patient in the Lloyd Davies position is used to mobilise the involved pelvic viscera and define the upper extent of the sacral division. The patient is then turned into the prone jackknife position and an incision is placed over the midline of the sacrum and continued to encompass any involved perineum (Figure 7.6).

The neurosurgical member of the team clears the spinous processes of the sacral vertebrae and the point of sacral division is confirmed. The sacral laminas are removed to expose the epidural space and the dural sac. The neural elements running to the specimen to be excised are divided and the dural sac closed. The sacrotuberous and sacrospinous ligaments are divided and the pelvic cavity entered. The body of the selected sacral vertebrae is divided with an osteotome and the tumour mass, involved pelvic viscera, and sacrum removed en bloc. After securing hemostasis and reconstructing the perineum, the patient is repositioned supine, the midline wound is reopened, and the appropriate stomas brought out through the anterior abdominal wall. An alternative to this is that the stomas are created initially prior to turning the patient for the sacral excision.

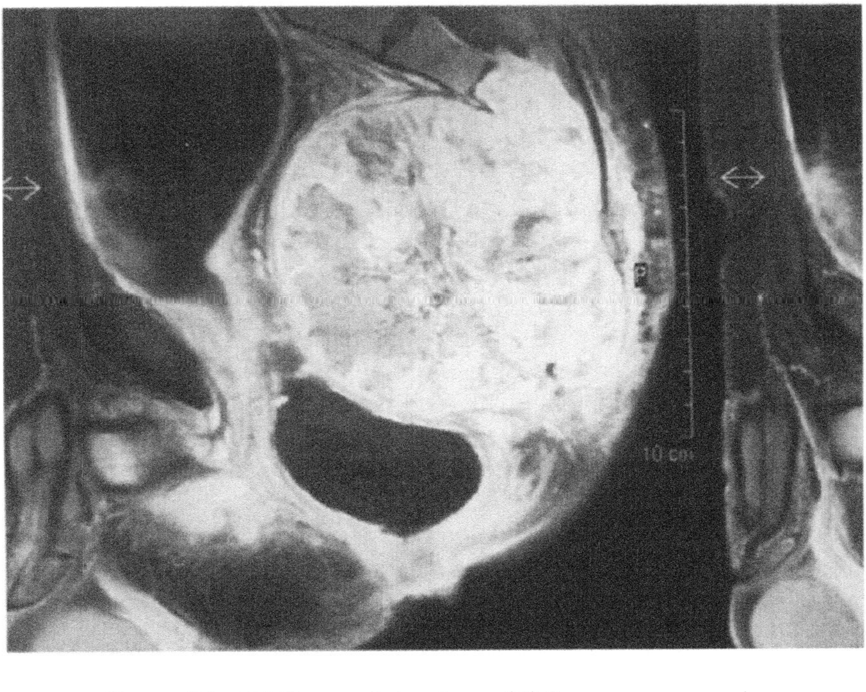

A

FIGURE 7.6. (A) Presacral chordoma. (B) Sacrectomy wound.

B 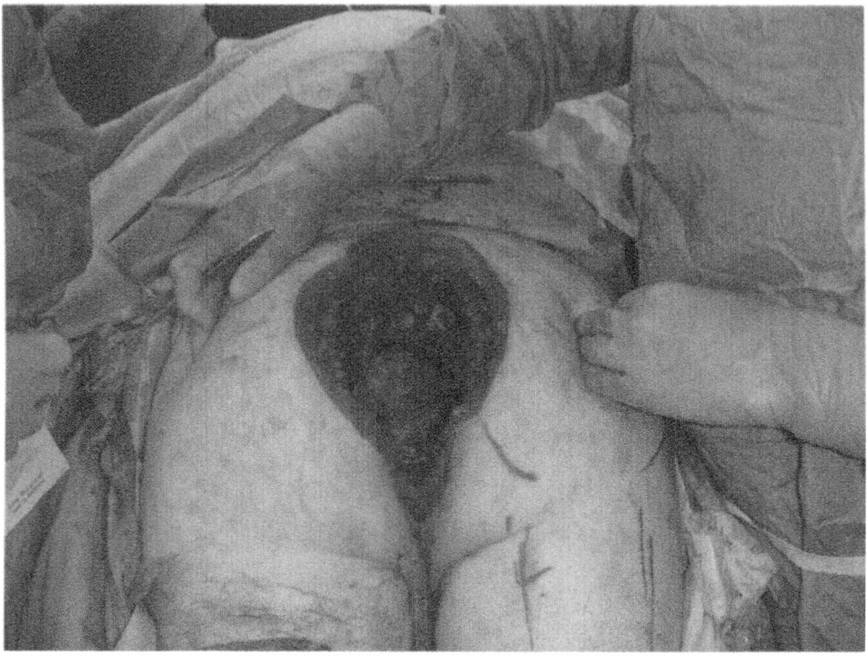

FIGURE 7.6. *Continued*

5. Reconstructive Problems

5.1. Intestinal Reconstruction

If, at the end of the pelvic excision, the anal canal and its innervation are both still intact, there is the prospect of re-establishing intestinal continuity under control of the anal sphincter and so avoiding a permanent stoma. A neorectal reservoir is desirable if the anastomosis is directly attached to the anal canal by either cross-stapled anastomosis or by mucosectomy and hand-sutured anastomosis to the dentate line [20].

In these circumstances, the gut is mobilised as a pedicled flap to reach down to the pelvic floor. Obesity is a substantial impediment to the tension-free movement of a gut pedicle to the anal canal. Not only does the fatty bulk of the mesentery impede its reach, but in addition the mechanical strength of a fatty mesentery is poor and excessive tension can tear the mesenteric fat and the enclosed blood vessels with disastrous consequences. For adequate reach in ileoanal pouch construction, the small bowel may need to be mobilised over the duodenum and the head of the pancreas. Elongation of the mesentery is assisted by incising the covering peritoneum and selectively dividing ileocolic vessels. But despite these measures, it must be accepted that in some cases an ileoanal pouch cannot be successfully constructed due to technical difficulty [21].

Similarly, obesity and arteriopathy can make it impossible to bring a viable length of left colon or transverse colon down the left paracolic gutter to the pelvic floor. This is particularly the case if a high inferior mesenteric tie devascularises the left colon. In many patients, the best option is to consider a permanent colostomy. Alternative strategies include bringing the transverse colon through the small-bowel mesentery or turning the right colon down the right paracolic gutter to effect a coloanal anastomosis.

5.2. Perineal Myocutaneous Reconstruction

Formal myocutaneous reconstruction of the perineum is required if a large perineal defect is left at the end of the surgical excision and/or there is reason to anticipate wound-healing problems such as those following extensive preoperative radiotherapy. The rectus abdominis muscle can be to provide a generous myocutaneous flap; based on the inferior epigastric vessels such a flap will fill the pelvis and the perineal defect [22,23]. This reconstruction is of value in excisional procedures for both recurrent rectal cancer and extensive perianal Crohn's disease removed as part of a proctectomy. Combined abdominoperineal access makes this reconstruction particularly appropriate.

In some patients, however, previous abdominal incisions and bilateral stoma placement can render the rectus muscles unavailable for perineal reconstruction. In these circumstances bilateral myocutaneous flaps based on both gracilis muscles are available along with local rotational flaps to bridge the perineal defect (Figure 7.7). In extreme cases, free flaps based

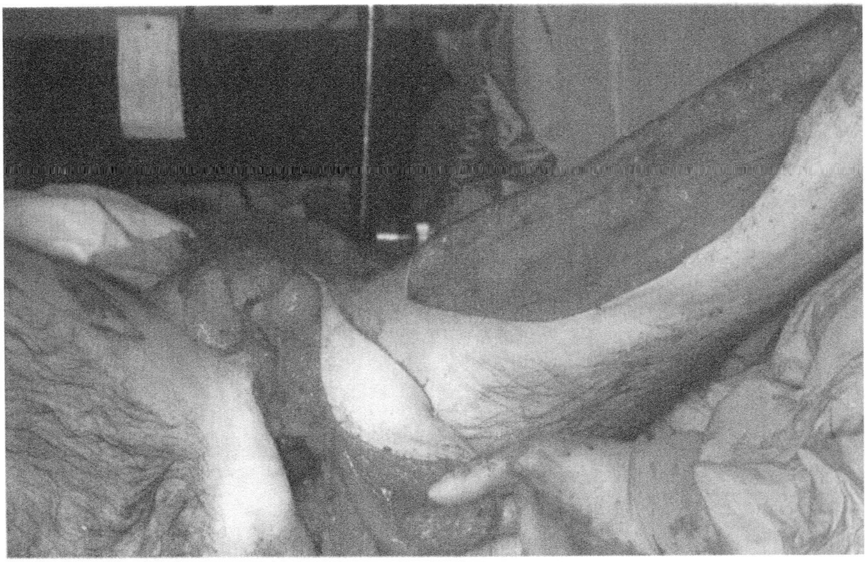

A

FIGURE 7.7 (A) Crohn's gracilis. (B) Hamstring sacral defect.

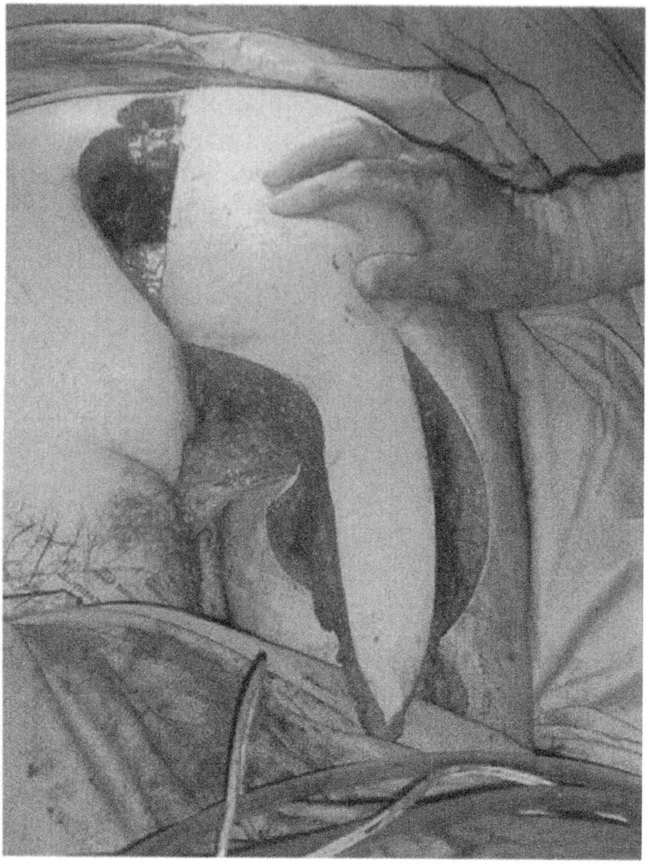

B

FIGURE 7.7. *Continued*

on the latissimus dorsi can be used in pelvic floor reconstruction. Involvement of a plastic surgeon in perineal reconstruction can add several hours to the procedure, but immediate myocutaneous closure of these wounds is associated with the reduced need for reoperation and readmission [24].

References

1. Magrini S, Nelson H, Gunderson LL, Sim FH. Sacropelvic resection and intraoperative electron irradiation in the management of recurrent anorectal cancer. *Dis Colon Rectum.* 1996;39:1–9.
2. Qinyao W, Weijin S, Yuoren Z, et al. New concepts in severe presacral hemorrhage during proctectomy. *Arch Surg.* 1985;120:1013–1020.
3. Bissett I, Hill G. Extrafascial excision of the rectum for cancer: a technique for the avoidance of the complications of rectal mobilization. *Semin Surg Oncol.* 2000;18:207–215.

4. Nivatvongs S, Fang D. The use of thumbtacks to stop massive presacral hemorrhage. *Dis Colon Rectum.* 1986;29:589–590.
5. Lucarotti M, Armstrong C, Bartolo D. Control of presacral bleeding in rectal surgery. *Ann R Coll Surg Engl.* 1991;73:289–290.
6. Timmons M, Kohler M, Addison W. Thumbtack use for control of presacral bleeding, with description of an instrument for thumbtack application. *Obstet Gynecol.* 1991;78:313–315.
7. Khan F, Fang D, Nivatvongs S. Management of presacral bleeding during rectal resection. *Surg Gynecol Obstet.* 1987;165:274–276.
8. Stolfi V, Milsom J, Lavery I, Oakley J, Church J, Fazio V. Newly designed occluder pin for presacral hemorrhage. *Dis Colon Rectum.* 1992;35:166–169.
9. Metzger PP. Modified packing technique for control of presacral pelvic bleeding. *Dis Colon Rectum.* 1988;31:981–982.
10. Finan MA, Fiorica JV, Hoffman MS, et al. Massive pelvic hemorrhage during gynecologic cancer surgery. "Pack and go back." *Gynecol Oncol.* 1996;62:390–395.
11. Andersson A, Bergdahl L. Urologic complications following abdominoperineal resection of the rectum. *Arch Surg.* 1976;111:969–971.
12. Beahrs J, Beahrs O, Beahrs M, et al. Urinary tract complications with rectal surgery. *Ann Surg.* 1978;187:542–547.
13. Fry D, Milholen L, Harbrecht P. Iatrogenic ureteral injury. *Arch Surg.* 1983;118:545–457.
14. Higgins C. Ureteral injuries during surgery: a review of 87 cases. *J Am Med Assoc.* 1967;199:118–124.
15. Lindsey I, Mortensen NJMc. Iatrogenic impotence and rectal dissection. *Br J Surg.* 2002;89:1493–1494.
16. Kusunoki M, Shoji Y, Yanagi H, et al. Current trends in restorative proctocolectomy: introduction of an ultrasonically activated scalpel. *Dis Colon Rectum.* 1999;42:1349–1352.
17. Maruta F, Sugiyama A, Matsushita K, et al. Use of the Harmonic Scalpel in open abdominoperineal surgery for rectal carcinoma. *Dis Colon Rectum.* 1999;42:540–542.
18. Scott NA, Schofield PF. Cytoreductive surgery for ovarian carcinoma. *Br J Surg.* 1990;77:481–482.
19. Wanebo HJ, Antoniuk P, Koness RJ, et al. Pelvic resection of recurrent rectal cancer: technical considerations and outcomes. *Dis Colon Rectum.* 1999;42:1438–1448.
20. Berger A, Tiret E, Cunningham C, Dehni N, Parc R. Rectal excision and colonic pouch-anal anastomosis for rectal cancer: oncological results at five years. *Dis Colon Rectum.* 1999;42:1265–1271.
21. Browning SM, Nivatvongs S. Intraoperative abandonment of ileal pouch to anal anastomosis—the Mayo Clinic experience. *J Am Coll Surg.* 1998;186:441–445.
22. Lavery IC, Lopez-Kostner F, Pelley RJ, Fine RM. Treatment of colon and rectal cancer. *Surg Clin North Am.* 2000;80:535–569.
23. Brough WA, Schofield PF. The value of the myocutaneous flap in the treatment of complex perineal fistula. *Dis Colon Rectum.* 1991;34:148–150.
24. Radice E, Nelson H, Mercill S, Farouk R, Petty P, Gunderson L. Primary myocutaneous flap closure following resection of locally advanced pelvic malignancies. *Br J Surg.* 1999;86:349–354.

8
Functional Reconstruction of the Perineum and Pelvic Floor

Alan D. McGregor

1. Introduction

The pelvis and perineum house closely related anatomical structures belonging to the urinary, reproductive, and gastrointestinal systems. Diseases, whether inflammatory or neoplastic, can spread readily from one organ to another. As a consequence, removal of the structure in which a disease has arisen may, under certain circumstances, entail concomitant removal of part or all of other related organs. Thus, for example, it may be necessary to remove a portion of vaginal wall as part of the abdominoperineal resection of Crohn's disease or rectal cancer.

All the structures in this part of the human body are highly specialised and it is possible to dispense with some without the need for sophisticated reconstruction. An end colostomy or an ileal conduit will replace rectum and anus or bladder adequately. What the end result of each lacks in aesthetics, it makes up in technical simplicity and ease of management for the patient. Of greater significance is the fact that each of these problems can be resolved by the same surgeon who carries out the resection of the diseased viscus.

The experience and technical range of individual surgeons varies, but overall tends to be limited by the scope of the training syllabus and the boldness of the trainers. Even allowing for a degree of overlap between specialties, neither gynaecologist, urologist, nor colorectal surgeon has the training or experience to reconstruct every defect he is likely to create in resecting the more complex diseases with which he is confronted. Whatever his (or her) specialty, the surgeon working in this field who is involved in treating extensive diseases will inevitably have to cooperate in the planning of surgery with colleagues in related surgical disciplines.

The need to reconstruct presupposes the existence of a defect. Some defects can be repaired readily by the surgeon who created it. A good example is the pelvic floor after an abdominoperineal resection for bowel cancer. Other defects demand the expertise of a reconstructive surgeon trained in techniques of plastic surgery. While it is fair to say that most surgeons have experience of some reconstructive techniques, that exposure is inevitably limited and is invariably restricted to a narrow range of techniques. These may be appropriate for a significant proportion of reconstructive problems, but not all. Every method has its limits and, with experience, every operator learns what these are. As a result, situations will arise when it is either necessary to push the technique of repair as far as or beyond the limits of its tolerance or to compromise the resection in order to permit reconstruction to take place. Whichever, the potential for disaster is considerable.

The experienced surgeon can estimate with reasonable certainty which resections are likely to create a defect requiring sophisticated repair. Collaboration with a reconstructive plastic surgeon has two distinct advantages for the colorectal surgeon. The first is the importation of knowledge and experience of all the possible reconstructive techniques that may be required. The second is that the resection can be carried out without concern for the defect that may result. This liberating effect means that the disease is treated properly with whatever margins of excision may be required. Put bluntly, the norm is FIRST MAKE THE HOLE, THEN FILL IT! This can be expanded to "the first team makes the hole and the second team fills it."

In this field of surgical practice, the macho individual who believes that he can do it all himself is a self-deluding dinosaur. The multidisciplinary team approach has everything to commend it. The ideal team contains a gynaecologist, a urologist, a colorectal surgeon, a clinical oncologist, and a reconstructive plastic surgeon. This blend works well in practice because, individual personalities apart, there is little overlap but each complements the others.

2. General Philosophy

The elements of reconstruction can be subdivided conveniently into those that address the issue of function and those that restore appearance. On occasions there is a degree of overlap. Some aspects of function are dependent on the effects of the resection. For example, sexual function in the male after pelvic surgery is dependent in large measure on preservation of autonomic nerve supply—if this has to be sacrificed, it cannot be reconstructed. Similarly, it may not be necessary to reconstruct bladder or bowel because diversion via the anterior abdominal wall may be satisfactory. The uterus is often sacrificed and cannot be replaced.

Reconstruction of pelvis and perineum is required only under certain circumstances. These are (a) (extended) skin loss, (b) partial (rarely complete) vaginal removal, (c) perineal proctectomy, (d) pelvic floor loss, and (e) excision after radiotherapy.

Each of these, singly or in combination, can be anticipated at the planning stage before surgery. No surgeon can be absolutely confident under all circumstances about what the postexcisional defect will be. As a consequence, the reconstructive surgeon is rarely able to counsel any patient with confidence prior to surgery about what form reconstruction will take. Paradoxically, this uncertainty, born of experience, has a reassuring effect upon patients as a general rule. Patients in this position recognise that any surgeon who is prepared to make such a statement is one who has both knowledge of his subject and judgement.

3. Anatomy and Function

The pure and applied anatomy of the pelvic floor and the perineum are, relatively speaking, minor considerations in the context of repairing the defect resulting from abdominoperineal excision of the rectum in cases of rectal carcinoma. The cutaneous perineal incision is made close to the anal margin, dissection of the bowel is in a plane close to the wall of the viscus and the pelvic diaphragm, pelvic floor and the cutaneous wound can be repaired directly with sutures. The intervening space may be drained. Although overall the management of the postexcisional defect barely merits the description of reconstruction, that is precisely what has been performed, albeit in its simplest form.

The colorectal surgeon, in closing his postexcisional defect in the standard manner, is recognising the implicit function and role of the pelvic diaphragm and the skin. It is, consequently, appropriate to consider the relevance and importance of each in relation to function and the need for reconstruction. This needs to be considered both in the context of why reconstruction is necessary, what form this may take, how the anatomy of each helps, hinders, or obviates the need for reconstruction, and the consequences of failure to undertake proper functional repair.

Put simply, the principal role of the pelvic diaphragm is to support the abdominal and pelvic viscera and to prevent prolapse of these organs into the perineum. Some organs pass through the pelvic diaphragm—removal of any of these requires repair of the resultant defect to restore the integrity of the pelvic floor and prevent prolapse or the feeling of dragging or "something coming down" of which patients with this problem complain. Because the muscles and fascia are draped in a bowl-shaped configuration, repair by direct suture is usually not a problem. Tension-free closure and a good blood supply invariably lead to problem-free healing with a good functional result.

The skin of the perineum has a considerable degree of inherent laxity that allows a wide range of flexion/extension and abduction at the hip. In the midline the skin is more closely adherent to underlying structures. The skin lies immediately over the fat in the base of the ischiorectal fossa where it is extremely mobile. As a consequence skin will move medially without excessive tension being placed on it. Advantage of this mobility is routinely taken in obtaining tension-free closure after simple rectal incision. Even if skin suture appears to be under tension with the hips in a position of abduction, the tightness is invariably relieved (or, at worst, reduced to an acceptable level) when the thighs are brought into a position of adduction at the end of the operation.

On occasion, however, direct skin closure becomes impossible due to the need to extend the cutaneous excision margin further laterally. Such wider excision is invariably required due to the need to resect diseased tissue, on occasion aggravated by previous excisional surgery. As a general rule, a wide skin excision margin is an intrinsic element in an extended resection of the rectum and, more often than not, a wide resection of the pelvic floor. Thus, the above-mentioned anatomical and functional areas, although separate in theory, tend to form part of a single reconstructive problem—exceptions are procedures such as perineal proctectomy in which pelvic floor reconstruction is not a problem.

The problem for the reconstructive surgeon (who invariably has no more than a concept of what the eventual problem confronting him is likely to be) is whether transfer of one or of more than one tissue is likely to be required. He is, however, fortunate that the usual surgical positioning of the patient in the modified Lloyd Davies position places at his disposal all the tissues he is likely to use without the need to prepare other parts of the body. In addition, it is possible to have two teams working simultaneously on the abdomen and the perineum, which results in a considerable saving in total anaesthetic and operating time.

4. Tissues for Reconstruction

When contemplating repair and reconstruction the surgeon must remember what he is trying to achieve: (a) pelvic floor repair, (b) skin integrity, and (c) obliteration of the intervening surgical dead space.

The tissues that have proved to be of value are those that are, at best, similar to or, at worst, analogous to those that are undergoing reconstruction. Ideally, they can provide a rigid repair for the pelvic floor, fill space, and provide skin. In practice, those that have been found to have a useful role are the rectus abdominis flap, in either myofascial or myocutaneous form, gracilis muscle, either as a muscle flap or myocutaneous flap, omentum, and split skin graft.

Other sources of tissue have been used on occasion, in particular when the more customary methods have been precluded. Consequently, the above list should be regarded as a list of best options rather than an exclusive list. Each of these tissues, furthermore, has an anatomical position and blood supply which lie outside the pelvis and perineum. As a consequence, they are not at risk of exposure to therapeutic pelvic or perineal radiation. Each is potentially available for reconstructive purposes whatever the position at the end of resection may be.

4.1. Rectus Abdominis

Flap repair using rectus abdominis in one of its variant forms has been described for pelvic floor and perineal repair [1,2] (See Figure 8.1). This is

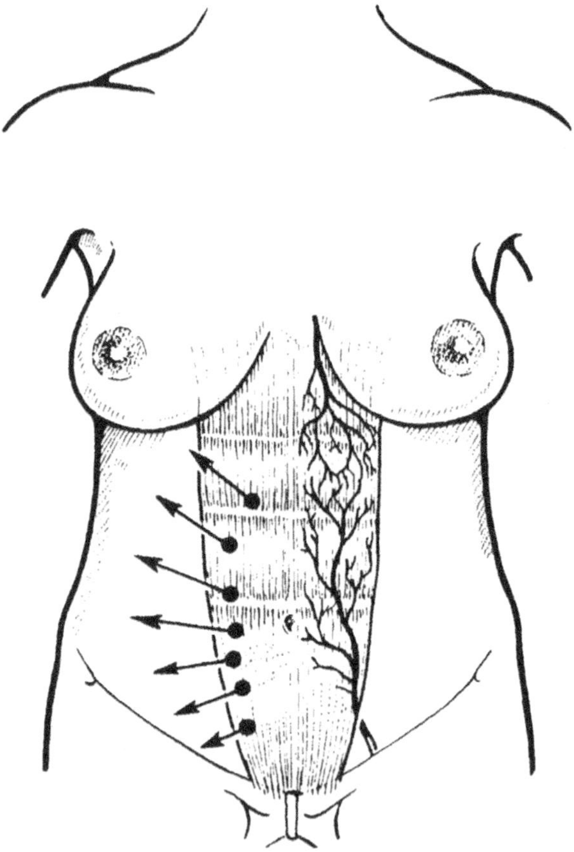

FIGURE 8.1. Illustration of the rectus abdominis muscles showing both the inferior and superior pedicles and the site of the perforators (arrows) that supply the overlying abdominal skin. (Reproduced with permission from McGregor AD, McGregor IA. *Fundamental Techniques of Plastic Surgery*. 10th ed. London: Churchill Livingston; 2000:66.)

hardly surprising because it is an extremely versatile muscle to which access is readily obtained in the routine course of intra-abdominal surgery.

The rectus abdominis muscles run vertically on each side of the midline from the xiphisternum and adjoining costal cartilages to the pubic crest, enclosed within the anterior and posterior layers of the rectus sheath formed by the aponeuroses of the other anterior abdominal muscles. Along its medial border, the two layers of the sheath fuse with one another and with their fellows on the opposite side to form the linea alba, a largely avascular structure. The formation of the sheath differs in the upper and lower abdomen. In the upper two-thirds, the aponeurosis of internal oblique splits to form its anterior and posterior layers, the anterior layer being reinforced by the aponeurosis of the external oblique, the posterior layer by the aponeurosis of transversus abdominis. In the lower third, the aponeurosis of all 3 muscles passes superficial to the rectus muscle, forming the anterior sheath. The posterior sheath is replaced by a filmy layer of fascia, the transversalis fascia, and the junction line of the lower border of the posterior sheath and the fascia is referred to as the arcuate line. The rectus muscle has 3 tendinous intersections that are adherent to the anterior sheath; posteriorly it lies free within the sheath.

Accompanying the segmental nerves that supply the rectus muscle, a pattern of arteries and veins, running in the plane between internal oblique and transversus abdominis, reaches the muscle by piercing the posterior sheath. The muscle is supplied by the superior and inferior epigastric arteries (and their accompanying veins). The inferior artery is usually the larger. In approaching one another from the above and below, each set of vessels runs vertically on the deep surface of rectus abdominis inside the rectus sheath for several centimetres before entering the substance of the muscle, anastomosing with its fellow at about the level of the umbilicus.

Branches are given off from the combined system that supply the muscle and the overlying skin, the latter by a series of segmental perforating vessels that reach the superficial fascia following their emergence from the anterior rectus sheath. These perforators determine to a considerable extent the shape of the skin islands that are designed to exploit them [2].

Based on the inferior epigastric vessels, which are branches of the external iliac vessels, flaps of varying designs can take advantage of the rectus abdominis anatomy to achieve repair of pelvic floor and perineum. The most obvious and the easiest route is to place the flap retropubically. This avoids the need to detach the pubic end of the rectus muscle which has a protective value in limiting the tension placed on the vascular pedicle during and at the completion of flap transfer.

Rectus flaps used in this way can be transferred as muscle, myofascial (muscle with rectus sheath), or myocutaneous flaps according to the precise needs of the individual case. Some features in the technique of raising the flap are common to all 3 of these variants. First, the anterior rectus sheath should be preserved below the arcuate line to prevent either subsequent incisional hernia or the need to use synthetic mesh to repair the anterior abdominal musculature. The anterior sheath can be incised vertically at any point and can be reflected from the rectus muscle by sharp dissection. Above the arcuate line, the anterior sheath, with or without overlying skin, can be raised with the muscle with impunity because the posterior rectus sheath alone is strong enough to prevent development of incisional hernia.

Raising the rectus in this way results in division of its segmental nerve supply and the lateral and superior sources of blood supply. Following transfer, the muscle undergoes denervation atrophy with diffuse interstitial fibrosis. Consequently, it provides an excellent source of tissue for pelvic floor reconstruction as it can be readily sutured to pubic rami anteriorly and to the sacrum posteriorly. Harvesting of anterior rectus sheath provides a very strong layer to suture to bone, and skin for perineal repair can be incorporated into the flap if required, though the amount of skin should not exceed what can be closed by direct suture on the abdominal wall, otherwise closure with a split skin graft becomes necessary.

Although it has all the attributes desirable in a readily accessible multipurpose flap, the applications for this reconstruction are extremely limited in practice. It has no role in pelvic floor repair after total pelvic exenteration because of the need to retain both rectus abdominis muscles in situ for diversion of bowel and bladder. It has little use in repair of posterior pelvic floor defects in which anterior pelvic structures (bladder and uterus) remain because retropubic transfer of the rectus muscle is not easy, and pelvic floor repair becomes extremely difficult.

The only practical application for the rectus flap in pelvic floor repair is following anterior exenteration with preservation of rectum and anus such that only one rectus muscle need be preserved for urinary diversion, and the other can be used as a flap reconstruction in one of the above forms as dictated by circumstances. These circumstances are rare indeed.

4.2. Gracilis

Although described as suitable for transfer as a muscle flap or, with overlying skin, as a myocutaneous flap [3], experience has shown that the skin perfusion via the muscle is poor and unpredictable. As a consequence, gracilis flap transfer is a reliable technique only when in its muscle form. If skin is required in association with this, it is best provided by means of a split skin graft. (See Figure 8.2–Figure 8.5.)

Gracilis lies on the posteromedial aspect of the thigh in the adductor group of muscles. It has a segmental pattern of blood supply, usually with 3 pedicles spaced at even distances along the muscle at the junction of each quarter. The proximal pedicle is the largest and beside it lies its solitary nerve supply. Though broad and fairly flat proximally, it becomes thinner and more rounded distally. A tendon arises in the lower thigh that crosses the knee deep to the long saphenous vein and inserts into the tibia. The

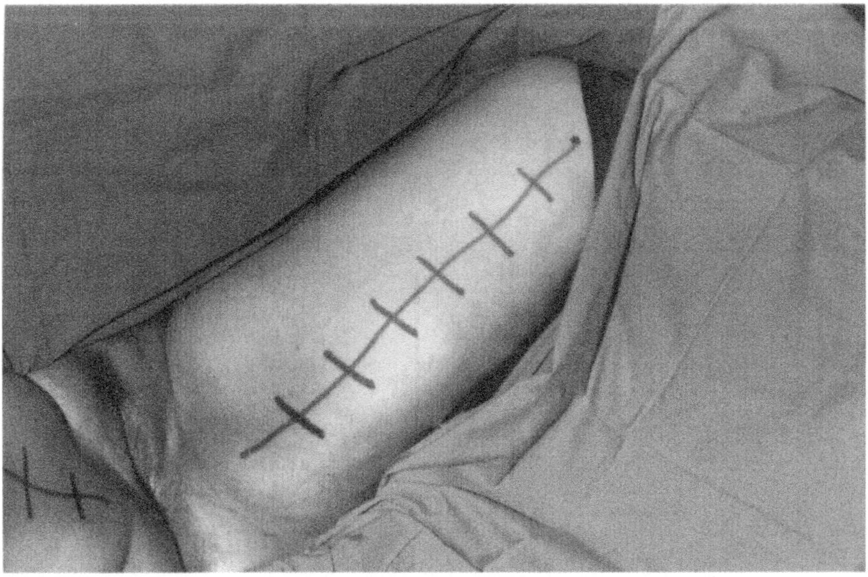

FIGURE 8.2. The pattern of incision on the thigh for harvest of the gracilis muscle flap. The precise positioning of the incision is not critical.

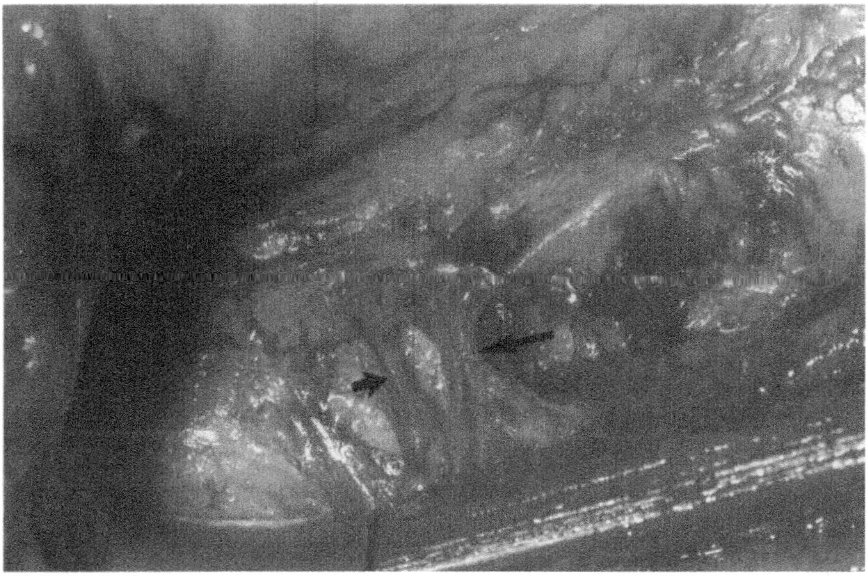

FIGURE 8.3. The nerve to gracilis (small arrow) and the dominant vascular pedicle (large arrow) are shown. The nerve always lies proximal to the vessels.

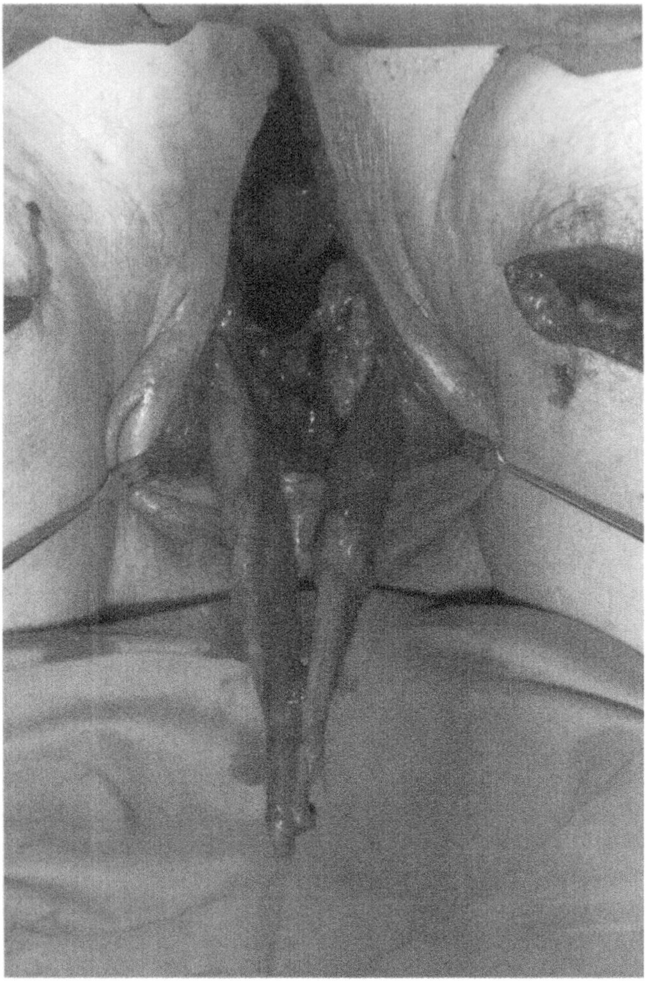

FIGURE 8.4. The gracilis muscles have been raised and tunneled subcutaneously. They have been brought out through the perineal wound.

tendon is readily palpable and is often covered in part distally by the muscle fibres of vastus medialis. Proximally, the muscle arises from an aponeurosis extending from the body of the pubis along the inferior ramus to reach the ramus of the ischium. Its principal blood supply is from the profunda femoris vessels [3]. Although it is technically possible to mobilise the dominant pedicle to increase the reach of a gracilis muscle flap, the gain achieved in this way is surprisingly small and, once performed, tends to ensure that the pedicle is under maximum tension, thereby enhancing the likelihood of circulatory problems and subsequent complications. As a general rule it is wiser to accept the anatomy as it is and to plan accordingly.

The dominant pedicle enters the muscle at a point one quarter of the length of the muscle from its origin to its insertion. If the muscle is raised throughout its length and all skin and soft tissue are mobilised from the muscle as far as its origin, the muscle can be turned back and tunnelled subcutaneously into the perineum and pelvic floor with ease. A length of muscle equivalent to the second quarter of its length comes to lie between pedicle and origin. This leaves the distal half of the muscle available for reconstructive use. The fact that this part is thinner and tendinous becomes

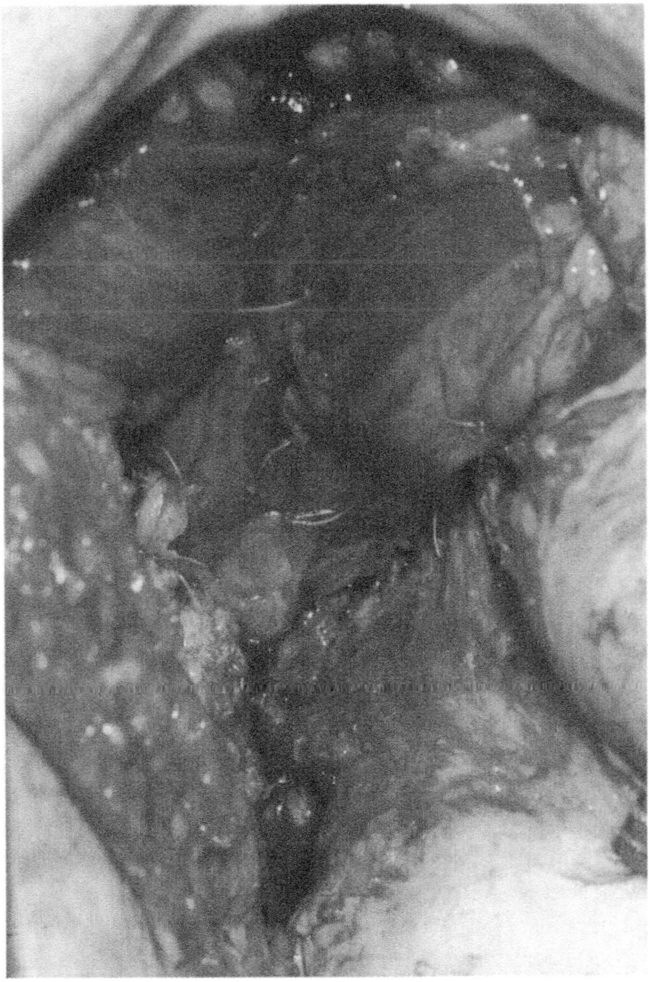

FIGURE 8.5. The appearance of the pelvic floor repair. Both gracilis muscles have been sutured to the sacrum and around the margins of the pubic rami to occlude the communication between the abdominal cavity and the perineum.

extremely useful because the tendon will reach as far as the symphysis pubis anteriorly and the sacrum posteriorly. The precise alignment of muscle and tendon can be decided according to the local anatomy and the exact defect requiring repair. It is wise to anchor tendon to bone in any event.

It is customary to fashion a skin incision along the posteromedial aspect of the thigh to obtain access to raise the gracilis muscle. The incision need not extend as far as the knee. The tendon can be mobilised and divided distal to the knee without difficulty. The quality of the resulting scar is this flap's greatest drawback. The scar tends to stretch and quality is poor. Hypertrophy is not uncommon, especially in younger women.

It is exceptional for one gracilis flap to be sufficient for primary pelvic floor or perineal repair. Both are usually necessary. Whether closure over the muscles with perineal skin is possible can often only be determined at the end of the procedure. As a routine, it is wise to divide the nerve supply to gracilis prior to transfer because this prevents unwanted muscle contraction and minimises the risk of separation at the site of tendon and muscle suture. If skin closure cannot be obtained, repair with a skin graft is required. When necessary, this is best applied as a delayed graft, usually 48–72 hours later. Whether this is in the form of sheet or mesh graft is at the discretion of the operator. The immobility resulting from denervation provides the ideal bed for uncomplicated graft take—unfortunately, the rest of the patient tends to be rather less immobile, consequently use of a bolus tie-over dressing has much to commend it.

4.3. Omentum

Another vascularised tissue outside the field of previous pelvic radiotherapy, with definite application and a useful role, either solely or in combination with other techniques, is omentum (Figure 8.6). While its usefulness is undoubted, doubly so because the abdomen is usually opened in the course of pelvic surgery resulting in the need for reconstruction, its general applicability is limited by uncertainty about its size [4] and about the effects upon it of previous surgery and previous abdominal disease. Another potential disadvantage is the concern about its reusability in the event of further surgical treatment following its use for pelvic floor or perineal repair. How best to use what omentum is available singly or in combination with other tissues is a matter for judgement born of experience. It is not a subject for which easy generalisations or guidelines can be given. As a general rule, however, omentum is better used for reconstruction of small defects. Larger defects are usually better repaired using omentum in combination with other techniques, although the surgeon can, on occasion, strike it lucky in finding an unusually generous omentum.

Omentum granulates rapidly and effectively, rapidly adhering to any surface to which it is applied. In preparing the omentum for transfer, it is

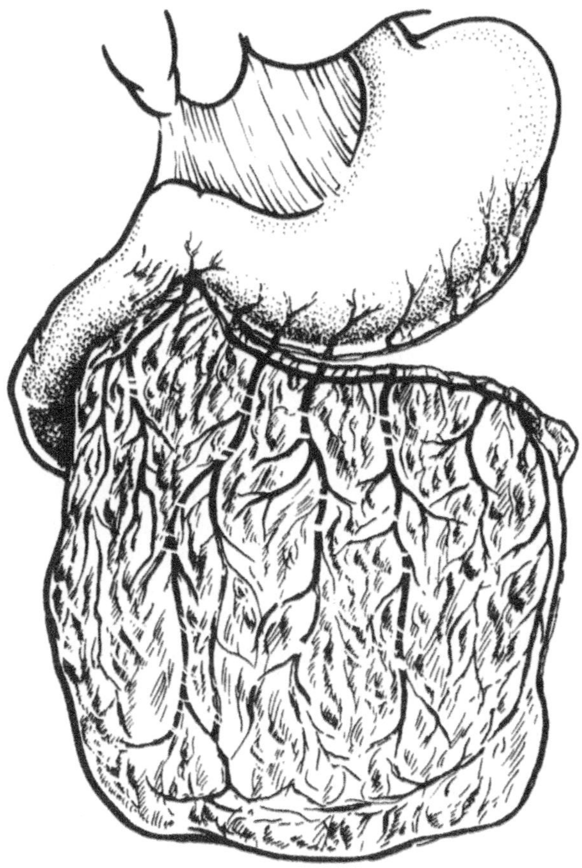

FIGURE 8.6. Illustration of the omental flap which has been pedicled on the right gastroepiploic vessels. (Reproduced with permission from McGregor AD, McGregor IA. *Fundamental Techniques of Plastic Surgery*. 10th ed. London: Churchill Livingston; 2000:111.)

first freed from its avascular attachments to the transverse colon, leaving it attached along the greater curvature of the stomach. It is vascularised from branches of the gastro-epiploic vessels that form a series of loops in the direction of its free border. To reach the pelvis, it is necessary to pedicle the omentum on the right or left gastro-epiploic vessels [5,6] (although it is technically easier to base the flap on the left gastro-epiploic pedicle [7]), the branches to the stomach being divided to allow it to be mobilised and thereby enhance its reach. Its looped vascular pattern allows it to be lengthened without losing its vascularity. Depending on the degree of adiposity of the patient, omentum can vary from a very substantial to a seemingly insubstantial structure. Whichever, if too small to reach the pelvis (and some are), the surgeon must accept the fact with good grace and select an alternative method of repair.

4.4. *Split Skin Graft*

Many colorectal surgeons have some experience of harvesting, applying, managing, and assessing skin grafts. Few do so regularly and the specialty as a whole could say little more than that they are occasional skin grafters. Nurses on colorectal units have even less experience. The perineum is a difficult and problematic area for obtaining good skin-graft healing. Nevertheless, a few general principles can be expounded. Delayed grafting tends to be more successful than primary grafting and mesh grafts tend to be more successful than sheet grafts. Complete, 100% take is the exception rather than the rule.

The perineum is moist and exposing the area to minimise maceration and maximise aeration is difficult, even with a cooperative patient. Moisture predisposes to bacterial growth and graft slippage, even when the graft margins are sutured to the skin edges. The most successful approach has been use of a bolus tie-over grafting technique [8] for 5 days, after which the dressing is removed and the patient takes daily baths. With this regime the perineum has been found to heal by a mixture of graft take, contraction of the wound, and epithelialisation, usually within 2–3 weeks.

5. Specific Repairs

5.1. *Perineum After Extended Skin Loss or Removal*

When confined to the perineum, removal of tissue is usually limited to skin and subcutaneous fat. Such problems are most commonly encountered by the colorectal surgeon in the context of treating inflammatory conditions of bowel or skin, or in managing localised skin neoplasia. Provided tissue removal does not encroach upon the anal margin, surgical repair need not necessarily be undertaken. This is an area in which subcutaneous and ischiorectal fat granulate well. As a consequence, areas of skin loss or removal heal quickly with acceptable results.

This is fortunate because alternative forms of repair have considerable drawbacks. Skin grafts require close immobile contact with a suitable bed before take can be achieved. This is a difficult area to immobilise, contamination with faecal organisms is virtually impossible to avoid, incomplete take is the rule, and the grafts tend to contract thereafter. Grafting has little advantage in the short term and the longer term appearance is often poorer. Function is not noticeably better.

Use of local skin flaps for repair of large wounds has been described, especially in the form of fasciocutaneous flaps from the thigh [9]. The resultant scarring is, however, extensive and usually poor in quality. These flaps offer little advantage.

5.2. *Partial Vaginal Repair*

Total vaginal repair is beyond the remit of this review. Not infrequently, however, whether as part of a resection for fistulating primary bowel disease or as part of an extended resection for malignancy, it is necessary to resect part of the vagina. Most commonly, this entails resection of the posterior wall but can extend to one or both lateral walls, thereby converting partial to subtotal vaginal excision. Whether vaginal reconstruction is undertaken is not merely a function of whether the patient is, and wishes to remain, sexually active—it is also of relevance to repair of an epithelial surface and restoration of perineal integrity without the risk of fistula formation. Resections of this sort are invariably one element in complex, major excisions. In the context of colorectal surgery, these invariably involve an abdominoperineal excision of the rectum and anus with the creation of a pelvic floor defect that cannot be repaired primarily. As a general rule the problem of vaginal reconstruction can be solved as an integral part of the pelvic floor repair by the importation of healthy vascularised tissue that can be sutured to the margins of the retained vaginal remnant. The tissue selected should possess 3 characteristics: it should granulate, heal to the vagina, and allow migration of vaginal epithelium over the granulating surface. Such an approach is preferable to use of skin grafts or flaps that provide a good stratified squamous epithelial surface but one that continues to keratinise and desquamate in contrast to the normal nonkeratising vaginal epithelium. Experience, admittedly limited, has been that use of omentum brought down anterior to gracilis muscles flaps (for pelvic floor repair) will tube and provide a close analogue to a neovaginal posterior wall, on occasion sufficient to allow vaginal intercourse. In the absence of a suitable omentum, gracilis muscle flaps can be raised and sutured to the residual vaginal wall, this in combination with pelvic floor repair. Under these circumstances, in particular, if it is necessary to repair the perineum with a skin graft, it is difficult to know how much of the exposed muscle to graft and how much to leave to epithelialise. This is a matter for peroperative judgement.

5.3. *Perineal Proctectomy*

Reconstruction after perineal proctectomy is most frequently required for closure of the postexcisional presacral dead space following extensive excision of fistulating disease arising from a large-bowel remnant that was retained (or not resected) because of surgical difficulties inherent in a previous colectomy. Adequate removal of fistulating disease, when present, requires that the excision margins be greater than otherwise might be expected. The surgeon must ensure that every vestige of epithelialised tracks and of disease is removed thoroughly. This inevitably creates a larger defect, usually pyramidal in shape, with a wide base and a long narrow apex. Surgical repair of the defect demands obliteration of the dead space at the apex—failure to achieve this creates a cavity that cannot readily close by fibrosis in the longer term and which is the ready focus for collection of secretions in the early postoperative phase. Suction drainage cannot close the space. At best, fluid drainage will persist unabated. This is a focus for infection which, at worst, will lead to wound breakdown and persistent low-grade discharge.

Because resection is confined below the pelvic floor, laparotomy is inappropriate. As a consequence, the omentum is not available for obliteration of the cavity at the apex of the surgical field. In these circumstances, gracilis muscle flaps are the repair of choice. The long narrow tendons hold sutures well and can be anchored to rigid structures at the apex of the pyramid. The bulkier central portion of the muscle provides volume to close the lower or middle part of the wound, and the muscle as a whole readily accepts a split skin graft for rapid restoration of skin continuity in the perineum in the event that there is a postexcisional deficiency of skin.

5.4. Pelvic Floor Loss

Loss of pelvic floor that requires reconstruction can arise under 3 sets of circumstances, all requiring extended colon resection at this level: invasive extracolonic malignancy, extensive fibrosing or fistulating inflammatory bowel disease, and after radiotherapy.

Reconstruction is required when the residual pelvic floor cannot be approximated and sutured without tension. The defect in the pelvic floor can be viewed as a problem in isolation or can be merely one element of a composite reconstruction of pelvic floor and perineum.

The first tissue to consider for pelvic floor repair is the greater omentum. It is the first choice because its use avoids the need for additional incisions and it is often present in sufficient quantity to be used to repair any perineal defect in addition. Its use for these purposes requires mobilisation on a unilateral pedicle following which it will usually extend as far as may be required to achieve the desired repair. On occasion, however, there is insufficient omentum to achieve satisfactory repair. Whether only part of the repair can be completed with omentum or none, the deficiency can be made good by using gracilis muscle flaps. Invariably both muscles are required. This has the disadvantage of creating scarring on both thighs, but the advantage that the repair is solid. Both techniques have the undoubted merit of using tissue coming from nonirradiated fields, thereby minimising wound healing problems in patients who have had previous radiotherapy. Either omentum or gracilis muscle will take a split skin graft if direct perineal closure cannot be obtained.

5.5. Surgery After Radiotherapy

Surgical repair of the pelvic floor and perineum is influenced most by whether the patient has been exposed to previous radiotherapy. The extent and nature of the disease being treated is largely irrelevant inasmuch as the surgically created defect is what remains after appropriate excision of diseased tissue. Radiotherapy creates significant problems because of its influence on intrinsic wound healing mechanisms, because of its extended effect on muscles and fasciae, and because of the changes seen in small and medium-sized arteries in particular. The vascular effects and, one assumes, the other effects, plateau at about 6 months after therapy is completed. Up to that point, the effects are of a more inflammatory nature with a degree of oedema and slightly greater difficulty in establishing tissue planes. Sutures tend to hold less well. Consequently, surgery is best carried out as soon after therapeutic radiation as possible. If radiotherapy is radical with the aim of being curative, the 6-month period after completion of treatment has invariably passed before persistence of disease becomes apparent. At this point, the surgeon has to contend with all the unwanted side-effects of radiation and must plan accordingly.

After radiotherapy, it is the general rule that formal reconstruction of pelvic floor and perineal wounds is necessary because tissues tend not to granulate, contract, or epithelialise in the normal way. In addition, the blood vessels within the pelvis, especially those derived from the internal iliac artery and its daughter branches, cannot be relied upon to support tissue transfer due to the direct effects of radiation on the vessels and due to the effects of fibrosis on tissue and vessel pliability and mobility. As a consequence, tissues under consideration for use to reconstruct and the blood vessels supplying those tissues must originate outside the irradiated field. Failure to observe this will result in importation of tissues with reduced healing capacity, reduced plasticity, a poorer blood supply, and an inherently greater capacity for wound healing problems.

Although the underlying physiological problems may be different, the approach to repair is the same as that outlined in Section 5.4 above, but with one difference. It is the almost invariable rule that the pelvic floor cannot be repaired directly after radiotherapy. Consequently, pelvic floor reconstruction should be regarded as the norm rather than the exception.

References

1. Tobin GR. Rectus abdominis flaps in vaginal and pelvic reconstruction. In: Strauch B, Vasconez LO, Hall-Findlay EJ, eds. *Grabb's Encyclopedia of Flaps.* 2nd ed. Philadelphia: Lippincott-Raven; 1998:1479–1484.

2. Taylor GI, Corlett RJ, Boyd JB. The versatile deep inferior epigastric (inferior rectus abdominis) flap. *Br J Plast Surg.* 1984;37:330–350.
3. Heckler FR. Gracilis myocutaneous and muscle flaps. *Clin Plast Surg.* 1980;7: 27–44.
4. Das SK. The size of the human omentum and methods of lengthening it for transplantation. *Br J Plast Surg.* 1976;29:170–174.
5. Alday ES, Goldsmith HS. Surgical technique for omental lengthening based on arterial anatomy. *Surg Gynecol Obstet.* 1972;135:103–107.
6. Yamamoto T, Mylonakis E, Keighley MRB. Omentoplasty for persistent perineal sinus after proctectomy for Crohn's disease. *Am J Surg.* 2001;181:265–267.
7. Topor B, Acland RD, Kolodko V, Galandiuk S. Omental transposition for low rectal anastomoses. *Am J Surg.* 2001;182:460–464.
8. McGregor AD, McGregor IA. *Fundamental Techniques of Plastic Surgery*. 10th ed. London: Churchill Livingston; 2000:52.
9. Yii NW, Niranjan NS. Lotus petal flaps in vulvo-vaginal reconstruction. *Br J Plast Surg.* 1996;49:547–554. (Also contains a good review of the literature.)

9
The Management of Inoperable Rectal Cancer

Sarah T. O'Dwyer

1. Introduction

Rectal cancer accounts for more than 160,000 global cancer deaths per annum with over 10,000 new cases diagnosed each year in the United Kingom [1]. Over recent years an increased interest in the management of rectal cancer has occurred as a consequence of the debate surrounding the incidence of local recurrence following resection of primary rectal tumours and the adoption of total mesorectal excision (TME) [2,3]. The TME debate has led to a heightened awareness of the variability of outcome following treatment of rectal cancer but has also prompted greater interest in preoperative local staging of the disease. The recognition and assessment of advanced tumours has been supported by major improvements in radiological imaging, allowing more objective determinants of staging and better planning for multimodality treatment [4]. Whether an advanced tumour is deemed resectable is subject to many variables but the consequences of a surgeon labeling a patient inoperable are profound. Living with a rectal cancer in situ, especially in the absence of metastatic disease, inevitably leads to a miserable state of uncontrollable pain, tenesmus, discharge, and infection. The importance of careful preoperative assessment, awareness of therapies that may downstage the tumour, and an understanding of the potential and pitfalls of radical surgical resection need to be explored.

2. Patient Assessment

Evaluation of the patient differs little whether one is dealing with an advanced primary rectal tumour or a recurrence. A key difference, however, is that there are likely to be less treatment options for recurrent disease as patients may have already received chemoradiotherapy. It is important to establish an accurate record of previous treatments including doses, methods, and timing of administration for drugs and radiation, in addition to copies of previous surgical operative records. Increasingly, patients present with new primary rectal cancers following previous radiotherapy for other pelvic tumours and this may preclude further radiation to the field. It is useful to document accurately the patient's symptoms including pelvic, perineal, or sacroiliac pain, urinary symptoms, and discharge that may indicate an established or imminent fistula. Recurrent fevers may occur secondary to fistulae, tumour necrosis, pelvic collections, and abscesses. The symptoms may indicate a need for urgent stoma formation or drainage procedures prior to future treatments aimed at downstaging the disease. Elimination of sepsis is essential so that aggressive chemoradiotherapy can be employed safely with minimal morbidity. As with any patient who is being considered for intensive multimodality cancer treatment, it is important to identify comorbid conditions and assess general performance status, including psychological and social factors that can influence an individuals' ability to progress through the treatment plan.

Clinical assessment requires an examination under anaesthetic (EUA) by a surgeon experienced in managing advanced disease. In the author's practice, a pelvic surgical team comprising colorectal and urological specialists undertake a joint evaluation. Fixity of the tumour to the sacrum, pelvic side walls, and adjacent organs must be determined and differentiated from tethering. Palpation peranum, pervaginum, and inspection, including proctoscopy, vaginoscopy, and cystoscopy with biopsy of irregularities, are mandatory for determining invasion. Frank invasion of soft tissues of the pelvic floor and perineum needs to be mapped in order to plan for reconstruction following excision in continuity with the tumour. In the author's experience, this detailed examination with intraoperative endo–anal ultrasound (EAUS) where appropriate, complements radiological assessment of local invasion leading to the most accurate clinical evaluation of T staging (Table 9.1) [4]. It must be remembered that an advanced rectal tumour may in itself be operable particularly where invasion is limited to pelvic organs and soft tissues rather than the bony pelvis or pelvic side walls. In such circumstances, resection may necessitate radical surgery with removal of adjacent organs and exentrative procedures that are beyond the scope of individual surgeons who have limited experience in dealing with advanced tumours. Seeking a second opinion on behalf of the patient reflects professional competence rather than defeat. Categorising a tumour as inoperable following EUA should really be reserved for cases fixed to the sacrum or

TABLE 9.1. Staging of rectal cancer.

TX	Primary tumour cannot be assessed
T0	No evidence of primary tumour
T1	Tumour invades submucosa
T2	Tumour invades muscularis propria
T3	Tumour invades through muscularis propria into subserosa or perirectal tissues
T4	Tumour perforates the visceral peritoneum or directly invades other organs or structures

bulky tumours with lateral extension to the pelvic side walls and limited mobility.

3. Radiological Imaging

Much has been written on the relative merits of different imaging modalities for evaluating primary rectal tumours with EAUS, spiral computed tomography (CT), and magnetic resonance imaging (MRI) all being supported [5–7]. For advanced T3 and T4 tumours, it may be necessary to use all 3 modalities to gain the most accurate picture in an individual patient. It is essential that the radiologist has experience in evaluating pelvic malignancy and is familiar with changes that result from previous surgery and radiotherapy. It is helpful if the radiologist is made aware of prior resections and treatments and given information of the findings at EUA [4]. The radiologist is a crucial member of the multidisciplinary team managing the patient. Although some radiologists claim that the newer CT scanners with multiplanar image reconstruction are equivalent to MRI in determining local extent and staging of rectal tumours, in the author's experience MRI remains superior for imaging advanced pelvic disease and is particularly useful in evaluating recurrent tumours (Figure 9.1). It is essential, however,

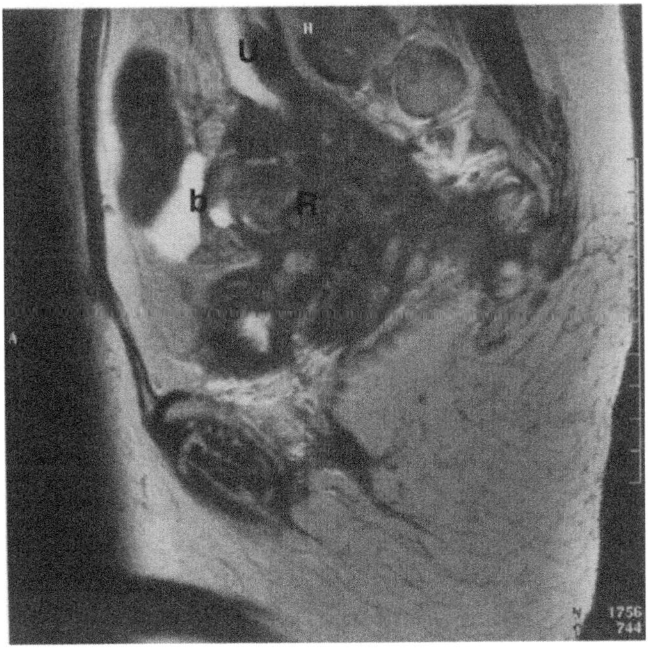

FIGURE 9.1. MRI showing recurrent rectal tumour (R) extending to the pelvic side wall and involving the left ureter (U) and bladder (b).

to perform CT imaging of the abdomen, liver, and thorax to screen for and quantify metastatic disease. The presence of hydronephrosis and hydroureter indicates the need for functional assessment with renography and potential intervention including nephrostomy and positioning of ureteric stents to protect renal function during therapy prior to surgery (Figure 9.2). Positron emission tomography (PET) can be useful in identifying occult metastatic disease and differentiating local recurrence from postsurgical or radiotherapy changes in the pelvis [8], but access to this imaging modality is at present seriously limited in the United Kingdom.

4. Therapeutic Strategies

Inoperable rectal tumours can be downstaged and rendered operable following treatment with radiotherapy alone or combined chemoradiotherapy (CRT). The extent of surgery required may be reduced significantly, allowing organ salvage or even reconstruction after tumour resection. Radical

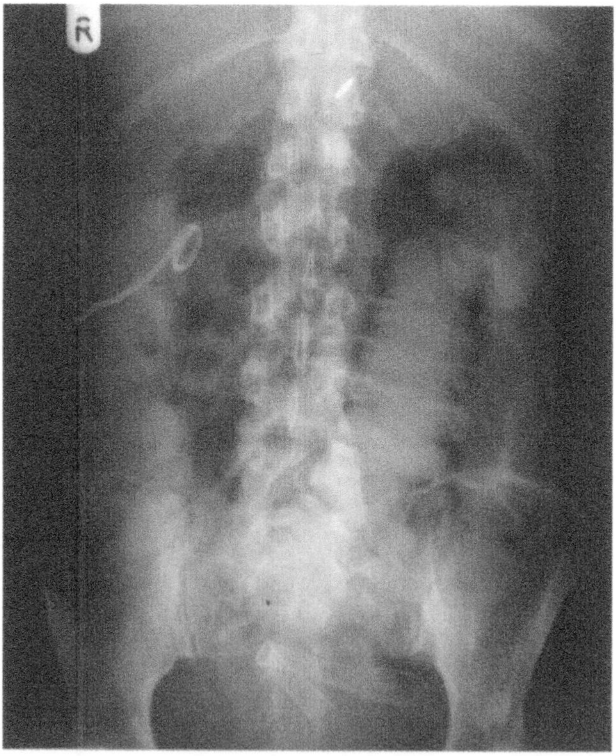

FIGURE 9.2. CT image showing a nephrostomy tube in the right renal pelvis and a stent at the rectosgmoid, both inserted prior to preoperative chemoradiotherapy.

surgery, however, may still be necessary after CRT and it is essential that the patient has confidence in the oncological team and appreciates the concept of a treatment package that together offers best outcome.

4.1. Preoperative Radiotherapy

Different groups offer a variety of radiotherapy regimens, but treatment generally consists of a total dose of 45–50 Gy to include the tumour bed, perirectal soft tissues, and pelvic side walls, but may not include all iliac nodes. Fractionation of the dose varies in different institutions, but usually consists of 20–30 fractions over 5–6 weeks (often described as long-course radiotherapy, in contrast to the 4–5 fractions of adjuvant preoperative radiotherapy used in less advanced disease). An early response to treatment includes increased vascularity and tissue oedema, hence in a circumferential tumour there is a risk of precipitating obstruction. Joint management is essential and if the tumour is in the upper rectum or at the rectosigmoid, stent insertion may be possible. Lower tumours are more problematic as positioning and retention of the stent is difficult; encroachment on the dentate line leads to severe discomfort and often requires stent removal. If at EUA a stenotic or obstructing tumour is recognised and stenting is impractical, there should be a low threshold for fashioning a defunctioning stoma to avoid the danger of tipping the patient into obstruction during radiotherapy.

Many series have demonstrated that using radiotherapy alone, tumours are downstaged [9], inoperable tumours can be rendered operable [10], and, on occasion, no histological evidence of tumour remains in the resected specimen. It has been noted, however, than even when the primary tumour has had a complete response to radiotherapy, there may be positive nodes in the resectate, hence excisional surgery is usually advised even when dramatic responses are noted on postradiotherapy treatment scans [11]. The timing of surgery following long-course radiotherapy has never been subjected to rigorous evaluation, but most groups leave an interval of at least 6 weeks to allow downsizing of the tumour. Re-evaluation with EUA and MRI is helpful to assess the expected extent of surgical resection. Overall, 45%–65% of fixed rectal tumours can be downsized and resected following radiotherapy alone, but almost half will develop local recurrence [12]. Failure to achieve local control and curative resection naturally led to the adoption of additional treatment modalities in advanced tumours. Some groups have had improved response using proton and neutron therapy [13,14], but the use of combined chemotherapy and radiotherapy has become the preferred approach.

4.2. Chemotherapy

In oncological practice it has been recognised for some time that chemotherapeutic agents potentiate the effects of radiotherapy. The last decade has seen the introduction of new chemotherapy agents directed toward metastatic colorectal cancer and current trials are evaluating the use of combined chemoradiotherapy treatments in advanced and inoperable rectal tumours [15–17]. Evidence of efficacy was initially generated from randomised studies of postoperative adjuvant CRT based on radiotherapy with or without bolus 5-fluoruracil (5FU) at the start and end of treatment [18,19]. A reduction in local recurrence by 34% and mortality by 29% was evident in patients receiving the 5FU boost. A subsequent larger study of 660 patients demonstrated survival benefits of infusional versus bolus 5FU in conjunction with postoperative radiotherapy [20]. Consequent to such studies, a number of groups have investigated the potential of using combinations of 5FU, cisplatin, and mitomicin in addition to radiotherapy before resection of the tumour. Although each study is relatively small (range of 7–64 patients), the results indicated that the combined treatments were feasible, and effective, particularly in locally advanced rectal tumours where 90% were downstaged and more than one half had potentially curative resections [21].

Phase I studies using tomudex ran into difficulties due to a high mortality in patients receiving combined treatments and increased toxicity also led to an unacceptable number of patients being unable to complete the radiotherapy program. Subsequent analysis suggested that dose reduction may have prevented a significant number of deaths and further evaluation is now underway in MRI staged T3/4 node-positive tumours, with early reports of 80% response and over 60% R0 resectability rates (Saunders, personal communication). In addition, the European Organization for Research and Treatment of Cancer (EORTC) 22921 study is evaluating the independent effects of preoperative radiotherapy and chemotherapy, with and without postoperative 5FU. Phase II studies are also underway using oxaliplatin, irinotecan, raltitrexed, and capcitabine in combination with radiotherapy.

Overall, the evidence suggests that for patients with good performance status and limited comorbidity, CRT leads to shrinkage of T3/4 tumours, offering the potential for less radical and more curative resections in locally advanced disease [22–25]. The course of CRT effects needs to be appreciated so as to gain maximal advantage of tumour response prior to surgical intervention. Although it can be difficult for the patient and family to accept, it is best to delay surgery for at least 8 weeks following treatment.

4.3. Intraoperative Radiotherapy

Despite full-dose preoperative CRT, some tumours extend to the surgical boundaries at the time of excision. Leaving residual frank macroscopic tumour or when the surgeon is concerned that microscopic resection margins are likely to be positive, additional strategies need to be employed to optimise the chance of eliminating pelvic disease. A few centers have facilities for intraoperative radiotherapy (IORT), where a radiation boost can be applied directly to the site under question. In a study of patients with fixed rectal tumours undergoing preoperative radiotherapy and radical resection alone, versus additional IORT, local recurrence was reduced from 11% to 3% [26]. Although the hardware is relatively expensive, IORT should be available in specialist centres where a significant caseload of locally advanced and recurrent pelvic tumours are managed.

5. Surgical Approaches

Reassessment of the patient 8 weeks following CRT includes repeat EUA and MRI of the pelvis. The extent to which the tumour has regressed can be mapped and operability checked. Tumour bulk may have decreased and sometimes this allows a better appreciation of fixity. Difficulties can arise, however, due to radiation fibrosis, particularly when dealing with recurrent disease where patients have had radiotherapy many months earlier. In such cases careful scrutiny of the MRI may assist in defining tumour infiltration from fibrosis. Unfortunately, there will be cases where doubt remains and only surgical exploration will ultimately reveal whether resection is feasible. It is important in such cases that the patient understands that despite undergoing surgery the tumour may not be resectable and it is useful to consider whether palliative procedures could benefit the patient so that they can be performed at this stage. The role of radical surgery as palliation, particularly where there is documented extrapelvic disease remains controversial. In the author's opinion, radical excisional surgery is justifiable particularly where the metastatic load is minimal and the patient is physically well. It must be remembered that excision may be the best means of achieving pain relief and eliminating sepsis, hence, providing the objectives of surgery are agreed with the patient, palliative excision can be considered. For any team taking on this work, morbidity and mortality must be carefully audited and minimised. A reasonable caseload is required in order to achieve best outcomes and evaluate the effects of multimodality treatments on recurrence, survival, and quality of life [27–29].

In the male, total pelvic exenteration (TPE) is usually required, particularly in anterior or circumferential tumours where attempts at dissection in the standard plane leaves tumour on the back of the seminal vesicles and prostate and is associated with early recurrence (Figure 9.3). In selected cases, it is possible to do a proctectomy or abdominoperineal rectal resection with an en-bloc radical prostatectomy achieving clearance without breaching the oncological plane. Reconstruction of the urinary tract avoids the need for an ileal conduit and second stoma. Female patients have the advantage of the gynaecological barrier and posterior clearance is often feasible, particularly if the patient has not had a hysterectomy. It is usually

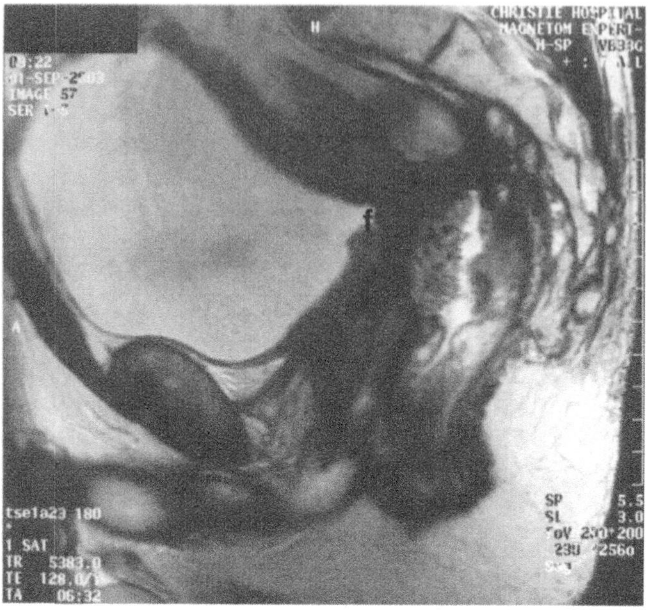

FIGURE 9.3. Large rectal tumour fistulating anteriorly into the bladder in the male. Despite the advanced nature of the disease, central tumours can be excised by TPE with good results.

possible to preserve the anterior vaginal wall, opening the vagina anteriorly separating the mid- and posterior pelvic organs.

Reconstruction is usually necessary in such cases to aid perineal wound healing and avoid future perineal hernia. Mobilisation and placement of the omentum in the pelvis and fashioning myocutaneous flaps should be standard practice for the pelvic surgical team undertaking these procedures. Both rectus abdominis (TRAM) flaps and gracilis flaps can be used, the advantage of the latter being retention of the anterior abdominal-wall musculature for support of stomas.

5.1. Intestinal Obstruction

The majority of patients with advanced unresectable rectal tumours will require a stoma for relief or prevention of impending obstruction. Planning which portion of bowel to use for a stoma is essential if there is a chance that gastrointestinal continuity could be restored after future excision of the tumour. Loop stomas are not favored by the author, as spillover remains a problem even if the loop is fashioned trying to avoid this problem. Prolapse is frequent in transverse loop stomas and the surgeon must recognise that a significant percentage of patients may not proceed to further excisional surgery. Generally, it is better to separate the bowel, fashioning a working end stoma and a mucous fistula. Should imaging suggest that small bowel is adherent to the tumour, a defunctioning ileostomy may be a satisfactory option. The same stoma can then be used in the future to defunction a low coloanorectal anastomosis after resection. Trephine and laparoscopically assisted stoma formation are acceptable and, on occasion, useful techniques, although a minilaparotomy allows the surgeon to assess fixity of the tumour should there be serious doubt that the patient may not complete the preoperative CRT treatment to allow downstaging of the disease.

The use of stents in tumours of the upper rectum and at the rectosigmoid has proved increasingly useful, particularly in the presence of advanced extrapelvic disease where disease progression is more likely to be determined by the systemic tumour than by local spread [30]. Mid- and low rectal tumours are usually not suitable for stent insertion due to the proximity of the anal canal and a tendency for the stent to migrate, causing pain and tenesmus due to the presence of the stent rather than the tumour.

Patients with circumferential tumours need careful evaluation for potential obstruction prior to embarking on radiotherapy, as oedema and tissue swelling during treatment can tip the patient into obstruction. Perforation and necrosis proximal to the tumour is uncommon during therapy, but when this occurs it is disastrous, as most patients loose their chance of downstaging and if they survive an emergency procedure few will go on to resection.

5.2. Resection: Surgical Principles

The surgical procedure will vary depending on disease extent and whether the tumour is confined to the posterior pelvis or involves the central and anterior pelvic structures (Figure 9.4). Lateral extension is associated with a poor prognosis and has a low resectability and cure rate [31].

Despite the radicality of the surgery often required, in experienced hands outcomes are good. Careful selection and preoperative planning are the cornerstones for success. Optimisation of respiratory and renal function and involvement of an anaesthetist experienced in such procedures is crucial. Antiembolic thromboprophylaxis in these high-risk patients should include low-molecular-weight heparin in addition to on-table intermittent calf compression. After surgery, calf compression continues on the critical care unit for at least 24 hours, and unless there are specific contraindications such as peripheral vascular disease, patients are encouraged to wear graduated-compression thigh-length stockings until they are fully mobile (even after discharge from hospital).

Protecting the patient from pressure or traction injuries on the operating table is the responsibility of the surgeon in charge, and with care brachial, lateral popliteal, and femoral nerve injuries can be avoided. It is

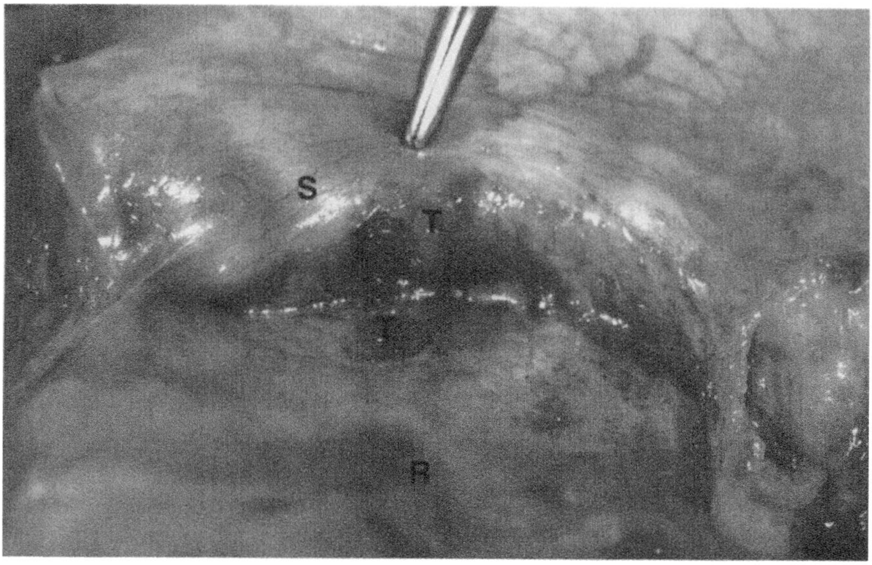

FIGURE 9.4. Tumour nodules (T) identified at operation involving the peritoneal reflection between the seminal vesicles (S) and rectum (R).

advisable to position the legs using supports with foot boots rather than Lloyd Davis stirrups so as to prevent pressure on the calf and avoidance of lower-limb injuries. It is important in lengthy procedures to minimise periods of head-down tilt with the feet elevated, as lower-limb perfusion can be compromised. Rarely, compartment syndrome may develop in the early postoperative period and, if not recognised, severe disability and even loss of limb can result. Intermittent changes of the patient's position by altering the operating table will assist in avoiding such complications.

High-dose intravenous antibiotics (cephalosporin and metronidazole 1.5 g) are given at induction of anaesthesia with a second dose given intraoperatively if the procedure is prolonged beyond 6 hours. Postoperative antibiotics are necessary when the procedure includes the urinary tract with diversion or bladder reconstruction. In such cases, gentamicin is also administered as introperative and postoperative boluses.

5.3. Surgical Techniques

Although the author recognizes that the pelvis can be accessed using a variety of abdominal incisions, a long midline approach is preferred so as to leave the rectus abdominal muscles undisturbed for stomal support and/or transposition flaps. In cases of recurrent tumour, entering the abdominal cavity may be difficult and time consuming. Dissection of the bowel from the anterior abdominal wall is often best performed using sharp dissection with a scalpel rather than scissors. Careful dissection, avoiding enterotomies, requires patience but full mobilisation can usually be achieved. Once the abdominal wall is free, palpation of the liver complements preoperative imaging in the accurate clinical staging of the disease. In doubtful cases, and where radical resection would be contraindicated by the presence of hepatic disease, the addition of intraoperative ultrasound can be helpful. It should be recognised, however, that in young fit patients, an aggressive approach to pelvic resection followed by delayed hepatic resection can be justified. Inspection of the general peritoneal cavity is also important as peritoneal surface deposits may also lead to an early decision to avoid radical resection. If such decisions are being considered, frozen-section positive biopsy is most helpful, but if not available, formal tissue biopsy must be taken to support future treatment plans.

Following previous pelvic surgery, loops of small bowel often prolapse into the pelvis and if the patient received postoperative radiotherapy, bowel loops may be densely adherent to the pelvic organs and side walls. In some cases, a dependant loop of mid small bowel or the terminal ileum is attached to the tumour and can be isolated by dividing the mesentery and stapling the efferent and afferent limbs to allow an en-bloc resection. Small-bowel anastomosis should be deferred until a decision is taken regarding the urinary tract, as the site may prove satisfactory for isolating an ileal conduit for urinary diversion.

Once the small bowel has been mobilized from the pelvis, it is often useful to perform a bimanual assessment of the tumour with one hand in the pelvis and the other from the perineum. This maneuver allows the operator to best assess fixity to the bony pelvis and aid in the definition of organ involvement. Entry to the posterior pelvis should begin from the lateral abdominal wall in the left iliac fossa. Mobilisation of the sigmoid colon and reflection of the colon to the midline and right-hand side will allow early identification of the ureter. If the patient has had a previous anterior resection, the colon and its mesentery may be adherent to the posterior abdominal wall and a higher approach may be necessary. Once identified, a loose sling should be placed round the ureter as gentle traction on the sling often aids further identification of the ureteric path through the pelvis. The use of ureteric stents should be considered where the preoperative radiology indicates close adherence of the ureter or dilatation, proximal to a pelvic tumour or nodal mass on the pelvic side wall. If the ureter cannot be safely identified and stents have not been inserted before laparotomy, the operator should abort the dissection until intraoperative placement of stents has occurred. Rarely, if a stent cannot be advanced cystoscopically it may be necessary to open the bladder.

Mobilisation of the colon to the pelvic brim allows separation of the lateral peritoneal fold and identification of the presacral fascia and mesorectal plane. It is important not to divide the blood supply to the bowel until one is certain that resection is possible. The anatomical position of the tumour may dictate the extent of resection required. Posterior and lateral tumours can be resected following a TME dissection with some modification. Rectal dissection proceeds along the mesorectal plane although the areolar avascular plane is usually lost as a consequence of radiation therapy and/or previous surgery. The tissues are usually thickened and fibrosed with areas of fusion to the presacral fascia, pelvic side walls, and pelvic floor. In addition, neovascularisation occurs following long-course radiotherapy and aberrant vessels may be part of the advanced disease. Venous bleeding is a major risk and care has to be taken to control vessels while the dissection proceeds as large losses can occur rapidly. Venous drainage may involve both internal and external iliac channels, and, if large veins are identified, it is usually safer to dissect from the pelvic brim following a path lateral to the ureter identifying the iliac vessels, allowing proximal formal ligation if and when required. Haemodynamic control must be maintained and constant interaction between anaesthetist and surgeon is essential. Access to bleeding points may be limited until the tumour can be removed, hence, packing and compression may be necessary while mobilisation continues. The inferior limit of dissection will often be determined by the bulk of the disease in addition to the actual anatomical position in the mid- or low rectum. In male patients, it may not be possible to resect a bulky tumour without resorting to an abdominoperineal approach. Where there has been a marked response to CRT it may be possible to get below a tumour, apply a staple, and preserve the anal canal. A coloanal or ultra-low colorectal anastamosis must be defunctioned, preferably with a loop ileostomy.

5.4. Exenterative Procedures

The principles of surgery will be outlined, but for a more detailed description and illustrations refer to Rob and Smith's *Surgery of the Colon, Rectum, and Anus* [32]. In the male, bulky tumours may be difficult to assess until mobilisation of the bladder with division of the superior and middle pedicles on one side has been performed. Further bimanual assessment will help in deciding operability and if the decision is to proceed division of the rectosimoid, using a linear stapler isolates the pelvic organs when TPE is deemed necessary for tumour clearance. This approach brings the operator onto the vesical pedicals that are ligated. The endopelvic fascia is opened anteriorly and the dorsal vein complex controlled and ligated.

In low tumours and in many cases of recurrence, there may be lateral extension and involvement of the pelvic floor. To achieve tumour-free margins dissection must proceed more laterally than in a standard anterior resection/TME. A combined abdominoperineal approach is often necessary to avoid breaching the oncological plane, with the abdominal operator guiding the perineal dissection posteriorly and laterally. With careful dissection using both standard and argon diathermy, blood loss can be minimised. Perineal dissection can be kept relatively dry using 1:400000 adrenaline in saline infiltration. Once the tumour has been removed, further hemostasis can be achieved. Occasionally, it is possible to avoid the formal perineal dissection. Once the prostatic urethra has been divided, the prostate and bladder can be reflected cranially and the anorectal plane identified. With the tumour superior, it can be possible to apply a stapling gun, preserving a short anorectal cuff. If gastrointestinal continuity is possible, complete mobilisation of the left colon and splenic flexure is required to allow a safe low pelvic anastomosis that should be defunctioned.

More commonly an end stoma is necessary. Shortening of the mesentery is another problem following long-course radiotherapy, hence, it often requires mobilisation of the left colon and splenic flexure to fashion a satisfactory stoma. Following mobilisation of the colon, however, an isolated vascularised colonic loop can be used as an alternative to small bowel for the urinary conduit bladder replacement. Using the colon has the advantage of limiting the number of anastomotic suture lines. If, however, small bowel has already been divided as described earlier, a standard ileal conduit is fashioned. Ureteric stents are left in situ for 10 days and the pelvic drain remains until the stents have been removed.

If performing a posterior clearance in the female, it is necessary to open the peritoneum anteriorly and mobilise the posterior wall of the bladder from the vagina. If the patient has had a hysterectomy, the vaginal vault is often fused either to the bladder or to the anterior rectal wall. Introduction of a swab into the vagina from the perineum can aid in the identification of the vaginal vault and once mobilisation has started, further elevation of the vagina using this maneuver assists dissection along the vaginal wall anteriorly. Care must be taken to identify the position of the ureters, particularly when the uterus is absent, as they may be injured at the lateral edge of the dissection at the angle of the vaginal vault. As indicated earlier, a liberal use of ureteric stents aids identification and protects against occult injury. The vagina is opened anteriorly below the level of the cervix and the vaginal wall is divided, taking a sleeve of the posterior vaginal wall in continuity with the uterus and rectum. It may be possible to identify a plane between the vagina and low rectum, preserving the anal canal.

Following formal exenteration, perineal reconstruction is usually necessary to aid wound healing and avoid future perineal hernias. Mobilisation and placement of the omentum in the pelvis and fashioning myocutaneous flaps should be standard practice for the pelvic surgical team undertaking these procedures. Both TRAM and gracilis flaps can be used, the advantage of the latter being retention of the anterior abdominal-wall musculature for support of stomas.

5.5. *Abdominosacrectomy*

When preoperative assessment has indicated involvement of the sacrum, in selected patients sacral excision can be performed en bloc. If proceeding with this radical resection, the operators must be sure there is no evidence of extrapelvic disease. It is generally accepted that involvement above S2 renders a patient inoperable as the morbidity, including lower-limb paralysis, is unacceptable. Although some have described anterior sacrectomy, that is, removing the anterior sacral cortex in continuity with the tumour, few consider such an approach practicable for the majority of cases.

The pelvic dissection proceeds as for standard exentrative surgery, dividing the blood supply to the organs in continuity with the tumour. Ligation of the middle rectal artery is performed after identification during the anterolateral dissection. Meticulous haemostasis is required and the surgeons must be satisfied that a dry pelvis has been achieved before proceeding with sacrectomy. Stomas can be fashioned at this stage or be deferred until the tumour has been removed.

The patient is turned into the jackknife position and the perineal incision is extended onto the sacral area between the buttocks. The skin flaps are elevated laterally to the sacraliliac joint. The parasacral muscles are divided with diathermy. The sacrum is divided bellow the S2 level in order to avoid opening the dural sac. The caudal limit of the sac is variable and if the sac is opened it must be formally ligated. The sciatic nerve is avoided laterally, the nerve roots are identified, and the sacral bone elevated. Anterior sacral vessels may need formal ligation at this stage, although full control may not be possible until the tumour and sacral bone have been removed in continuity. Closure of the wound is best performed using myocutanous flap reconstructions.

5.6. *Additional Procedures*

Even with preoperative CRT and the extended nature of the surgery described some patients will have tumours that remain unresectable. The use of isolated pelvic perfusion for a variety of advanced pelvic malignancies has been modified using balloon occlusion catheters positioned under fluoroscopic control. Using these techniques, 9 of 16 patients with unresectable rectal tumours had significant tumour regression and the tumours were excised [33]. While not without complications, such treatment may be useful for patients with extensive disease confined to the pelvis and may be helpful in palliation of pain associated with unresectable tumours.

6. Outcome of Chemoradiotherapy and Surgery

When considering the results of aggressive management of fixed or inoperable rectal tumours, there is a notable variation in the published literature. For locally advanced primary tumours, 5-year survival is reported as 40%–80%, morbidity as 30%, and operative mortality less than 10% [34–38]. Outcomes will clearly vary when considering primary rather than recurrent disease and more accurate and objective pretreatment staging will hopefully allow better comparison in future [39,40]. In a large series of 83 cases of recurrent cancer recently reported by Yamada, of the 60 patients that had resection, 5-year survival was dependant on the pattern of pelvic invasion [41]. Where the disease was confined to the central pelvis, there was a 38% 5-year survival, compared with 10% where there was sacral involvement and with no survivors at 5 years where the disease extended to the lateral pelvis. Similar conclusions have been drawn from other experience which reveals significant morbidity and short survival in laterally advanced recurrent disease [42,43]. The psychological effects of extensive and exentrative surgery must always be recognized by groups that undertake this work and ongoing support and counselling must be offered to patients and their families to achieve the best outcome [44].

7. Palliative Treatments and Procedures

For some patients tumour removal will prove impossible despite attempts at downstaging advanced disease using the methods described. Others have advanced metastatic disease or have significant comorbidity that limits an aggressive approach with CRT and excisional surgery. There is much to offer such patients as treatment will be customised to individual needs and structured around palliation of symptoms. The main problem for patients with an unresectable pelvic tumour is pain and discharge, while obstruction, external fistulae, bleeding, and chronic infection may require intervention. Close working relationships between surgeons, oncologists, and palliative care teams allows a care plan to be developed that responds to the ever-changing needs of these patients.

7.1. Pain Management

Severe and relentless pain in the sacroiliac region, across the buttocks, and in the perineum is often a consequence of a tumour growing along the sacral nerve routes or infiltration into the sacral bone. The patient is distressed, cannot sit, and may not sleep. Everything must be done to relieve such pain and combinations of oral, transdermal, and infusional agents may be required [45]. Older patients have a fear of opiate drugs that must be addressed early in the management to allow them access to the full range of pharmacological options. Combined therapy using opiates and anti-inflammatory preparations are generally associated with best responses.

A sudden increase in pain may indicate additional complications such as pathological fracture. Radiological confirmation is important as additional palliative radiotherapy to the site may be possible, particularly if it is outside the original radiotherapy field. Alteration in the pattern of pain may also indicate additional complications such as local infection or abscess formation following perforation or tumour necrosis. Magnetic resonance imaging may identify a collection worthy of drainage either radiologically or surgically.

In a small number of patients with persistent local disease and minimal metastaic cancer, increasing sedative effects may be an unacceptable complication and consideration of epidural analgesia may be necessary. In the United Kingdom, the majority of such patients are managed in a hospice setting although improved community services increasingly allows home support in individual cases.

7.2. Discharge

The presence of a rectal tumour usually results in recurrent discharge, initially from the anal canal but as the tumour progresses free discharge may occur through the vagina or from the bladder. Most patients will require a stoma to divert the faecal contents and decrease the incidence of infection. It is important, however, that the patient does not misunderstand and believe that fashioning a stoma will relieve them of all discharge. Once the faecal stream has been diverted, other methods of trying to locally control the tumour discharge can be applied.

Radiotherapy not only reduces the tumour volume but can limit the discharge, albeit temporarily. Application of varying energy sources to ablate the tumour are all successful. Common treatments include simple diathermy, laser and argon ablation, or attempts at more radical endoanal resection of mucosal tumour [46,47]. Each can be offered where most appropriate for relief of symptoms.

7.3. Bleeding and Infection

Some blood loss is almost inevitable from tumours that remain in situ, and although patients worry about the presence of blood in the toilet rarely is the bleeding significant. It is important to reassure patients and to check blood counts from time to time. Should there be a significant bleed, usually with loss of clots, endoscopic inspection may reveal an area suitable for argon or laser treatment that can successfully control local bleeding points. If the patient has not received radiotherapy, it can be useful after immediate control of the acute bleed has been established. Some have advocated application of adrenaline-soaked gauze in these circumstances and found it helpful particularly if there is a general bleed from the tumour. The majority of patients can be supported with hematinics and transfusion as required.

Pelvic infection may result from local perforation of the tumour or necrosis. Occasionally a small-bowel or urinary fistula may contribute to the generation of a pelvic collection and in such cases careful clinical evaluation and MRI will help to define the anatomy. In the majority of cases, the collection is walled off but may track from the pelvis along tissue planes into the perineum, buttocks, thigh, or even the knee, presenting as an inflammatory fluctuant soft-tissue swelling. In order to prevent systemic sepsis, local infection needs to be drained and eradicated. Chronic pelvic sepsis may contribute significantly to increasing pelvic pain, intermittent discharge, or a deterioration disproportionate to the progression of the disease. Wherever possible, collections should be drained and systems defunctioned, following which the patient's general state will improve. Radiological drainage may be possible, but when patients have had previous surgery, the standard approaches may be impossible and a joint approach under general anaesthesia with on-table imaging can be successful. When a urinary fistula is present, both nephrostomy and direct catheter drainage may be required.

8. Conclusions

The miserable outcome for patients whose rectal tumours cannot be resected drives the pelvic cancer team to strive wherever possible to downstage tumours and resect even when this may be with palliative intent. Careful clinical assessment and radiological imaging allows a treatment plan to be formulated using combined chemoradiotherapy and subsequent surgery. Radical resections such as total pelvic exenteration and sacrectomy can be successfully performed in appropriately selected patients. Experienced teams can obtain reasonable outcomes with acceptable levels of morbidity and low operative mortality. For patients who have to live with a tumour in situ, palliative approaches can offer incremental improvements with control of pain and discharge being a key component in improving and maintaining quality of life.

References

1. Parkin DM. Global cancer statistics in the year 2000. *Lancet Oncol.* 2001;2: 533–541.
2. MacFarlane JK, Ryall RD, Heald RJ. Mesorectal excision for rectal cancer. *Lancet* 1993;341:457–460.
3. Kapiteijn E, Marijnen CA, Nagtegaal ID, et al. Preoperative radiotherapy combined with total mesorectal excision for resectable rectal cancer. *N Engl J Med.* 2001;345:638–646.
4. Robinson P, Carrington B, Swindell R, O'Dwyer ST. Accuracy of MRI in predicting disease extent in recurrent and advanced rectal cancer. *Clin Radiol.* 2002;57:514–522.
5. Hunerbein M. Endorectal ultrasound in rectal cancer. *Colorect Dis.* 2003;5: 402–405.
6. Bartram C, Brown G. Endorectal ultrasound and magnetic imaging in rectal cancer imaging. *Gastroenterol Clin North Am.* 2002;31:827–839.

7. Beets-Tan RG, Beets GL, Borstlap AC, et al. Preoperative assessment of local tumour extent in advanced rectal cancer: CT or high resolution MRI. *Abdom Imaging.* 2000;25:533–541.
8. Heubner RH, Park KC, Shepherd JE, et al. Meta analysis of PET imaging for recurrent colorectal cancer. *J Nucl Med.* 2000;41:1177–1189.
9. Sebag-Montefiore D. Treatment of T4 tumours: the role of radiotherapy. *Colorect Dis.* 2003;5:432–435.
10. James RD, Schofield PF. Resection of 'inoperable' rectal cancer following radiotherapy. *Br J Surg.* 1985;72:279–281.
11. Medich D, McGinty J, Parda D, et al. Preoperative chemoradiotherapy and radical surgery for locally advanced distal rectal adenocarcinoma. *Dis Colon Rectum.* 2001;44:1123–1128.
12. Frykholm GJ, Pahlman L, Glimelius B. Combined chemo and radiotherapy vs radiotherapy alone in the treatment of primary, non respectable adenocarcinoma of the rectum. *Int J Radiat Oncol Biol Phys.* 2001;50:433–440.
13. Isacsson U, Montelius A, Jung B, Glimelius B. Comparative treatment planning between proton and X-ray therapy in locally advanced rectal cancer. *Radiother Oncol.* 1996;41:263–272.
14. Engenhart-Cabillic R, Debus J, Prott FJ, et al. Use of neutron therapy in the management of locally advanced nonresectable primary or recurrent rectal cancer. *Recent Results Cancer Res.* 1998;150:113–124.
15. James R, Price P, Valentini V. Ralitrexid (Tomudex) concomitant radiotherapy as adjuvant treatment for patients with rectal cancer: preliminary results of phase 1 studies. *Eur J Cancer.* 1999;35(suppl 1):S19–S22.
16. Myerson RJ, Valentini V, Birnbaum EH, et al. Phase I/II trial of three-dimensionally planned concurrent boost radiotherapy and protracted venous infusion of 5FU for locally advanced rectal carcinoma. *Int J Radiat Oncol Biol Phys.* 2001;50:1299–1308.
17. European Organization for Research and Treatment of Cancer (EORTC). EORTC publication 22921.
18. Krook JE, Moerrtel CG, Gunderson LL, et al. Effective surgical adjuvant therapy for high risk rectal cancer. *N Engl J Med.* 1995;324:709–715.
19. Bosset JF, Magnin V, Maingnon P, et al. Preoperative radiochemotherapy in rectal cancer: long term results of a phase II trial. *Int J Radiat Oncol Biol Phys.* 1995;46:323–327.
20. O'Connell MJ, Martenson JA, Wieand HS, et al. Improving adjuvant therapy for rectal cancer by combining protracted infusion fluorouracil with radiation after curative surgery. *N Engl J Med.* 1994;331:502–507.
21. Videtic Gm, Fischer BJ, Perera FE, et al. Preoperative radiation with concurrent 5-fluoruracil continuous infusion for locally advanced unresectable rectal cancer. *Int J Radiat Oncol Biol Phys.* 1998:42:319–324.
22. Mohiuddin M, Hayne M, Regine WF, et al. Prognostic significance of post chemoradiation stage following preoperative chemotherapy and radiation for advanced/recurrent rectal cancers. *Int J Radiat Oncol Bio Phys.* 2000;48:1075–1080.
23. Onaitis MW, Noone RB, Hartwig M, et al. Neoadjuvant chemoradiation for rectal cancer: analysis of clinical outcomes from a 13 year institutional experience. *Ann Surg.* 2001;233:778–785.

24. Sanfilippo NJ, Crane CH, Skibber J, et al. T4 rectal cancer treated with preoperative chemoradiotherapy to the posterior pelvis followed by multivisceral resection: patterns of failure and limitations of treatment. *Int J Radiat Oncol Biol Phys.* 2001;51:176–183.
25. Gohl J, Merkel S, Rodel C, Hohenberger W. Can neoadjuvant radiochemotherapy improve the results of multivisceral resection in advanced rectal carcinoma? *Colorectal Dis.* 2003;5:436–441.
26. Sadahiro S, Suzuki T, Ishikawa K, et al. Intraoperative radiation therapy for curatively resected rectal cancer. *Dis Colon Rectum.* 2001;44:1689–1695.
27. Begg CB, Cramer LD, Hoskins WJ, Brennan MF. Impact of hospital volume on operative mortality for major cancer surgery. *JAMA.* 1998;280:1747–1751.
28. Guren MG, Wiig JN, Dueland S, et al. Quality of life in patients with urinary diversion after operation for locally advanced rectal cancer. *Eur J Surg Oncol.* 2001;27:645–665.
29. Mannaerts GH, Schijven MP, Hendrikx A, et al. Urologic and sexual morbidity following multimodality treatment for locally advanced primary and locally recurrent rectal cancer. *Eur J Surg Oncol.* 2001;27:265–272.
30. Khot U, Wenk Lang A, Murali K, et al. Systematic review of the clinical evidence on colorectal self expanding metal stents. *Br J Surg.* 2002;89:1096–1102.
31. Yui R, Wong SK, Cromwell J, et al. Pelvic wall involvement denotes a poor prognosis in T4 rectal cancer. *Dis Colon Rectum.* 2001;44:1676–1681.
32. Cohen AM. Pelvic exenteration and other extended operations. In: Rob, Smith, eds. *Surgery of the Colon, Rectum and Anus.* 5th ed. Woburn, MA: Butterworth-Heinemann; 1993.
33. Wanebo HJ, Belliveau J, Begossi G, Levy A. Isolated chemotherapeutic perfusion of the pelvis for advanced rectal cancer. *Colorectal Dis.* 2003;5:508–514.
34. Lehnert T, Methner M, Pollock A, Schaible A, Hinz U, Herfarth C. Multivisceral resection for locally advanced primary colon and rectal cancer: an analysis of prognostic factors in 201 patients. *Ann Surg.* 2002;235:217–225.
35. Moriya Y, Akasu T, Fujita S, Yamamoto S. Aggressive surgical treatment for patients with T4 rectal cancer. *Colorectal Dis.* 2003;5:427–431.
36. Crowe PJ, Temple WJ, Lopez MJ, Ketcham AS. Pelvic exenteration for advanced pelvic malignancy. *Semin Surg Oncol.* 1999;17:152–160.
37. Law WL, Chu KW, Choi HK. Total pelvic exenteration for locally advanced rectal disease. *J Am Coll Surg.* 2000;190:78–83.
38. Myerson GH, Rutten HJ, Martijn H, et al. Abdominosacral resection for primary irresectable and locally recurrent rectal cancer. *Dis Colon Rectum.* 2001;44:806–814.
39. Meterissian SH, Skibber JM, Giacco GG, el-Naggar AK, Hess KR, Rich TA. Pelvic exenteration for locally advanced rectal carcinoma: factors predicting improved survival. *Surgery* 1997;121:479–487.
40. Temple W, Saettler EB. Locally recurrent rectal cancer: role of composite resection of extensive pelvic tumors with strategies for minimizing risk of recurrence. *J Surg Oncol.* 2000;73:47–58.
41. Yamada K, Ishizawa T, Niwa K, Chuman Y, Akiba S, Aikou T. Patterns of pelvic invasion are prognostic in the treatment of locally recurrent rectal cancer. *Br J Surg.* 2001;88:988–993.
42. Zacherl J, Schiessel R, Windhager R, et al. Abdominosacral resection of recurrent rectal cancer in the sacrum. *Dis Colon Rectum.* 1999;42:1035–1039.

43. Garcia-Aguilar J, Cromwell JW, Marra C, Lee S, Madoff R, Rothenburger DA. Treatment of locally advanced recurrent rectal cancer. *Dis Colon Rectum.* 2001; 44:1743–1748.
44. Turns D. Psychological issues: pelvic exenterative surgery. *J Surg Oncol.* 2001;76:224–236.
45. Beretta GD, Pessi MA, Poletti P, Mosconi S, Labianca R. New drugs and combinations in palliative treatment of colon and rectal cancer. *Eur J Surg Oncol.* 2001;27:595–600.
46. Zaman A, Vassilev S, Mateev M, Mazgalov L, Filev F. Superiority of Nd: YAG laser to cryosurgery in treatment of rectal carcinoma. *J Clin Laser Med Surg.* 1994;12:79–83.
47. Mischinger HJ, Hauser H, Cerwenka H, et al. Endocavity Ir-192 radiation and laser treatment for palliation of obstructive rectal cancer. *Eur J Surg Oncol.* 1997;23:428–431.

10
The Role of the Oncologist in the Treatment of Colorectal Cancer

SHIBANI NICUM, RACHEL MIDGLEY, and DAVID J. KERR

1. Introduction

It is becoming increasingly clear that modern cancer care will be delivered by a multidisciplinary team that includes surgeons, clinical and medical oncologists, radiologists, pathologists, and specialist nurses. Implicit in this is the notion that each of the specialists has some contribution to make to the patient's management. Chemotherapy and radiotherapy have established roles in the treatment of colorectal cancer and can contribute to cure rate, prolongation of survival, reduction of local rates of recurrence, and enhanced quality of life in patients with advanced disease. The pool of patients eligible for either of these treatment modalities is increasing as new trial data become available, for example, it has been estimated that up to as many as 80% of primary rectal-cancer patients would benefit from radiotherapy, 35% of colon-cancer patients from chemotherapy in the adjuvant setting, and 75% of patients who relapse or present with metastatic disease. The purpose of this chapter is to provide the evidence base for chemotherapy and radiotherapy and discuss the potential therapeutic advances that may be offered by functional genomics.

2. Chemotherapy

Meta-analysis of 13 phase III randomised trials, including a total of 1365 patients, compared chemotherapy with best supportive care in patients with advanced colorectal cancer has demonstrated that palliative 5-fluorouracil–based therapy was associated with a 35% reduction in the risk of death (95% CI, 24%–44%). This translates into an absolute improvement in survival of 16% at 6 and 12 months and an improvement in median survival of 3.7 months [1] (Figure 10.1).

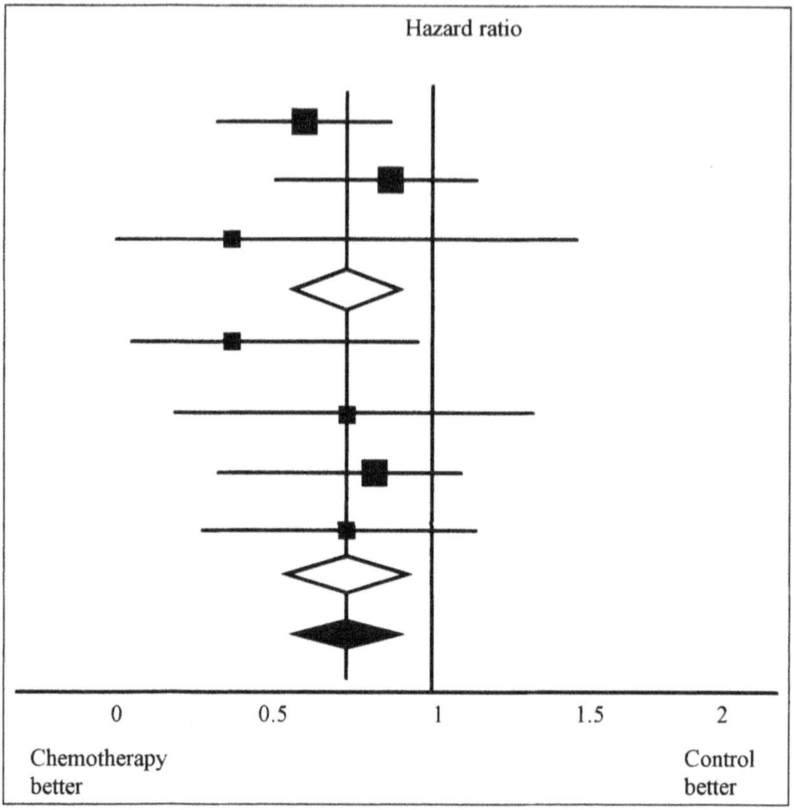

FIGURE 10.1. Pooled analysis of individual patient data for survival. Data grouped by systemic and regional administration of chemotherapy.

2.1. 5-Fluoruracil (5FU)

5-Fluoruracil is a prodrug whose active metabolites, after intracellular conversion, inhibit thymidylate synthase. This agent impairs DNA synthesis and is largely S-phase (replication) specific. However, metabolites of 5FU can also be falsely incorporated into DNA and RNA and interfere with cell protein production and growth. Meta-analysis demonstrated that overall response rates to 5FU alone in advanced disease were about 11% with a median survival of only 11 months [2]. The toxicities of 5FU-based regimens include nausea, vomiting, diarrhoea, mucositis, myelosuppression, and, more rarely, cardiac and neurological effects.

In an attempt to augment the efficacy of 5FU, various drugs have been coadministered, such as methotrexate, levamisole, and, to greatest effect, folinic acid (FA).

2.1.1. Biomodulation of 5FU with Other agents

2.1.1.1. 5FU with Folinic Acid (FA)

The cytotoxic effect of 5FU is due to the inhibition of DNA and RNA synthesis. 5-fluoro-2′-deoxyuridylate (FdUMP) is one of the active metabolites of 5FU, and thymidylate synthase (TS) is the target enzyme of FdUMP. Folinic acid, a precursor of 5,10-methylenetetrahydrofolate, a reduced folate, increases the degree of thymidylate synthase inhibition, preventing DNA synthesis, and thus inducing apoptosis (Figure 10.2). Meta-analysis has indicated that, in advanced colorectal cancer, 5FU/FA combinations led to improved response rates of 23% compared with 11% for 5FU alone. This means that 23% of patients had at least a 50% reduction in the volume of their disease as defined by a product of bidimensional perpendicular mea-

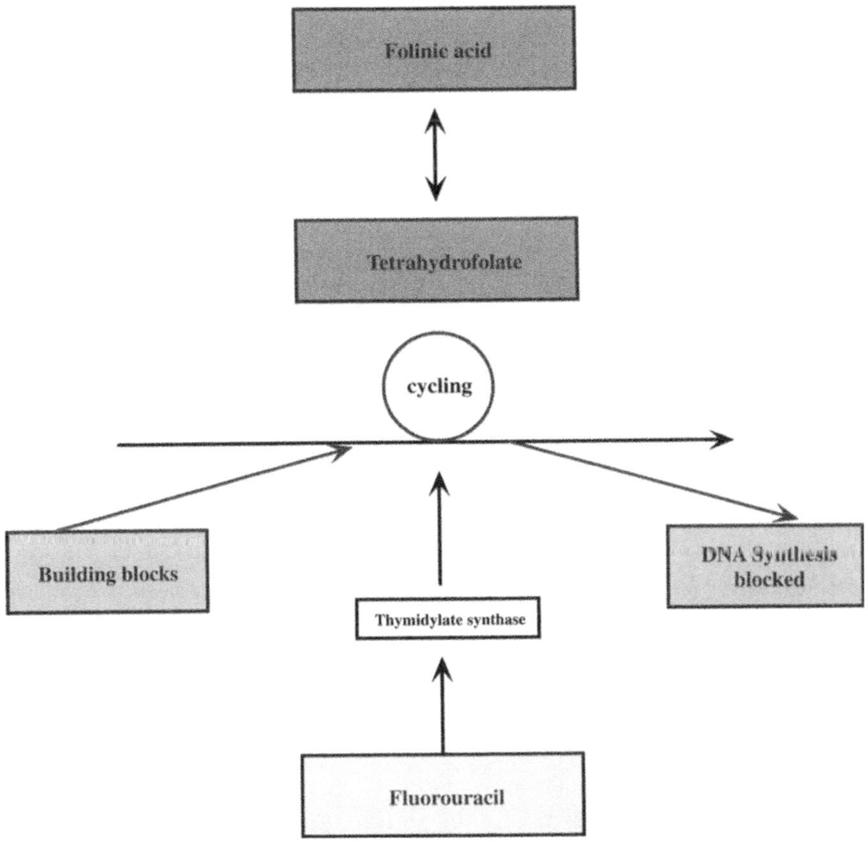

FIGURE 10.2. Intracellular metabolism and mechanism of action of fluorouracil and modulation by folinic acid.

surements on computed tomography (CT) or ultrasound scan. There was also a trend towards better overall survival (not statistically significant) [3].

Although there has been a tradition of use of high-dose folinic acid, results from the QUASAR (Quick and Simple and Reliable) trial suggest that in the adjuvant bolus 5FU setting, low-dose FA ($20\,mg/m^2$) is just as efficacious as high-dose FA ($200\,mg/m^2$) with a concomitant reduction in toxicity [4,5].

2.1.2. Modulation of 5FU by Regimen and Route of Administration

2.1.2.1. Continuous IV Infusion Versus Bolus IV 5FU

As 5FU has a half-life of 8–14 minutes, the rationale for infusional therapy is that a higher proportion of susceptible cells will enter the S phase of the cell cycle during the window of therapeutic plasma concentration with infusion compared to bolus administration. In practice, for tumours such as colorectal carcinomas, with a relatively slow doubling time, extending the period of infusion appears to be beneficial in terms of increased tumour response [6,7]. It has also been demonstrated that bolus administration of 5FU inhibits RNA synthesis, whereas continuous infusional (CI) therapy inhibits thymidylate synthase, the latter being more cytotoxic. Mechanisms of resistance may therefore be dependant on mode of administration [8].

Continuous infusional therapy permits increased total delivery of 5FU with lower peak bone-marrow concentrations. This alters the dose-limiting toxicity from myelosuppression and stomatitis to hand–foot syndrome.

A meta-analysis of 6 randomised trials included data from 1219 patients demonstrated that tumour response rates were significantly higher in patients assigned to 5FU CI than to 5FU bolus (22% vs 14%, $P = .0002$). Overall survival was also significantly higher in patients receiving 5FU CI ($P = .04$), although median survival times were not significantly different, (12.1 vs 11.3 months). All the trials confirmed that desquamation of palms and soles (hand–foot syndrome) was more frequent in the 5FU CI group (34% vs 13%, $P < 10^{-7}$), while grade 3 to 4 haematologic toxicity was more a feature of bolus 5FU (31% vs 4%). Performance status was the most important independent prognostic factor for response, followed by primary tumour site, rectal being more sensitive than colonic primaries [9]. However infusional patients require indwelling central catheters and the benefits may be offset by factors such as increased risks of infection and thrombosis.

2.1.2.2. Oral 5FU Analogues

There is growing interest in oral agents such as UFT (uracil/tegafur) and capecitabine (5FU prodrug) as the enteral route is more acceptable to patients and reduces costs in terms of staffing and admission rates. Four multicentre trials in patients with advanced colorectal cancer compared oral UFT plus FA or capecitabine with intravenous 5FU and demonstrated roughly equal efficacy and similar median survival times. There was less mucositis, neutropenia, and alopecia, but more hand–foot syndrome in the oral treatment group reflecting the prolonged plasma concentrations with oral agent administration that mirror those seen with infusional 5FU regimens [10–13].

2.1.2.3. Regional Administration of 5FU

Approximately 20% of patients who relapse after potentially curative surgery will have disease macroscopically confined to the liver. Resection of these metastases is only sensibly attempted in 10%–15% of these patients and only 25% of those undergoing resection are alive at 5 years. Hepatic arterial chemotherapy maybe a reasonable alternative to resection. Regional chemotherapy depends on the premise that most cytotoxic agents have steep dose-response curves and that high drug concentrations can be generated in target organs such as the liver because of differential drug clearance. Both 5FU and its derivative, fluorodeoxyuridine, have significant rates of hepatic arterial extraction, thus achieving high regional dose intensity with low systemic toxicity.

A meta-analysis of 6 randomised trials of hepatic arterial infusion demonstrated improved response rates of 41% compared with 14% for systemic therapy or supportive care, but the survival advantage was minimal [14]. At present, a large multicentre phase III trial performed in the United Kingdom is undergoing analysis. This randomised patients with advanced colorectal cancer confined to the liver to either hepatic arterial 5FU/FA or the intravenous de Gramont regimen. The doses were adjusted to give comparable systemic levels of 5FU and the trial is powered to detect a doubling in survival.

Technical complications of this particular modality include infection of the hepatic arterial catheter, thrombosis of the hepatic artery, and backflow of cytotoxic agents into the gastroduodenal artery, resulting in duodenitis. Patients are therefore treated prophylactically with warfarin and ranitidine.

2.3. Mechanistically Novel Cytotoxics

Recently, several new drugs such as irinotecan (IR) and oxaliplatin have been introduced that have a mechanistically novel mode of action, distinct from that of 5FU. However, the optimal way of integrating these compounds into therapy still needs to be determined. The situation may be clearer once the results of a trial comparing various combinations of 5FU/FA, irinotecan, and oxaliplatin for the first- and second-line treatment of metastatic colorectal cancer are available (Figure 10.3).

2.3.1. Irinotecan

Irinotecan, a camptothecin analogue, inhibits DNA topoisomerase I and induces single-stranded DNA breaks and replication arrest [15]. In phase

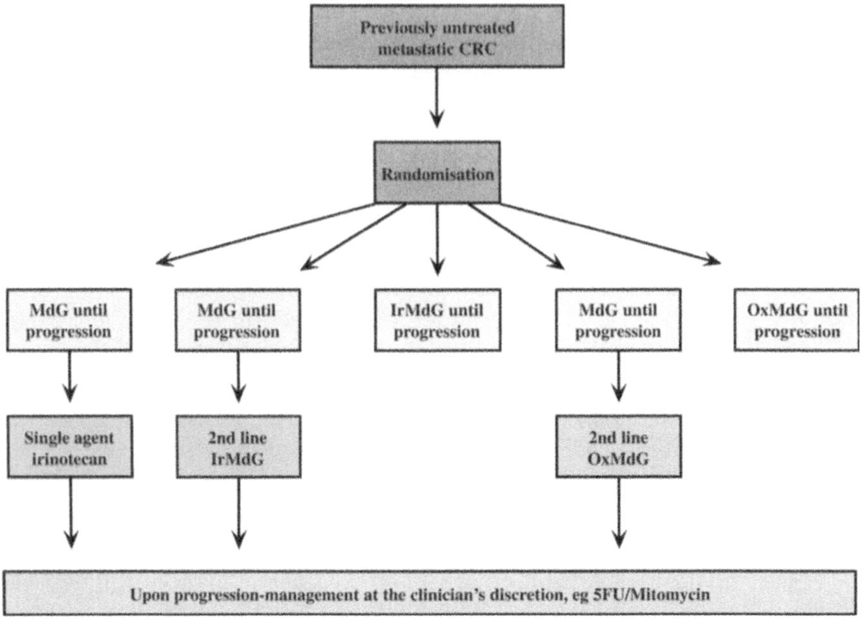

FIGURE 10.3. Schematic representation of the trial design of FOCUS/CR08.

II studies of patients with metastatic colorectal cancer, irinotecan had response rates of 11%–23% [16–19]. A further 40% of patients achieved disease stabilisation for a median period of 5 months [19]. Side effects include an early cholinergic syndrome consisting of bradycardia, diarrhoea, hypotension, and abdominal cramps, which can be prevented by intravenous or subcutaneous atropine; delayed effects including diarrhoea (22%), neutropenia (14%), vomiting (14%), and alopecia can occur about 5 days after treatment.

Two randomised trials have demonstrated the efficacy of irinotecan in patients with advanced colorectal cancer who have progressed despite treatment with bolus 5FU, eliciting improved survival, tumour-related symptoms, and quality of life (QOL). The first trial randomised 133 patients to irinotecan (350 mg/m^2 every 3 weeks) and 134 patients to continuous infusional 5FU. Patients treated with irinotecan lived significantly longer than the 5FU group ($P = .035$) with median survival of 10.8 and 8.5 months, respectively. Survival at 1 year was increased from 32% (5FU) to 42% in the irinotecan group. Median progression-free survival was also significantly longer with irinotecan (4.2 vs 2.9 m, $P = .030$) [20]. The second trial assigned 189 patients to receive irinotecan and 90 patients to supportive care alone. Overall survival was significantly better in the group receiving irinotecan ($P = .0001$), with median survival of 9.2 months in the irinotecan group and 6.5 months in the supportive care group. Survival at 1 year was

36.2% in those receiving irinotecan and 13.8% in the supportive care cohort [21]. These results clearly indicate that in the setting of metastatic colorectal cancer, those patients with reasonable performance status and liver function, who have progressed with standard 5FU/FA should be offered treatment with irinotecan.

Two recent trials have also confirmed the efficacy of irinotecan in the first-line treatment of advanced colorectal cancer, either in combination with 5FU/FA or alone. The first study randomised 387 chemo-naive patients with metastatic colorectal cancer to receive either a combination of irinotecan (IR, 180 mg/m^2) plus infusional 5FU/FA (de Gramont) or infusional 5FU/FA alone [22]. This trial demonstrated a significant advantage for the combination regimen of 5FU/FA and irinotecan, in terms of tumour regression (41% vs 23%), median time to tumour progression (7 m vs 4 m), and median overall survival (17 m vs 14 m, $P = .0031$).

These findings were confirmed by another large multicentre trial that randomly assigned 683 patients with previously untreated metastatic colorectal cancer to receive either irinotecan plus 5FU/FA weekly for 4 weeks every 6 weeks; 5FU/FA for 5 consecutive days every 4 weeks (Mayo regimen); or irinotecan alone weekly for 4 weeks every 6 weeks [23]. Patients treated with the first-line combination of 5FU/FA and irinotecan had a significantly higher probability of overall response compared to the groups receiving 5FU/FA or irinotecan alone (39% vs 21% vs 18%, respectively, $P < .001$), a significantly longer time to tumour progression (7 m vs 4 m vs 4 m, $P = .004$), and a better median survival (15 m vs 13 m vs 12 m, $P = .04$). The most prominent side effects were diarrhoea (22% for the combination of IR/5FU/FA vs 13.2% for 5FU/FA vs 31% for IR alone) and neutropenia (24% for IR/5FU/FA vs 42% for 5FU/FA vs 12% for IR alone), but 75% of the prescribed doses of irinotecan and 5FU could still be administered. Furthermore, the addition of irinotecan to the regimen of 5FU/FA did not compromise quality of life. The study concluded that weekly treatment with irinotecan and 5FU/FA was superior to the widely used Mayo regimen of 5FU/FA as first-line therapy for metastatic colorectal cancer in terms of overall and progression-free survival.

Both studies demonstrated a superiority of the 3-drug combination and worldwide this is now accepted as the new gold standard of care. The exact dosing and scheduling to maximise efficacy and minimise toxicity, for example, by administering drugs sequentially rather than concomitantly, still needs to be determined. The effect of irinotecan on survival is currently being evaluated in the adjuvant setting in patients with Dukes C colorectal cancer. The trial is comparing weekly 5FU/FA with weekly 5FU/FA and irinotecan as adjuvant therapy following curative resection of stage III colorectal cancer and will hopefully clarify whether the increased cost (financially and in terms of toxicity) can be justified in this setting. Finally, QUASAR II will assess the role of irinotecan/capecitabine in combination in the adjuvant treatment of colorectal cancer.

2.3.2. Oxaliplatin

Oxaliplatin is a third-generation platinum analogue that induces DNA cross-linkages and thus apoptotic cell death. It has been shown in vitro to have activity against human cancer cell lines and to act synergistically with 5FU [24]. Phase II studies with single-agent oxaliplatin in patients with advanced colorectal cancer demonstrated response rates of 10% in those with 5FU-resistant disease and 25% in chemotherapy naive patients. However, with intensive 5FU/FA/oxaliplatin combination regimens, response rates could be increased to 46%, even in patients previously treated with 5FU [25]. Two randomised trials have shown that combinations of oxaliplatin/5FU/FA used first line in the treatment of metastatic colorectal cancer increased the probability of tumour regression and slightly prolonged the time to tumour progression without significant effects on survival compared to 5FU/FA [26,27].

In the first study, 420 patients were randomised to receive a 2-weekly regimen of either infusional 5FU/FA alone or infusional 5FU/FA plus 85 mg/m^2 of oxaliplatin on day 1. The median progression-free survival was better in the oxaliplatin arm (39.6 wk vs 27.8 wk, $P < .001$), with response rates of 57% versus 26% respectively when interim analysis was performed on 200 patients [26]. The second study assessed the role of oxaliplatin plus chronomodulated 5FU/FA. In 200 patients receiving chronomodulated bolus 5FU/FA with peaks at 4:00 AM with or without oxaliplatin (125 mg/m^2 on day 1), the median progression-free survival was 7.9 months in the oxaliplatin arm and 4.3 months in the control arm ($P = .5$). There was no significant difference in the median overall survival between the two groups (17.6 m vs 19.4 m, respectively, $P = .82$) [27]. However, an analysis of the use of second-line chemotherapy and metastectomies in the two arms demonstrated that there was a higher incidence of both in the group treated with 5FU/FA alone, and this may account for the lack of significant survival benefit in the oxaliplatin arm. Oxaliplatin is currently being assessed in the adjuvant setting, comparing a weekly regimen of oxaliplatin/5FU/FA with 5FU/FA in patients with resected Dukes B and C colorectal cancer.

The predominant side effect of oxaliplatin is peripheral neuropathy which can take two forms—an acute, sometimes painful, neuropathy exacerbated by cold, also manifesting as laryngeal dysaesthesia and a chronic cumulative stocking-and-glove peripheral neuropathy. The acute neuropathy can be reversed by stopping or reducing the rate of the infusion; however, the cumulative neuropathy may not be fully reversible.

2.4. *Adjuvant Chemotherapy*

Despite improvements in surgical technique and postoperative care, colorectal cancer continues to kill 95,000 people in Europe alone each year. Eighty percent of patients will undergo potentially curative resection, but more than one half will subsequently develop recurrence and die of their disease [28]. This is thought to be due to the presence of micrometastases at the time of surgery and adjuvant therapy aims to eradicate these cells.

It has also been observed that the presence of a primary tumour inhibits the growth of metastases and its removal may therefore stimulate residual cell proliferation. This rise in the growth fraction may increase their susceptibility to the effects of chemotherapy in the immediate postoperative period and early adjuvant chemotherapy may confer greater benefit, although this has not been formally tested in randomised trials [29].

The route and form of adjuvant chemotherapy is based on the natural history of colorectal cancer. The tumour may spread to distant sites sequentially via the portal vein and portal venous infusional treatment maybe of value in the adjuvant setting. However, tumours may disseminate simultaneously via the blood and lymph to various organs and systemically administered cytotoxic therapy may therefore be more appropriate. For locally recurring tumours, such as rectal carcinoma, local agents such as radiotherapy maybe more beneficial (Figure 10.4).

Moertel et al. evaluated adjuvant chemotherapy after surgery in 318 patients with stage B colorectal cancer comparing surgery alone with surgery followed by fluorouracil and levamisole, 929 stage-C patients received surgery alone, surgery plus levamisole, or surgery plus fluorouracil and levamisole. This study demonstrated that only patients with Dukes C colorectal cancer who received surgery/5FU/levamisole had a 33% lower odds of death and 41% reduced recurrence risk than those treated with surgery alone [30]. Three large phase III trials have also shown improved disease-free and overall survival after adjuvant treatment with 5FU and folinic acid regimens. There is a decrease in the odds of dying from colon cancer by 25%–30% and an absolute survival benefit of 5%–6% compared to controls [31–33].

A prospective trial of treatment duration has shown that 4 years after adjuvant chemotherapy there was no significant difference at 6 months or

Site and stage	**Chemotherapy**	**Radiotherapy**
Dukes C Colon cancer	Established indication. 5FU/FA :6 lives saved per 100 treated. New agents currently being trialed.	No benefit.
Dukes B colon cancer	No firmly established indication. Particular patient subgroups may benefit.	No benefit.
Dukes B/C rectal cancer	Indication not firmly established.	Established indication. Pre-operative maybe superior to post-operative (less toxic and more efficacious).

FIGURE 10.4. Benefits of adjuvant therapy.

12 months for 5FU, folinic acid, or levamisole in terms of disease-free survival or overall survival [34]. Preliminary results of the QUASAR trial suggest that low-dose FA (20 mg/m^2) is as efficacious as high-dose FA (200 mg/m^2) and better tolerated [35]. This has significant cost implications for adjuvant chemotherapy. This study has also demonstrated that that the addition of levamisole does not delay recurrence or improve survival.

The majority of the trials to date have demonstrated a significant benefit for adjuvant chemotherapy in Dukes C colon cancer. However, for Dukes B colon cancer the indication remains uncertain and such patients should continue to be randomised into trials such as QUASAR 1 (Figure 10.5). Results of such trials are awaited to clarify the situation for patients with Dukes B colon cancer and Dukes B/C rectal cancer.

The gold-standard route of administration of chemotherapy in the adjuvant setting is intravenous. However, micrometastases (less than 3 mm) in the liver are thought to derive their blood supply from the portal vein, as opposed to macroscopic liver metastases that are dependant on the hepatic artery. Administration of chemotherapy directly into the portal vein should locally produce greater concentrations with fewer systemic side effects because of substantial first-pass metabolism. Meta-analysis from ten trials, including data from 4000 patients and 1557 deaths of portal vein infusion (PVI) 5–7 days after surgery compared with surgery alone, demonstrated a 4.7% survival benefit at 5 years (P = .006) [36]. However, the confidence intervals were wide and there was no definite evidence of a decrease in the number of patients who developed liver metastases. Furthermore, preliminary results from the largest study to date of PVI, the AXIS trial, which randomised 4000 patients after surgery to either PVI or observation alone suggest no significant differences in overall survival to date.

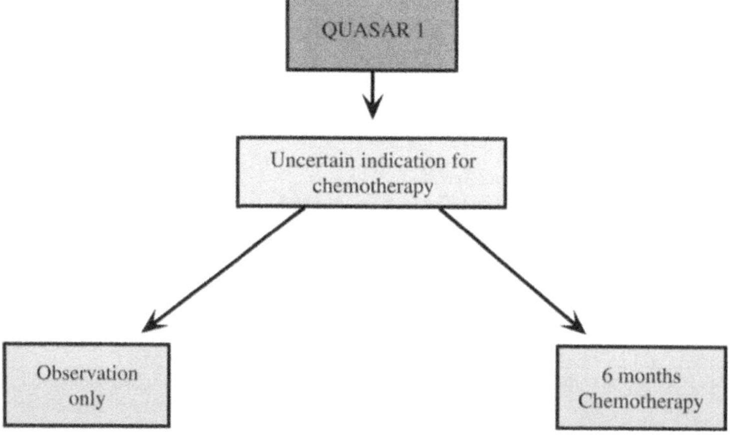

FIGURE 10.5. Schematic representation of the QUASAR 1 study.

3. Rectal Carcinoma and the Role of Radiotherapy

Data from Europe indicates that the 5-year survival rate for rectal cancer improved from 40% to 48% during the period from 1977–1989. This was mainly due to increased curative resections, fewer advanced cases, and decreased postoperative mortality. Despite potentially curative surgery, the 5-year survival rates are approximately 60%, varying from about 80% in patients with stage I disease to 30% in those with stage III disease, thus indicating that resection alone is adequate treatment only for patients with early disease [37]. Recurrence will occur locally within the pelvis in 50% of cases and radiotherapy has therefore formed the mainstay of treatment. Radiotherapy is also important in the symptomatic treatment of advanced rectal cancer, and can improve pain, haemorrhage, and tenesmus. In addition, one large study has demonstrated that radiotherapy can convert 35%–75% of locally advanced inoperable tumours to resectability [38].

Four randomised trials have assessed the role of adjuvant radiotherapy preoperatively. The largest trial administered 25 Gy in 5 fractions and demonstrated a significant improvement in overall survival (58% vs 48%) by a relative reduction in local recurrence rate of 61% [39]. The other 3 trials have also revealed significant decreases in the local recurrence rates of between 50%–63% [40–42]. The main disadvantage of preoperative radiotherapy compared to postoperative treatment is that there is possibly a group of patients, usually those patients with stage T1/2, N0, M0 disease who do not require any adjuvant treatment and who are therefore being overtreated. However, advantages of preoperative treatment include decreased tumour seeding at the time of surgery, increased radiosensitivity compared to postoperative fibrous wound areas, and improved rates of sphincter-sparing surgery. Currently, preoperative radiotherapy is recommended for patients with T3 or resectable T4 rectal cancer.

Postoperative radiotherapy even at higher doses has been shown to be less effective than preoperative treatment, possibly due to rapid tumour-cell repopulation after surgery and wound hypoxia reducing radiosensitivity. However, 3 trials have demonstrated that 40–50 Gy postoperatively significantly reduced rates of local failure compared to surgery alone [43–45]. The dose of radiation is important as dose response in radiation therapy follows a sigmoidal distribution and therefore a small decrease in dose can result in a large difference in local control. Of the 3 randomised trials, the National Surgical Adjuvant Bowel and Breast Project (NSABP) is the only trial to confirm that postoperative radiation therapy decreases local failure and it is the only trial which administered continuous course, full-dose therapy with modern techniques. A MRC study has also shown lower recurrence rates for radiotherapy after surgery than for surgery only (hazard ratio 0.54 [95% CI, 0.38–0.66], $P = .001$) [46].

There has only been one randomised trial comparing preoperative versus postoperative radiotherapy in patients with rectal cancer. The dose of radiation postoperatively was significantly higher, 60Gy compared to 25Gy presurgery, and despite this the study demonstrated a significantly lower rate of recurrence in patients treated preoperatively (12% vs 21%, $P < .02$) [47]. However, the results of this trial must be interpreted with caution as the local failure rates with surgery alone were higher than accepted rates in the United Kingdom and the United States.

In an attempt to reduce the frequency of inappropriate radiotherapy administration to patients with early stage disease, the CRO7 trial is randomising rectal cancer patients to either preoperative radiotherapy (25Gy) or selective postoperative radiotherapy (45Gy) if the circumferential resection margins are involved on histological inspection. Postoperative patients will receive chemoradiotherapy (Figure 10.6).

Animal studies have suggested that 5FU has the capacity to prime rectal-cancer cells and sensitise them to subsequent radiation. Indeed, one study has demonstrated a significant benefit for patients treated with a combination of 5FU chemotherapy and radiation compared with the cohort treated with radiotherapy alone [48]. However, only results of CRO7 and other trials will demonstrate whether or not a combination of chemotherapy and radiotherapy is both effective and safe in this setting and this combination can not be condoned as standard therapy at present.

4. New Approaches to the Treatment of Colorectal Cancer

4.1. Immunotherapy

Several immunotherapeutic techniques have been suggested for use in colorectal cancer. These include antibody-mediated therapies and immune-cellular–mediated therapies such as peptide vaccination with mutated ras peptides and dendritic-cell vaccination.

Over the past 10 years several clinical trials have assessed monoclonal antibodies as therapeutic agents for advanced solid tumours, and demonstrated no significant benefits. Explanations for the failures have included antigenic heterogeneity and poor accessibility of cells in advanced tumours. However, there seems to be more promise in the adjuvant setting. In a randomised trial, 189 patients with Dukes C colorectal cancer were assigned to receive either a monoclonal antibody, 17-1A, that binds a tumour-specific cell surface glycoprotein (17-1A) or observation only. Survival was significantly lengthened in the antibody treated group, with 5-year survival rates of 51% vs 36% ($P = .025$). Side effects included mild constitutional and gastrointestinal symptoms [49]. This antibody is currently being tested as a single agent in patients with Dukes B colorectal cancer and also in combination with 5FU/FA in Dukes C colorectal cancer following curative resection.

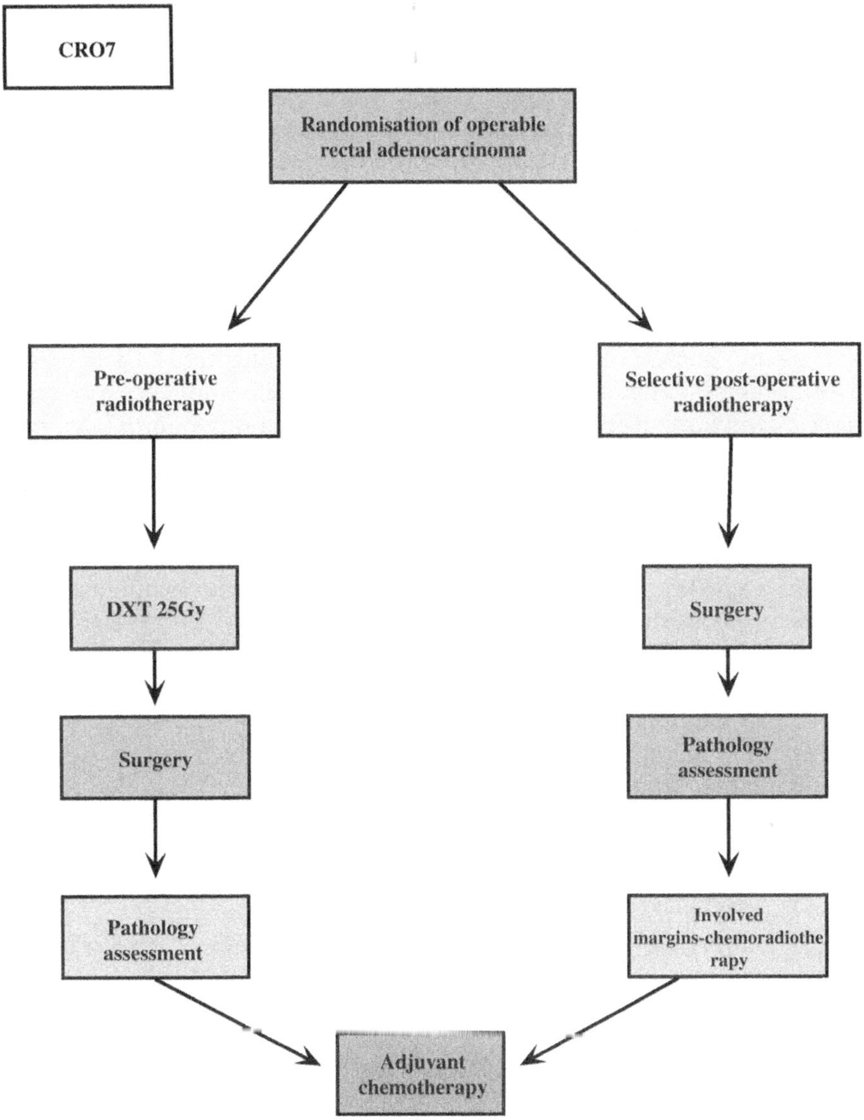

FIGURE 10.6. Schematic representation of the CRO7 trial.

4.1.2. Recombinant Virus Vaccines

CEA is a 180 kd cell-surface glycoprotein that appears to be involved in cellular adhesion, cell-to-cell interactions, and possibly glandular differentiation. It is a member of a family of glycoproteins that are expressed in the tumour cells of 85% of patients with colorectal cancer. A direct immunologic approach to carcinoembryonic-antigen (CEA)–bearing tumours has been developed using inoculation with a recombinant vaccinia virus which expresses the human CEA gene. Vaccinia virus is a member of the DNA containing Poxviridae family of viruses. These viruses replicate within the host cell's cytoplasm and can elicit both humoral and cell-mediated immune responses, therefore copresentation of human protein products with vaccinia may enhance immunogenicity to the protein and thus start or augment tumour rejection [50].

In a phase I study, 26 patients with advanced gastrointestinal, breast, and lung adenocarcinoma were administered with escalating doses of recombinant vaccinia–CEA vaccine. There was no serious toxicity and although a therapeutic immune response was not demonstrated, these patients generated cytotoxic T lymphocytes specific for CEA which would be expected to have a significant role in rejection of tumour cells positive for CEA [50].

4.2. Gene Therapy

Gene therapy encompasses various techniques in which viral and nonviral vectors are used to deliver to tumour cells, genes that encode cytokines, tumour-suppressor proteins, and proteins that sensitise cells to chemotherapy (such as p53). Following successful completion of phase I trials of adenovirus delivered p53 tumour-suppressor genes via the hepatic artery, phase II studies combining the virus with 5FU are now in progress [51].

Phase I trials of virus-directed enzyme prodrug therapy (VDEPT) are currently in progress. This novel technique involves insertion of genes into cells that transcribe enzymes capable of metabolising prodrugs into potent cytotoxic species. Adenoviral vectors that link the carcinoembryonic antigen (CEA) promoter to the structural gene for the bacterial enzyme cytosine deaminase have been developed [52]. Cytosine deaminase metabolises the prodrug 5-fluorocytosine to 5FU. Transduction of the gene hybrid should theoretically only occur in cells expressing CEA thus conferring tumour selectivity on the cytotoxic agent. This permits a 1000-fold higher concentration of 5FU in the tumour and the neighbouring cells (the bystander effect) than in the systemic circulation. This technique is currently being assessed in patients with advanced colorectal cancer, and if found to be efficacious it will be tried in the adjuvant setting.

Acknowledgments. The support of Cancer Research UK and the Medical Research Council is gratefully acknowledged.

References

1. Colorectal Cancer Collaborative Group. Palliative chemotherapy for advanced colorectal cancer: systemic review and meta-analysis. *BMJ.* 2000;321:531–535.

2. The Advanced Colorectal Cancer Meta-analysis Project. Meta-analysis of randomised trials testing the biochemical modulation of 5-fluorouracil by methotrexate in metastatic colorectal cancer. *J Clin Oncol.* 1994;12:960–969.
3. The Advanced Colorectal Cancer Meta-analysis Project. Modulation of 5FU by leucovorin in patients with advanced colorectal cancer; evidence in terms of response rate. *J Clin Oncol.* 1992;10:896–903.
4. Petrelli N, Douglas HO, Herrera L, et al. The modulation of 5FU with leucovorin in metastatic colorectal carcinoma: a prospective randomised phase III trial. *J Clin Oncol.* 1989;7:1419–1426.
5. Poon MA, O'Connell MJ, Wieand S, et al. Biochemical modulation of 5FU with leucovorin: confirmatory evidence of improved therapeutic efficacy in advanced colorectal cancer. *J Clin Oncol.* 1991;9:1967–1972.
6. Myers CE, Diaslo R, Eliot HM, et al. Pharmocokinetics of the fluoropyrimides: implications for their clinical use. *Cancer Treat Rev.* 1975;3:175–183.
7. Fraile RJ, Baker LH, Baroker TR, et al. Pharmocokinetics of 5FU administered orally, by rapid intravenous and by slow infusion. *Cancer Res.* 1980;40: 2223–2228.
8. Aschele C, Sobiero A, Faderan MA, et al. Novel mechanisms of resistance to 5FU in human colon cancer (HCT 8) sublines following exposure to two different clinically relevant dose schedules. *Cancer Res.* 1992;52:1855–1864.
9. Meta-analysis Group in Cancer. Efficacy of intravenous continuous infusion of 5FU compared with bolus administration in advanced colorectal cancer. *J Clin Oncol.* 1998;16:301–308.
10. Pazdur R, Douillard JY, Skillings JR, et al. Multicentre phase III study of 5FU or UFT in combination with leucovorin in patients with metastatic colorectal cancer [abstract]. *Proc Am Soc Clin Oncol.* 1999;18:1009.
11. Twelves C, Harper P, Van Cutsem E. A phase III trial (S014796) of Xeloda (capecitabine) in previously untreated advanced/metastatic colorectal cancer [abstract]. *Proc Am Soc Clin Oncol.* 1999;18:1010.
12. Carmichael J, Popiela T, Radstone D, et al. Randomised comparative study of ORZEL (oral uracil/tegafur) plus leucovorin (IV) versus parenteral 5FU plus leucovorin in patients with metastatic colorectal cancer [abstract]. *Proc Am Soc Clin Oncol.* 1999;18:1015.
13. Cox JV, Pazdur R, Thibault A, et al. A phase II trial of Xeloda TM (capecitabine) in previously untreated advanced/metastatic colorectal cancer [abstract]. *Proc Am Soc Clin Oncol.* 1999;18:1016.
14. Meta-analysis Group in Cancer. Re-appraisal of hepatic arterial infusion in the treatment of non-resectable liver metastases from colorectal cancer. *J Natl Cancer Inst.* 1996;88:252–258.
15. Bleiberg H. CPT-11 in gastro-intestinal cancer. *Eur J Cancer.* 1999;35:371–379.
16. Pitot HC, Wender DB, O'Connell MJ, et al. Phase II trial of irinotecan in patients with metastatic colorectal cancer. *J Clin Oncol.* 1997;15:2910–2919.
17. Rougier P, Bugat R, Douillard JY, et al. Phase II study of irinotecan in the treatment of advanced colorectal cancer in chemotherapy naïve patients and patients pre-treated with 5FU-based chemptherapy. *J Clin Oncol.* 1997;15: 251–260.

18. Rothenberg ML, Eckard JR, Kuhn JG, et al. Phase II trial of irinotecan in patients with progressive or rapidly recurrent colorectal cancer. *J Clin Oncol.* 1996;14:1128–1135.
19. Van Cutsem E, Rougier P, Droz JP, et al. Clinical benefit of irinotecan (CPT-11) in metastatic colorectal cancer resistant to 5FU [abstract]. *Proc ASCO.* 1997; 16:268a.
20. Rougier P, Van Cutsem E, Bajetta E. Randomised trial of irinotecan versus 5FU by continuous infusion after 5FU failure in patients with metastatic colorectal cancer. *Lancet* 1998;352:1407–1412.
21. Cunningham D, Pyrhonen S, James RD, et al. Randomised trial of irinotecan plus supportive care versus supportive care alone after 5FU failure for patients with metastatic colorectal cancer. *Lancet* 1998;352:1413–1418.
22. Douillard JY, Cunningham D, Roth AD, et al. Irinotecan combined with 5FU compared with 5FU alone as first line treatment for metastatic colorectal cancer: a multicentre randomised trial. *Lancet* 2000;355:1041–1047.
23. Saltz LB, Cox JV, Blanke C, et al. Irinotecan plus 5FU plus leucovorin for metastatic colorectal cancer. *N Engl J Med.* 2000;343:905–914.
24. Raymond E, Chaney SG, Taamma A, et al. Oxaliplatin, a review of preclinical and clinical studies. *Ann Oncol.* 1998;9:1053–1071.
25. DeGramont A, Vignoud J, Tournigant C, et al. Oxaliplatin with high dose leucovorin and 5FU 48 hour continuous infusion in pre-treated metastatic colorectal cancer. *Eur J Cancer.* 1997;32:214–219.
26. DeGramont A, Figer A, Seymour M, et al. Leucovorin plus 5FU with or without oxaliplatin as first line treatment in advanced colorectal cancer. *J Clin Oncol.* 2000;18:2938–2947.
27. Giacchetti S, Perpoint B, Zidani R, et al. Phase III multi-centre randomised trial of oxaliplatin added to chronomodulated 5FU-leucovorin as first line treatment of metastatic colorectal cancer. *J Clin Oncol.* 2000;18:136–147.
28. Abulfi AM, Williams NS. Local recurrence of colorectal cancer: the problems, the mechanisms, management and adjuvant treatment. *Br J Surg.* 1994;81:7–17.
29. De Wys WD. Studies correlating the growth rate of a tumour and its metastases and providing evidence for tumour related systemic growth retarding factors. *Cancer Res.* 1972;32:374–379.
30. Moertal CG, Fleming TR, MacDonald JS, et al. Levamisole and fluorouracil for the adjuvant treatment of resected colon cancer. *N Engl J Med.* 1990;322: 352–358.
31. IMPACT trial. Efficacy of adjuvant fluorouracil and folinic acid in colon cancer. *Lancet* 1995;345:939–944.
32. O'Connell M, Maillard J, Kahn MJ, et al. Controlled trial of fluorouracil and low dose leucovorin given for six months as post-operative adjuvant therapy for colon cancer. *J Clin Oncol.* 1997;15:246–250.
33. Wolmark N, Rockette H, Fisher, B et al. The benefit of leucovorin modulated 5 fluorouracil as post-operative adjuvant treatment for primary colon cancer:results from the National Surgery and Adjuvant Breast and Bowel Project Protocol C-03. *J Clin Oncol.* 1993;11:1879–1888.
34. O'Connell MJ, Lauie JA, Shepherd L, et al. A prospective evaluation of chemotherapy duration and regimen as surgical adjuvant treatment for high risk colon cancer: a collaborative trial of North Central Cancer Treatment group and

the National Cancer Institute of Canada Clinical trials Group [abstract]. *Proc Am Soc Clin Oncol.* 1996;15:209.
35. QUASAR Collaborative Group. Comparison of fluorouracil with additional levamisole, higher dose folinic acid, or both, as adjuvant chemotherapy for colorectal cancer: a randomised trial. *Lancet* 2000;355:1588–1596.
36. Liver Infusion Meta-analysis Group. Portal vein chemotherapy for colorectal cancer, a meta-analysis of 4000 patients in 10 studies. *J Natl Cancer Inst.* 1997;89:497–505.
37. Bosset JF, Mantion G, Lorchel F, et al. Adjuvant and neoadjuvant radiation therapy for rectal cancer. *Semin Oncol.* 2000;27:60–65.
38. Pahlman L. Pre-operative treatment of rectal cancer. In: *Management of Colorectal Cancer.* Bleiberg H, Rougier P, Wilke HJ, eds. London: Martin Dunitz, 1998:153–166.
39. Swedish Rectal Cancer Trial. Local recurrence rate in a randomised multicentre trial of pre-operative radiotherapy compared to surgery alone in resectable rectal cancer. *Eur J Surg.* 1996;162:397–402.
40. James RD, Haboubi N, Schofield PF, et al. Prognostic factors in colorectal cancer treated by pro-operative radiotherapy and immediate surgery. *Dis Colon Rectum.* 1991;34:546–551.
41. Gerard A, Buyse M, Nordlinger B, et al. Pre-operative radiotherapy as adjuvant treatment in rectal cancer. Final results of a randomised study of the EORTC Gastrointestinal Tract Cancer Co-operative Group. *Ann Surg.* 1988;208:606–614.
42. Stockholm Rectal Cancer Study Group. Preoperative short term radiation therapy in operable rectal carcinoma. *Cancer* 1990;66:49–53.
43. Balsler I, Pederson M, Teglbjaerg PS, et al. Postoperative radiotherapy in Dukes B and C carcinoma of the rectum and rectosigmoid: a randomised multicentre study. *Cancer* 1986;58:22–28.
44. Gastrointestinal Tumour Study Group. Prolongation of the disease-free interval in surgically treated rectal carcinoma. *N Engl J Med.* 1985;312:1464–1472.
45. Fisher B, Wolmark N, Rockette H, et al. Post-operative adjuvant chemotherapy or radiation therapy for rectal cancer: results from NSABP Protocol R-01. *J Natl Cancer Inst.* 1988;80:21–29.
46. MRC Rectal Cancer Working Party. Randomised trial of surgery alone versus surgery followed by radiotherapy for mobile cancer of the rectum. *Lancet* 1996;348:1610–1614.
47. Jansson-Frykholm G, Glimelius B, Pahlman L. Pre-operative or post-operative radiotherapy in adenocarcinoma of the rectum: final treatment results of a randomised trial and an evaluation of late secondary effects. *Dis Colon Rectum.* 1993;36:564–572.
48. O'Connell MJ, Martenson JA, Wieand HS, et al. Improving adjuvant therapy for rectal cancer by combining protracted infusion 5FU with radiation therapy after curative surgery. *N Engl J Med.* 1994;331:502–507.
49. Reithmuller G, Schneider-Gadicke E, Schmilok G. Randomised trial of monoclonal antibody for adjuvant treatment of resected Dukes C colorectal. *Lancet* 1994;343:1177–1183.
50. Kerr DJ, Midgley RS. Immunotherapy for colorectal cancer: potential application in an adjuvant setting. *Semin Oncol.* 2000;27(suppl 10):132–137.

51. Venook AP, Bergsland EK, Ring E, et al. Gene therapy of colorectal liver metastases using a recombinant adenovirus encoding WT p53 (sat 58500) via hepatic artery infusion: a phase I study. *Proc ASCO.* 1998;17:431a.
52. Huber BE, Austin EA, Good SS, et al. In vivo anti-tumour activity of 5FU on human colorectal cancer cells genetically modified to express cytosine deaminase. *Cancer Res.* 1993;53:4619–4626.

11 Investigation of Functional Bowel Disorders

PONNANDAI J. ARUMUGAM, JOHN BEYNON, and BHARAT PATEL

1. Introduction

Functional bowel disorders present a management challenge to coloproctologists, therefore, careful history taking, recording of symptomatology, and clinical assessment are essential in the evaluation of these patients (Table 11.1).

Patients may present with symptoms of rectal bleeding and tenesmus and it is vitally important that colorectal malignancy is excluded before attributing the patient's symptoms to functional disorders. This will entail an endoscopic or a contrast study of the colorectum before proceeding to comprehensive assessment of the clinical problem.

As patients with functional bowel disorders present with a variety of symptoms, it is important to be as objective as possible in documenting the symptoms that may be complemented by the use of specifically modified and validated quality-of-life questionnaires, in addition to those used to assess specific problems such as continence (e.g., Cleveland continence score). This role can be performed by a specialist colorectal nurse who is able to document the presenting complaints and has contact with patients following surgery or biofeedback.

Assessment is completed by a thorough clinical examination of the abdomen and anorectum. Anal tone and squeeze should be evaluated and gluteal recruitment, if present, is recorded as is the presence of rectocoele, external prolapse, and solitary rectal ulcer.

Pelvic-floor dysfunction is assessed routinely by evacuatory proctography, anal manometry, and endo–anal ultrasound (EAUS) [1,2]. Other complementary investigations such as magnetic resonance imaging (MRI) of the pelvic floor, electromyography (EMG), pudendal nerve terminal motor latency (PNTML), and colonic transit studies are useful. Although careful and thorough clinical examination can detect the majority of defects, the above investigations play an important role in determining the appropriate management for symptomatic patients.

Table 11.1. History and record of symptomatology.

Inquire about
• Presence of rectal bleeding, mucous discharge, or perineal pressure
• Type of incontinence: solid, liquid, or flatus
• Impact of symptoms: need for a pad, restriction of daily or sexual function
• Awareness of need to defaecate
• Presence/absence of obstructed defaecation/incomplete evacuation
• Need for digitation vaginally or rectally to evacuate
• Previous anal surgery: haemorrhoidectomy, sphincterotomy, or fistula surgery
• Anoreceptive Intercourse
• Urinary and sexual history

2. Evacuatory Proctography

Evacuatory proctography was first described by Burhenne in 1964 but was not widely used clinically for nearly 20 years [3]. This is a dynamic assessment of defaecation and can provide information on function of the pelvic-floor muscles and the rectum. A wide overlap exists in normal findings in asymptomatic subjects and different groups of symptomatic patients [4]. Further, it is difficult to differentiate controls from symptomatic patients based on proctographic findings alone [5,6]. Abnormalities demonstrated on the proctogram correlate poorly with symptomatology and manometric assessment, and the majority of radiologists rely on time taken to evacuate and completeness of evacuation [6,7]. Evacuatory proctography does, however, provide an understanding of pelvic-floor pathophysiology but this must be interpreted cautiously. A decision to proceed with surgery rather than conservative management must not be based on radiographic diagnosis alone but must include consideration of patient symptoms, clinical findings, and the results of other appropriate complementary investigations.

Karasick et al., in their study on the role of parity and hysterectomy, believed evacuatory proctography to be a useful tool in assessing pelvic-floor disorders, while Klauser et al. showed a good interobserver agreement in assessing rectocoele on proctography [8,9]. Mahieu et al. described variations in the technique while Bernier et al. and Ginai et al. contributed towards designing the commode used in this investigation [10–12].

Indications for evacuatory proctography for the assessment of functional disorders include (a) obstructed defaecation/incomplete evacuation, (b) constipation, (c) solitary rectal ulcer, (d) rectal prolapse or intussusception, and (e) anal incontinence.

The barium paste used is readily available commercially but can also be prepared from barium powder and potato/corn starch. This paste is usually delivered into the rectum by a commercially available gun. Most centers now use liquid barium to coat the lining of the rectum prior to injection of the thick viscous barium paste, which simulates stools. This examination does not provide the ideal natural environment to assess an individual's defaecation, but it is probably the closest method of simulating the real process. The vagina can be outlined using a water-soluble, contrast-soaked tampon, while some centers also use oral contrast medium to opacify the small bowel to aid in the diagnosis of enterocoele.

Radiation exposure can be of concern, especially in women of child-bearing age. The somatic dose index is in the order of 210 mrad for men and 100 mrad for women [4]. Videoproctography results in increased exposure time, however, newer subtraction and digital fluoroscopy techniques have been introduced to reduce the dose [13].

A radiolucent commode that can be safely attached to a fluoroscopic table is available commercially or can be designed by individual hospitals (Figure 11.1). Disposable plastic bags or trays are used to collect the evacuated barium paste.

Various techniques are available to record the defaecatory activity, with video proctography and digital fluoroscopy being increasingly used [14–17].

Balloon proctography has been used with a deflated balloon being introduced into the rectum and filled with barium. Lateral films are taken of the anorectum at rest and on straining [16]. A commercially available balloon can be used and can measure anal-sphincter pressures. Balloon proctography cannot, however, accurately demonstrate intussusception and there are discrepancies in the measurement of anorectal angle.

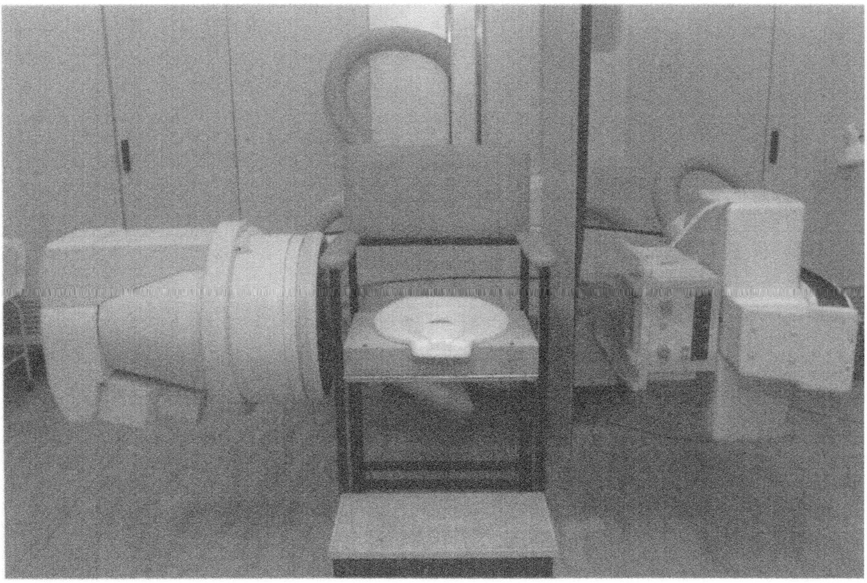

FIGURE 11.1. Radiolucent commode used for proctographic assessment can be safely attached to a fluoroscopic table and is available commercially or can be designed by individual hospitals.

In order to quantify rectal evacuation, patients are asked to evacuate 100 mL of barium paste into a disposable plastic bag lying on a weight transducer. The embarrassing nature of this form of assessment necessitates that studies should be performed in a quiet private environment with minimum personnel to reassure the patient. Several aspects of defaecation, such as maximum emptying and the proportion of barium evacuated, can be measured and can be used to monitor treatment [18].

No bowel preparation is required for the investigation. Liquid barium (30 mL) is introduced initially to coat the rectum; it is followed by the viscous barium paste introduced using a disposable enema tip and a caulking gun. Up to 250 mL barium paste is injected, until the patient has a sensation of rectal fullness. Continuous injection of the paste on the withdrawal of the enema tip will outline the anal canal to the anal verge, allowing assessment of the anal-canal length.

Lateral spot films and video recording are then obtained with the patient sitting upright on the commode at rest (Figure 11.2), squeezing (Figure 11.3), and straining without evacuation (Figure 11.4). Patients are also asked to cough to demonstrate potential incontinence. The patient is then instructed to evacuate with several spot films being obtained with a completion film on full straining (Figure 11.5, Figure 11.6).

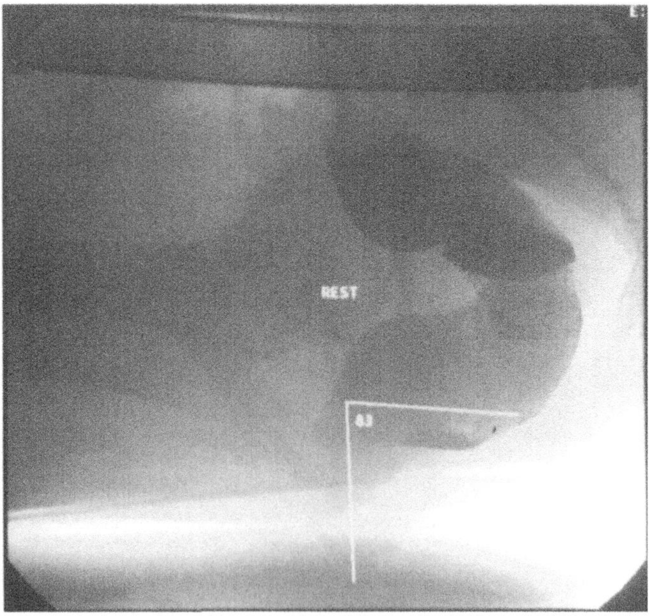

FIGURE 11.2. Lateral spot films with the patient sitting upright on the commode at rest.

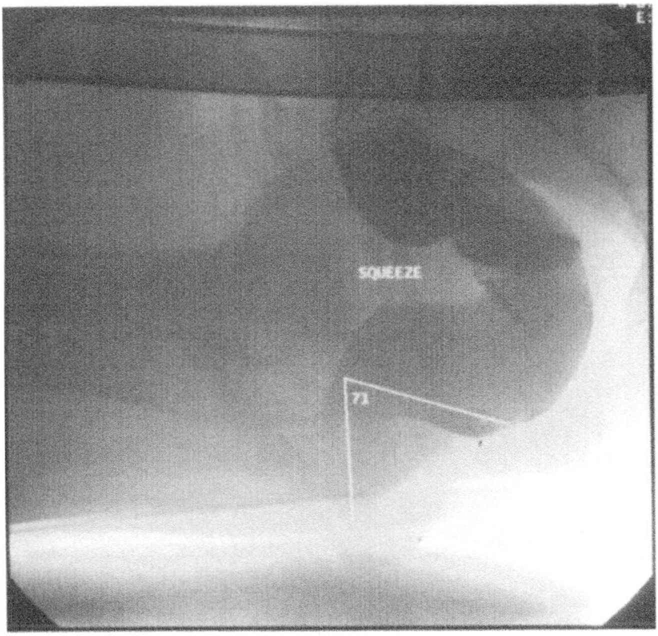

FIGURE 11.3. Squeeze assessment during proctography.

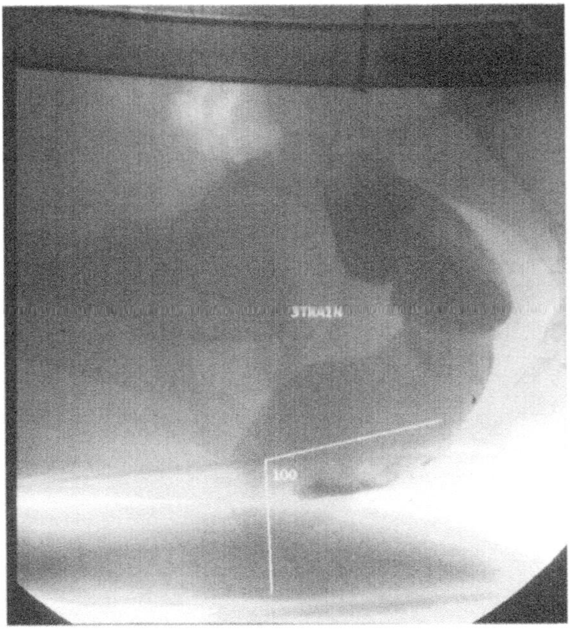

FIGURE 11.4. Straining without evacuation. Patients are also asked to cough to demonstrate potential incontinence.

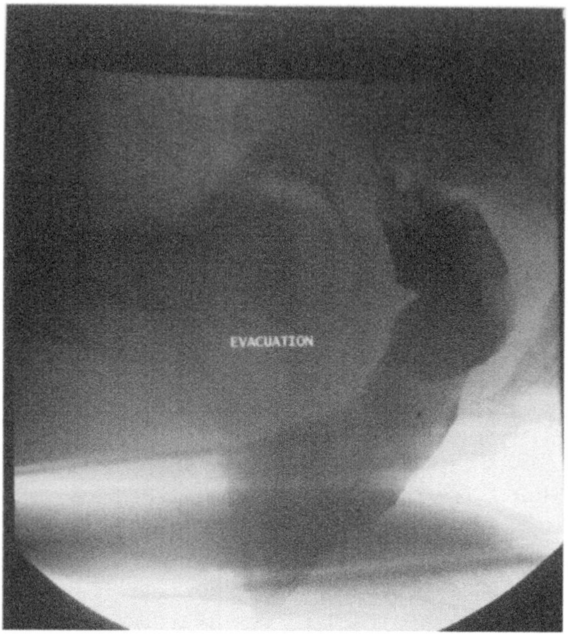

FIGURE 11.5. The patient evacuating with a completion film on full straining.

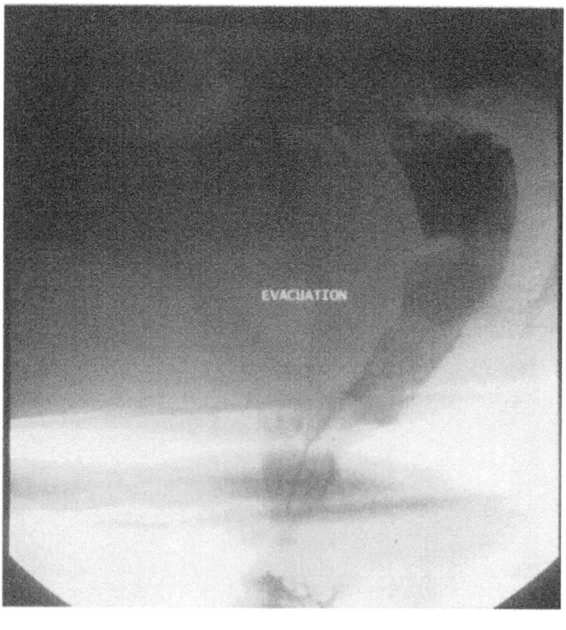

FIGURE 11.6. The patient evacuating with a completion film on full straining.

2.1. *Normal Appearances*

Bartram et al., Goei et al., and Shorvon et al. have contributed extensively in the understanding of the defaecatory process in normal individuals and have shown that pelvic-floor function deteriorates with age [4,15,19]. The majority of the patients studied were asymptomatic volunteers and despite this a variety of abnormalities were demonstrated. It is possible that these findings may be associated with pelvic-floor dysfunction, which may lead to symptoms in later life. The radiological findings must therefore be interpreted with caution and in association with the patient's symptomatology and clinical findings.

2.1.1. Anal Canal

The anal canal is usually closed at rest; however, it can be open in normal volunteers and this may be associated with cough incontinence [4]. The length of the canal is measured by the distance between the anal orifice and the point where the anal canal meets the cone-shaped walls of the distal rectum. The mean length in men is 2.2 cm and in women it is 1.6 cm [4]. The accuracy of this assessment must be questioned as there is a discrepancy between anal-canal length measured by anal manometry and evacuatory proctography, the former averaging around 4 cm [20].

The anorectal junction is usually related to the pubococcygeal line but in evacuatory proctography the inferior margin of the ischial tuberosity is used. Shorvon et al. [4] has shown a variation of the position of anorectal junction above the ischial tuberosity in men and women, and in elderly people.

2.1.2. Anorectal Angle

The anorectal angle is measured between the axis of the anal canal and a line drawn along the rectal floor, and is referred to as the posterior anorectal angle. A central anorectal angle has also been described; this is the angle between a line drawn through the center of the rectum and the axis of the anal canal. This angle is approximately 20° greater than the posterior anorectal angle [15].

The posterior anorectal angle varies from 65°–125° in men and 70°–135° in women, with some interobserver variation being observed [9].

Contraction of the pelvic-floor muscles due to squeezing will make the angle more acute, the mean decrease being approximately 20°. Elevation of the anorectal junction is seen almost in all normal subjects and is brought about by both pelvic-floor contraction and lengthening of the anal canal. Absence of elevation and failure of anorectal angle to become more acute indicates the likelihood of a pelvic-floor abnormality.

On straining without defaecating, the muscles should relax, increasing the anorectal angle and causing descent of the anorectal junction. However, it has been demonstrated that this may cause a paradoxical decrease in the anorectal angle in 30% of patients due to inappropriate contraction of puborectalis.

2.1.3. Pelvic-floor Descent

Pelvic-floor descent is defined as the distance the anorectal junction descends from its resting position. The normal range of pelvic floor descent is 2–3 cm while it can occasionally elevate from 1–2 cm [15,19]. Considerable variation in descent was observed in one series from 1.8 cm to 5.4 cm in men and from 0.7 cm to 5.9 cm in women [4].

2.1.4. Changes in the Rectal Wall

Rectocoeles are quite common in normal asymptomatic women and may also be seen in men [4,15]. They appear as a bulge of the rectal wall beyond the extrapolated line of the normal wall. When small (<2 cm) and when they do not retain barium, they should be considered a normal variant [4]. A depth of 2–4 cm is considered a moderate rectocoele (Figure 11.7) and greater than 5 cm, a large rectocoele. A 2-cm or more widening of the rectovaginal space signifies the presence of an enterocoele. Opacification of the small bowel will demonstrate an enterocoele in such cases. Herniation of the rectum, small bowel, or omentum into the space posterior to the

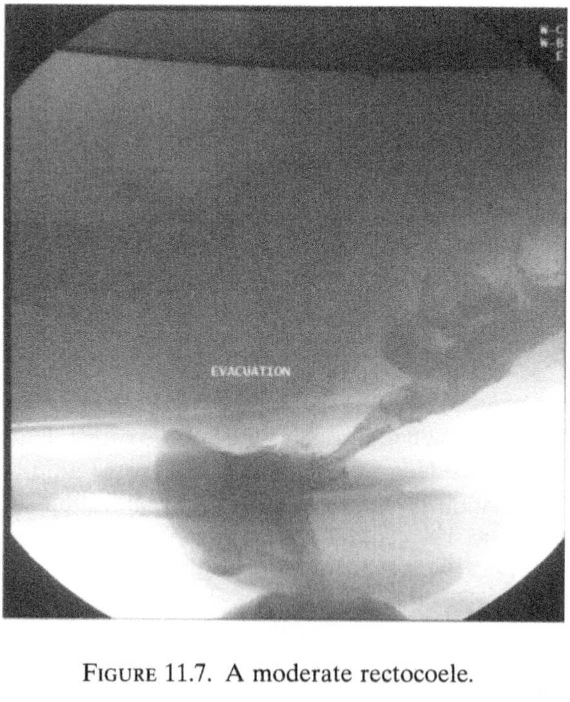

FIGURE 11.7. A moderate rectocoele.

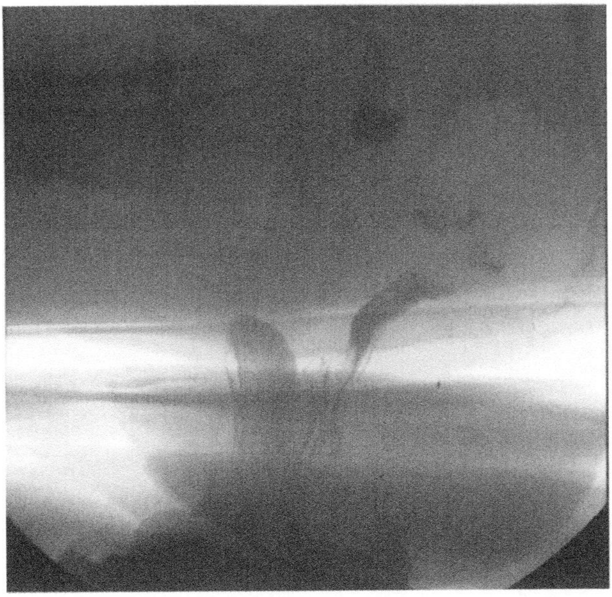

FIGURE 11.8. Prolapse of the intussusception resulting in frank external prolapse.

rectum is rare with the normal space between the rectal wall and sacrum at S3 level being around 10 mm. Any widening beyond this is regarded as abnormal and indicates posterior herniation.

Anterior mucosal rectal-wall prolapse is commonly seen in 50% of asymptomatic female volunteers and should be interpreted with caution [4].

Intrarectal intussusception is invagination of the rectal wall, which migrates distally towards the anal canal. Grade 1 and 2 represent infoldings in the wall of the rectum of less than 3 cm, and grade 3 is greater than 3 cm, but not circumferential. Grade 4 is circumferential intussusception and grade 5 is similar to grade 4 but abutting onto the internal anal orifice [4]. Prolapse of the intussusception into the anal canal is known as intra-anal intussusception and may be responsible for the solitary rectal ulcer syndrome. Prolapse of the intussusception beyond the anal verge results in frank external prolapse (Figure 11.8). Any degree of intussusception ranging from intrarectal to frank external prolapse may occur with or without the presence of a rectocoele. Frequently, intussusception and rectocoele coexist (Figure 11.9) and their recognition is of importance in the surgical management of these patients.

2.1.5. Perineometry

Perineometry is a valuable investigation in view of its simplicity and lack of radiation exposure, but is an indirect, external measure of actual pelvic

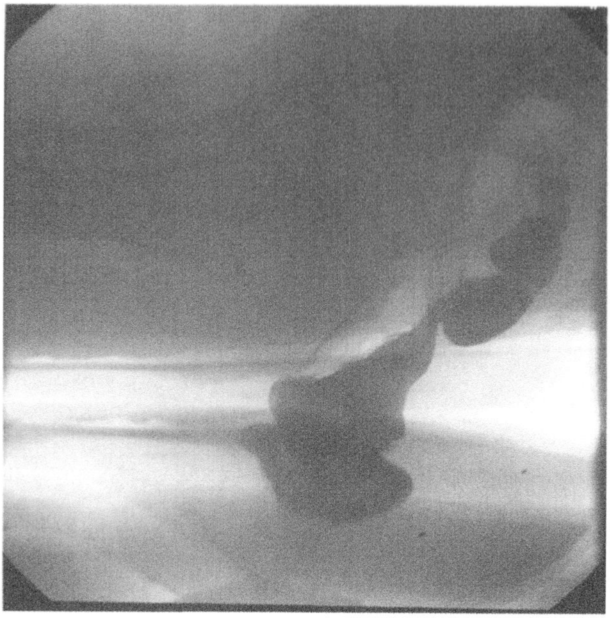

FIGURE 11.9. Coexisting rectocoele and intussception.

diaphragm descent. Since perineometry cannot be performed without being affected by normal shortening of the anal canal during straining or the variability in subcutaneous fat over the ischial tuberosities, it can often underestimate perineal descent by as much as 60% [20].

3. Anal Manometry

Manometric assessment of the anorectum is mandatory in the assessment of the patient with functional problems such as faecal incontinence, rectal prolapse, and constipation. It is also indicated in the assessment of patients with a variety of other clinical conditions including chronic anal fissures, especially in females [21], prior to complex fistula surgery, assessment of sphincter function before low anterior resection in the in the elderly, before pouch surgery to assess quality of sphincters (especially in middle-aged multiparous women).

A variety of tests are available to assess the anal sphincter and rectal sensation in clinical practice and those most commonly used are:

1. Resting anal pressure, reflecting internal anal sphincter activity (IAS).
2. Maximal squeeze pressure, reflecting external anal sphincter function and innervation (EAS).
3. Anal-canal length.

4. Anal-canal pressure in response to cough.
5. Rectoanal inhibitory reflex.
6. Sensory thresholds: first sensation, urge to defaecate, and maximal tolerated volume.
7. Rectal compliance and capacity.
8. Electromyography.
9. Pudendal nerve terminal motor latency (PNTML).

Various systems have been used recording single or multiple channels of data and utilising microballoons filled with water, water-perfused catheters, and microtransducers [22]. Unfortunately these differing techniques have lead to a variety of normal ranges, making comparison between studies difficult if not impossible. Azpiroz et al. in a review concluded anorectal manometry is useful but is limited by the absence of standardisation and normal data from healthy individuals [23]. Further interpretation of the data is complicated due to the patient's ability to compensate for their defects. The introduction of the more expensive microtransducers allowing multichannel recording has allowed a more comprehensive accurate reproducible assessment to be made. The data can be recorded both in the static position and with the patient ambulatory. When downloaded onto a personal computer, detailed analysis is possible. Synchronous assessment of mass electromyography (EMG) and multifibre EMG can also be performed.

Catheters or microtransducers can be connected to an automated withdrawal system or hand-held device. In a station pull-through the catheter is withdrawn in a stepwise fashion after insertion into the rectum, recordings are taken at 0.5–1-cm intervals. This allows an assessment to be made of anal-canal length, which varies according to gender. The length varies from 2–5.5 cm with the mean in women being 3.7 cm and men 4.6 cm.

There may be inaccuracies when radial pressure asymmetry is present. Studies have shown men have higher mean resting and squeeze pressures than women though they decline as age advances in both genders [24,25]. Normal mean resting pressure in adults is between 70–110 cm H_2O and is contributed to by both the internal and external sphincters though the exact contribution made by each is not certain. It is thought the internal sphincter is responsible for about 85% of resting tone. The resting tone gradually increases from cranial to caudal along the canal and the high-pressure zone is from 1–2 cm from the anal verge [26]. This zone is longer in men than women. In addition, resting pressure varies circumferentially in the anal canal: highest posteriorly at the top of the anal canal and lowest near the anal verge, while the reverse is the case for resting pressure anteriorly. The anal cushions also contribute to the resting pressure and these close the anal canal at rest. There is also a dynamic component of resting pressure observed by the presence of slow waves and ultra-slow waves which are observed on pressure recordings. Slow waves occur with a frequency of

10–20/min and with amplitude of 5–25 cm H_2O, while ultra-slow waves have frequency <3/min and amplitude of 30–100 cm H_2O.

The combined contraction of the EAS and puborectalis produces the squeeze pressure. The maximal squeeze pressure is 50%–100% above the resting pressure, ranging from 135–250 cm H_2O [26] (Figure 11.10, Figure 11.11). Squeeze pressure declines over time due to fatigue with the maximum pressure lasting <1 minute. The distribution of the squeezes pressure also varies due to the position of the muscles as follows:

Upper third—pressure highest posteriorly and lowest anteriorly.
Middle third—pressure equal radially.
Lower third—pressure highest anteriorly and lowest posteriorly.

Pressures are lower in incontinent patients compared to age- and sex-matched controls (Figure 11.12). However, there is extensive crossover between pressures recorded in patients and controls, with McHugh et al. finding 39% of women and 44% of men had normal resting pressures within the range of the matched controls [25–29]. Hallan et al. compared the accuracy of assessment between a well-trained finger and anal manometry [30].

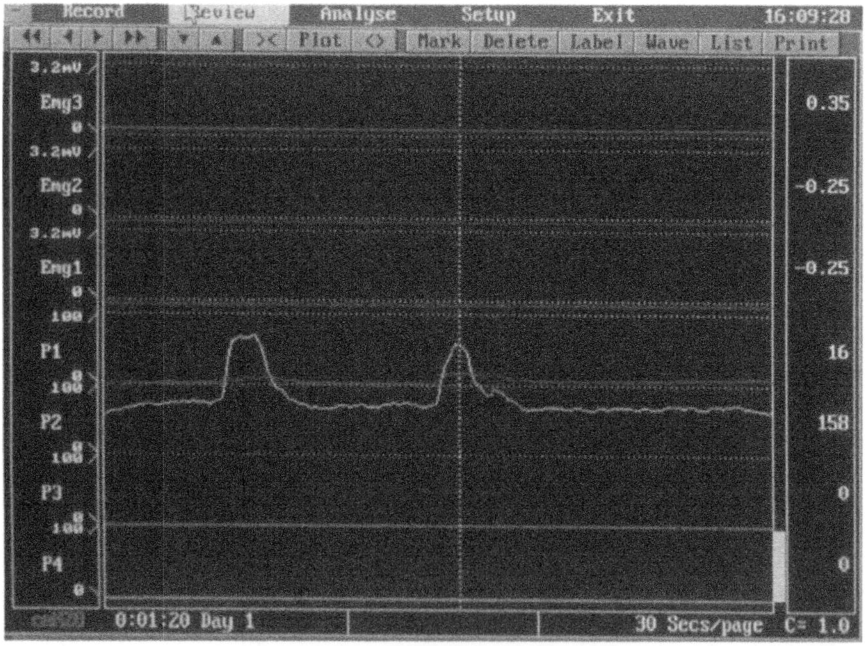

FIGURE 11.10. Resting anal pressure demonstrated on manometric assessment.

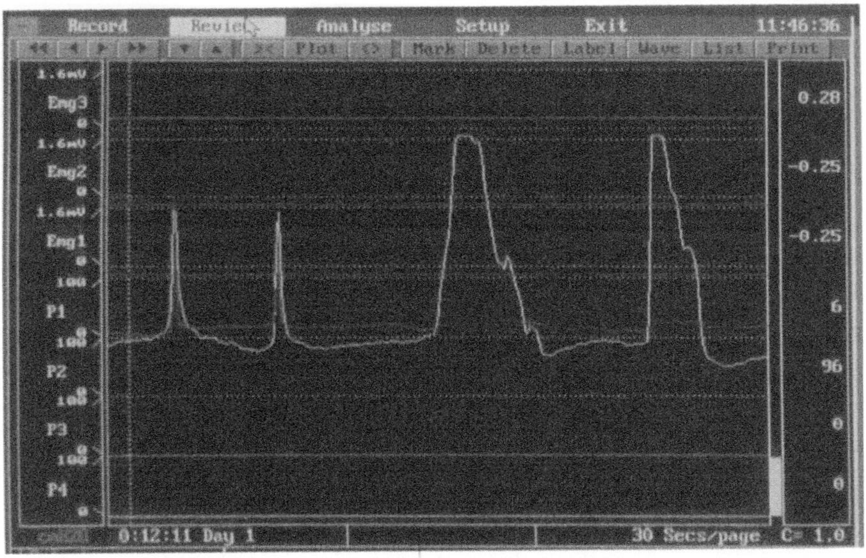

FIGURE 11.11. Maximal squeeze pressure.

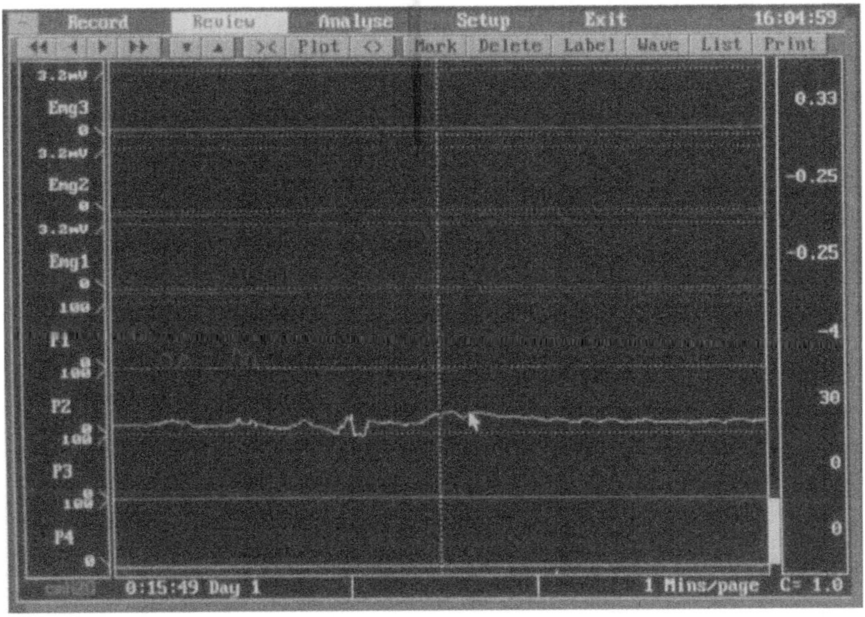

FIGURE 11.12. Low pressures in an incontinent patient.

3.1. Rectoanal Inhibitory Reflex

Rectal distension causes a reflex inhibition of internal anal sphincter (IAS) and contraction of the external anal sphincter (EAS). The mechanism of this reflex is as follows: as stool fills the rectum it eventually reaches the anorectal junction, as there is relaxation of the proximal anal canal. A spinal-cord reflex is initiated resulting in the relaxation of the IAS and the sensation of a call to stool. If there is a morphological damage to the EAS or it is denervated as in pudendal neuropathy, then incontinence occurs. The reflex, which is present in all healthy people, was first described by Gowers and is believed to be mediated by myentric plexus and stretch receptors in the pelvic floor [31]. The test is easily conducted by placing a manometry catheter in the high-pressure zone of the anal canal and a balloon within the rectum. The volume in the balloon is increased and then there is a rapid and profound decrease in resting pressure. It is initiated by a volume of 10 mL or less. It is absent in Hirschprung's disease, systemic sclerosis, and Chagas disease [32]. It has been shown to recover after a coloanal anastomosis [33]. This reflex allows the contents to be sampled by the transitional-zone mucosa to discriminate between solid, liquid, and air [34].

Saigusa et al. analysed 100 patients who underwent double stapled-pouch anal anastomosis and found presence of rectoanal inhibitory reflex in only 53% following surgery. There was no difference in the continence scores in patients with or without the reflex [35]. However, they noted a decreased incidence of nocturnal soiling if the reflex was present.

3.2. Vector Volume Manometry

Vector volume manometry allows a 3-dimensional reconstruction of the anal canal and has the ability to assess radial asymmetry. Sphincter defects are associated with indices of 0.6 or less and normal is a vector symmetry index (VSI) of 1.

Vector volume manometry is performed by a radially arranged 8-channel catheter, which records the pressure as the catheter is withdrawn and the software constructs the image. It is very useful in demonstrating a traumatic cause for faecal incontinence such as an isolated defect compared with global weakness of the external sphincter, which may denote a nerve-conduction defect [36]. However, the correlation with anal endosonography and EMG is not good with 11% and 13% of sphincter defects being detected, respectively [37].

3.3. Rectal Sensation

Rectal sensation is assessed using a water-filled balloon, which is gradually inflated. Rectal filling and sensation can be variable in individuals with a wide normal range with patients with obstructed defaecation having a very high rectal threshold volume [38]. Normal first perception starts between 10–30 mL while the urge to defaecate starts from 60–100 mL and the maximal tolerated volume ranges from 220–270 mL [39,40].

3.4. Rectal Compliance

From the change in volume and the associated pressure change, compliance can be calculated:

$$Compliance = \delta V/\delta P$$

This gives an indication of the distensibility of the rectum. Mean rectal compliance is between 4–14 mL/cm H_20 and is measured by a rectal balloon filled with water [40]. Rectal compliance is reduced in Behcet's disease, Crohn's disease and after radiotherapy. However, rectal compliance is found to be normal in incontinent patients.

3.5. Electromyography

Electromyography of the anal sphincter or levator ani can be used to show that a muscle has been denervated and that this is part of the clinical problem. Electromyography was used to map external-sphincter defects before surgery by either concentric-needle studies or single fiber studies but has been replaced by endo–anal ultrasound. Puborectalis EMG has been shown to demonstrate paradoxical contraction in obstructed defaecation but has been shown to be present in normal individuals [41].

Internal-anal-sphincter hypertonia has been shown to be associated with nonhealing fissures and can be demonstrated by EMG [42].

3.6. Pudendal Nerve Terminal Motor Latency

Pudendal nerve terminal motor latency is a simple nerve-conduction study used in the assessment of the pelvic floor. It is performed using a specially designed finger cot with a stimulating electrode at the fingertip and a recording electrode at the base of the finger. The latter electrode sits in the anal canal while the other is applied to the pudendal nerve as its passes around the iliac spine. The stimulus is applied at the iliac spine and the anal-canal electrode records the response. The nerve latency is measured from the stimulus to the motor response in the external sphincter and normal values range from 1.5–2.5 ms. Sato et al. have shown that there is physiologic variation in PNTML related to where it is recorded in the anal canal [43]. It is delayed with increasing age and is prolonged in 24% of patients with faecal incontinence. It is also prolonged in patients with rectal prolapse, solitary rectal ulcer syndrome, and severe constipation [44].

A prolonged PNTML is associated with a bad prognosis after an anterior anal sphincter repair for external sphincter defects [45].

Thomas et al. compared PNTML and EMG in 80 patients with faecal incontinence secondary to obstetric surgical trauma and found both PNTML and EMG were useful in providing additional information about the neurogenic basis of incontinence [46].

4. Magnetic Resonance Imaging of the Pelvis

Magnetic resonance imaging allows a multiplanar assessment which is non-invasive, quick, avoids ionising radiation, requires no preparation or contrast medium, and it is relatively non-operator–dependent. However, it is expensive, time consuming, and does not provide good mucosal images as seen on evacuatory proctography.

It is increasingly being used in obstructed defaecation (pelvic surface coil) and faecal incontinence (endo–anal MRI coil).

Healy et al., in a controlled study comparing obstructed defaecation patients with asymptomatic controls, showed MRI is useful in demonstrating more pelvic pathology compared to evacuatory proctography such as pelvic visceral descent, levator muscle, and plate descent [47]. They recommended MRI in symptomatic patients who were reported as normal following proctography.

Endo–anal coil MRI was compared with endo–anal ultrasound in assessing the sphincters in incontinent patients by Fletcher et al., who demonstrated the superiority of MRI in evaluating the thickness of the puborectalis and external sphincter [48]. MRI is also able to demonstrate degeneration of external anal sphincter with age. Both procedures were equally effective in identifying defects of the sphincters.

By comparing dynamic MRI with videoproctography, Matsuoka et al. have showed MRI is unable to detect rectocoeles and intussusception effectively [49]. Further, there were differences in the measurement of the anorectal angle and perineal descent compared with proctography. However, Lamb et al. believe dynamic MRI proctography to be a useful alternative to conventional proctography in a small study of 40 patients [50].

The evidence thus far supports the role of MRI in evaluation of faecal incontinence, either on its own or as an adjunct to endo–anal ultrasound; however, its role in assessing obstructed defaecation patients is still evolving.

5. Endo–anal Ultrasound

Endo–anal ultrasound (EAUS) is a minimally invasive easily accessible technique that provides detailed anatomy of the anal canal. It complements anal manometry and evacuatory proctography and is mandatory in the investigation of faecal incontinence. It also has a role in the management of obstructed defaecation and other functional bowel disorders.

Indications for EAUS assessment in the functional bowel disease patient include faecal incontinence, constipation and obstructed defaecation, post-surgical assessment, anal pain, and solitary rectal ulcer syndrome.

5.1. Technique and Instrumentation

Ideally, a 360-degree cross-sectional image is required, and this is obtained by using a mechanically rotating transducer. The most commonly used scanner is manufactured by Bruel and Kjaer (Figure 11.13), and uses an

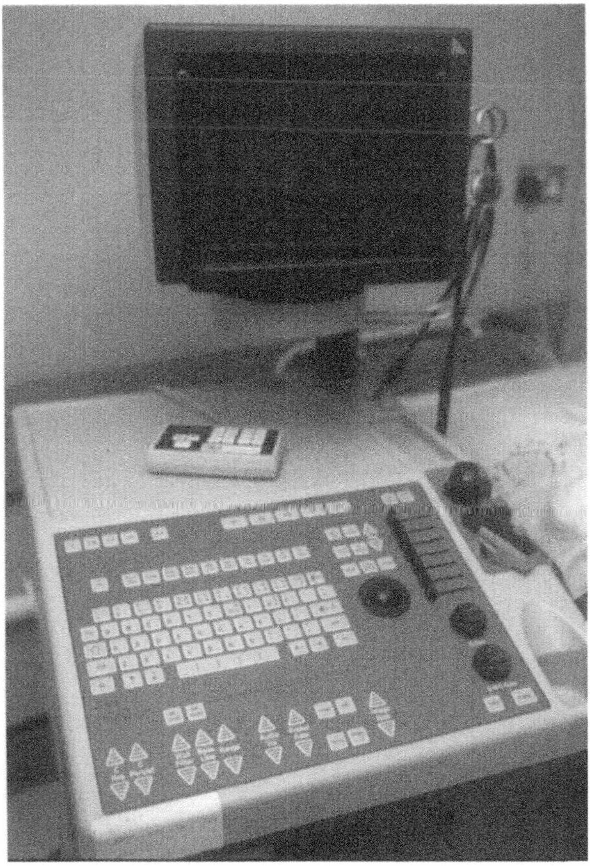

FIGURE 11.13. An endoanal ultrasound scanner by Bruel and Kjaer.

1850 endoprobe with a 10MHz transducer. The transducer is protected by a plastic cone with an outside diameter of 17mm (Figure 11.14) and filled with degassed water to prevent artifacts caused by air bubbles. The assembly is covered by a large condom with gel both inside and outside to provide acoustic coupling. Patients are examined in the prone position to avoid perineal asymmetry and the images are orientated such that anterior is uppermost and viewed from the feet of the patient. The anal canal is examined as a dynamic process and images are conventionally obtained at superficial, mid, and deep levels (Figure 11.15–Figure 11.17).

The various layers of the anal canal as depicted on EAUS examination are as illustrated in Table 11.2.

Variation in the anatomy of the anal canal is apparent between males and females, particularly in the external anal sphincter (Figure 11.18), and changes in the appearances of the sphincters with age are important in interpretation of the endosonic anatomy of the anal canal.

The thickness of the internal sphincter shows a positive correlation with age in the high- and middle-anal canal in the female asymptomatic nulliparous women [52]. However, the external sphincter shows a negative correlation with age at high-, mid-, and low-anal levels. There is no significant correlation between thickness of longitudinal muscle or puborectalis.

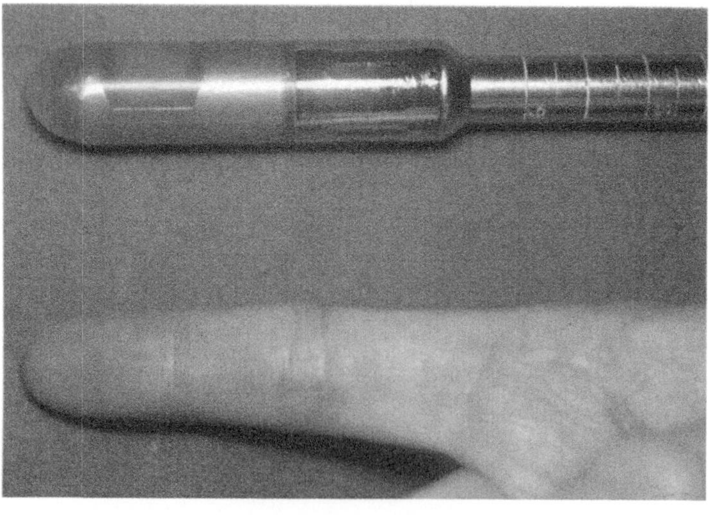

FIGURE 11.14. The transducer protected by a plastic cone.

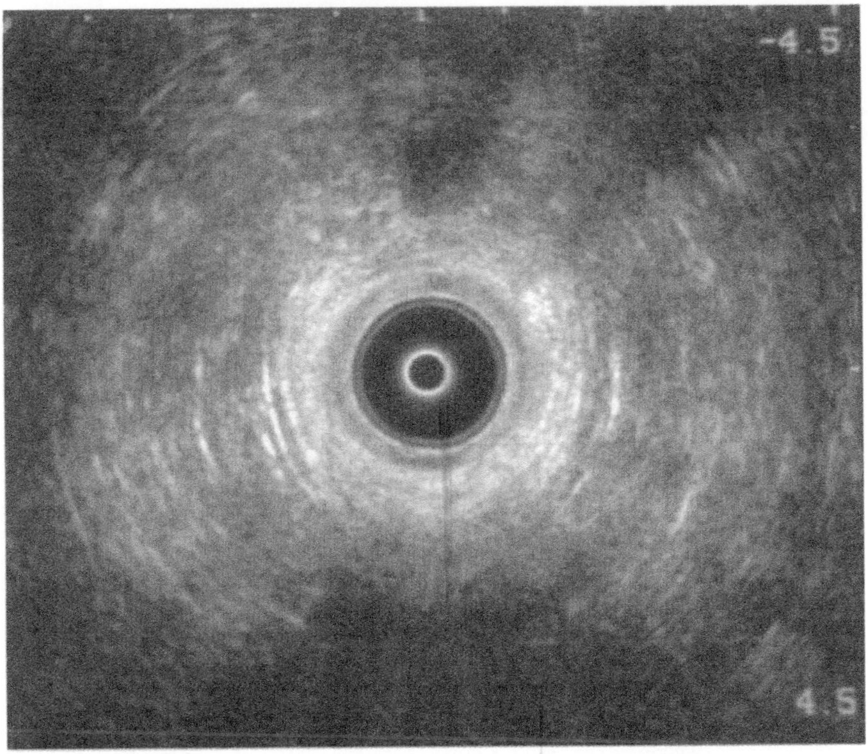

FIGURE 11.15. Endo–anal scan showing superficial level.

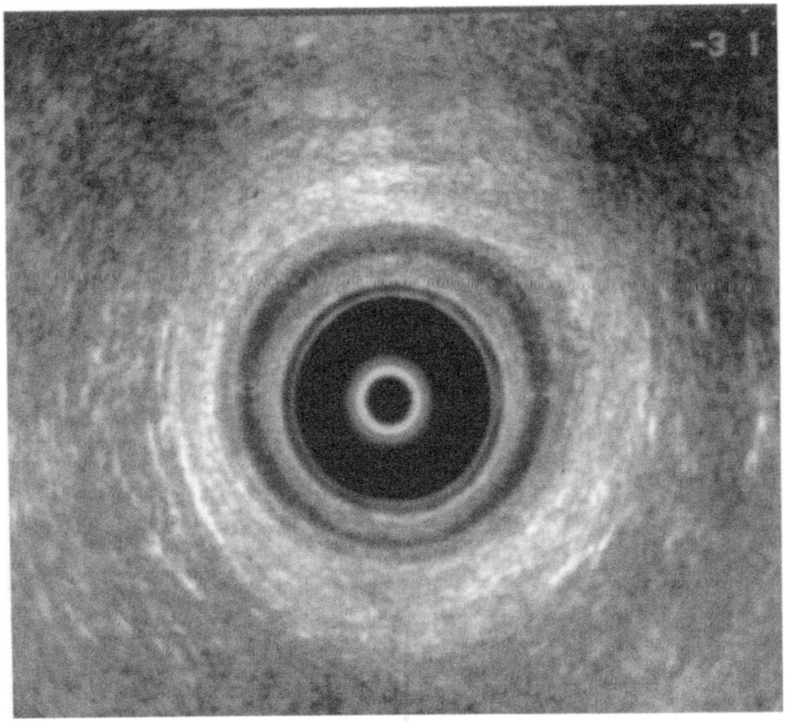

FIGURE 11.16. Endo–anal scan showing mid level.

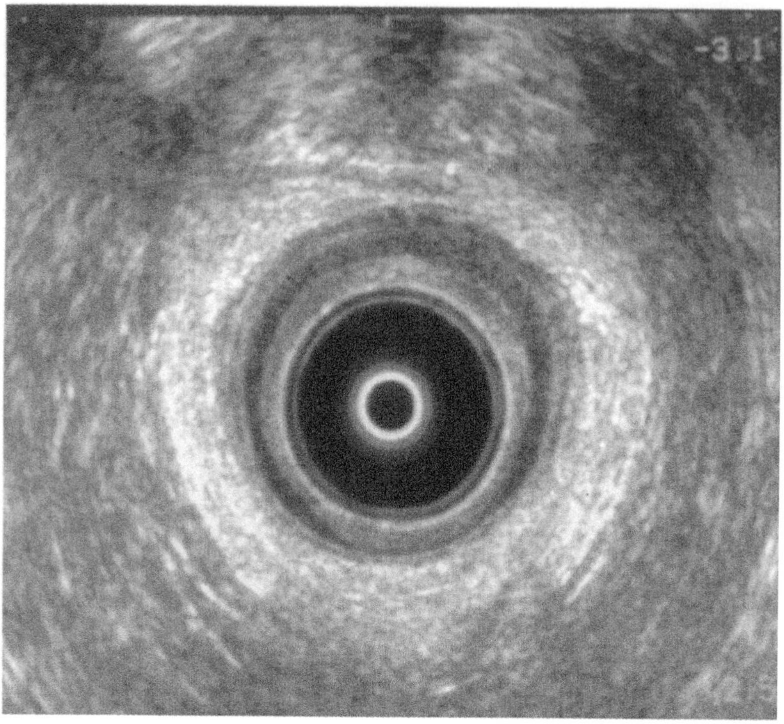

FIGURE 11.17. Endo–anal scan showing deep level.

In patients less than 55 years of age, the internal sphincter is between 2.4–2.7-mm thick, while above 55 years it is from 2.8–3.4-mm thick (Figure 11.19, Figure 11.20).

The conjoint longitudinal muscle coat surrounding the internal sphincter is continuation of the outer longitudinal muscle coat of the rectum. It forms a prominent hyperechoic layer between the internal and external sphincters. This layer is not sonographically uniform and thin short hypoechoic areas within it may be due to segments of smooth muscle devoid of connective tissue.

The external sphincter is complex and a trilaminar arrangement is accepted with deep, superficial, and subcutaneous parts. As the probe is

TABLE 11.2. Endosonographic layers of the anal canal.

1. Mucosa/cone interface, hyperechoeic layer
2. (Mucosa)–(hypoechoeic layer) not always seen
3. Subepithelial layer, hyperechoic layer
4. Internal anal sphincter, hypoechoiec layer
5. Longitudinal muscle, hyperechoic layer
6. External sphincter, mixed echogenicity layer

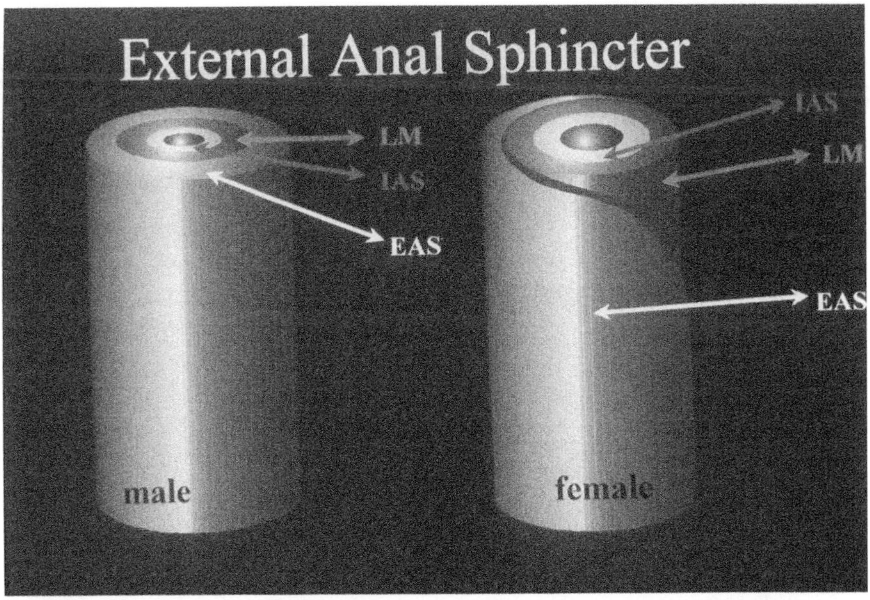

FIGURE 11.18. Diagrammatic representation of the variation in the anatomy of the anal canal in males and females.

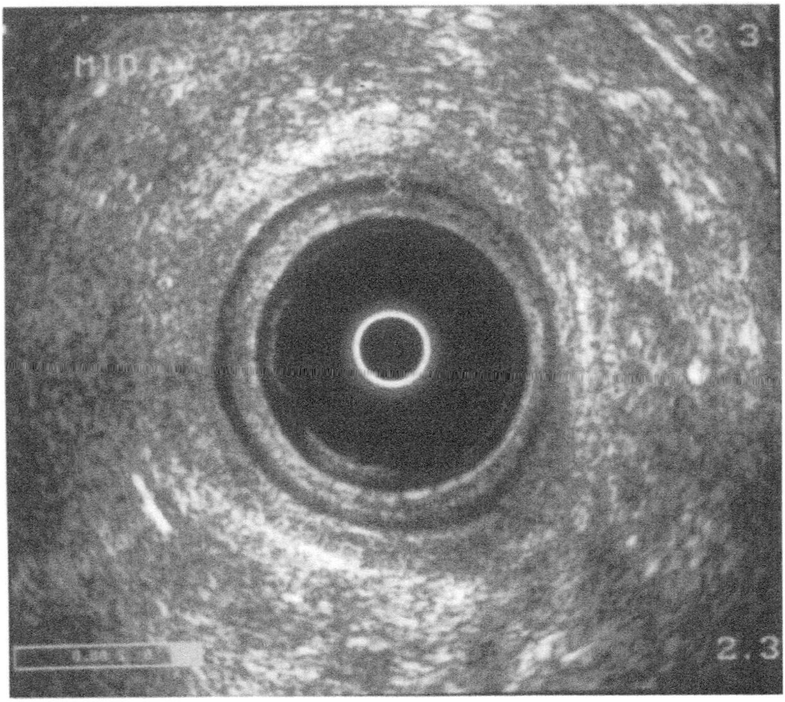

FIGURE 11.19. Variation in the thickness in the internal sphincter with age.

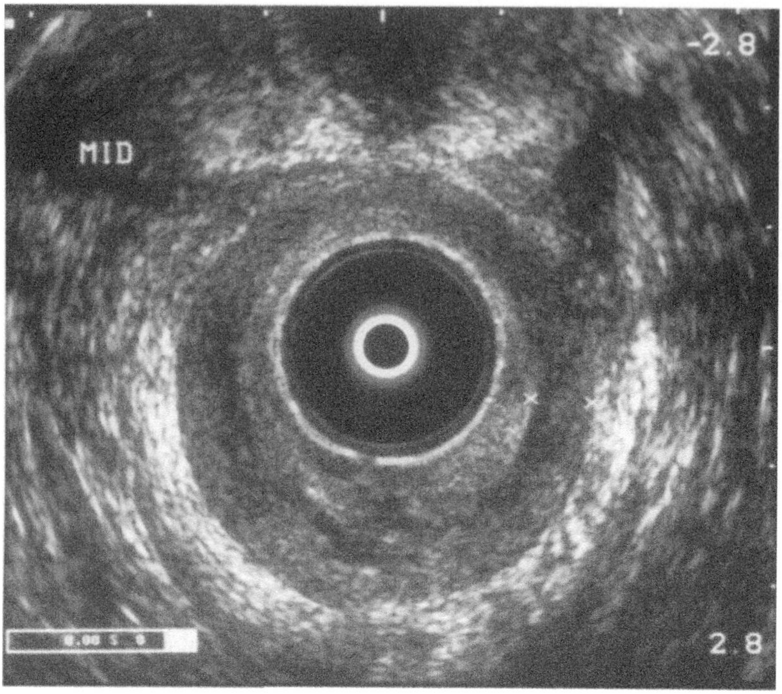

FIGURE 11.20. Variation in the thickness in the internal sphincter with age.

withdrawn, the hyperechoic U-shaped sling of puborectalis comes in view. The external sphincter is identified as converging fibres anteriorly as the probe comes down and they converge to form an annular ring [53]. In females, the external sphincter may be very thin anteriorly. In males, the external sphincter is more symmetrical and annular at all levels with an outer hypoechoic ring. In females, the echogenicity is identical and the layers are difficult to delineate and there is a natural deficiency anteriorly in the deep part of the anal canal.

Recently, 3-dimensional ultrasonography has been introduced [54]. Conventional axial imaging may not give the accurate length of a sphincter tear but 3-dimensional imaging allows visualisation of the sphincter complex in multiple planes (Figure 11.21).

5.2. *Faecal Incontinence*

Endo–anal ultrasound has been shown in various studies to be a useful tool in mapping sphincter defects. It distinguishes patients with sphincter defects from idiopathic faecal incontinence and allows the surgeon to manage this complex condition appropriately. Endo–anal ultrasound also has a role in

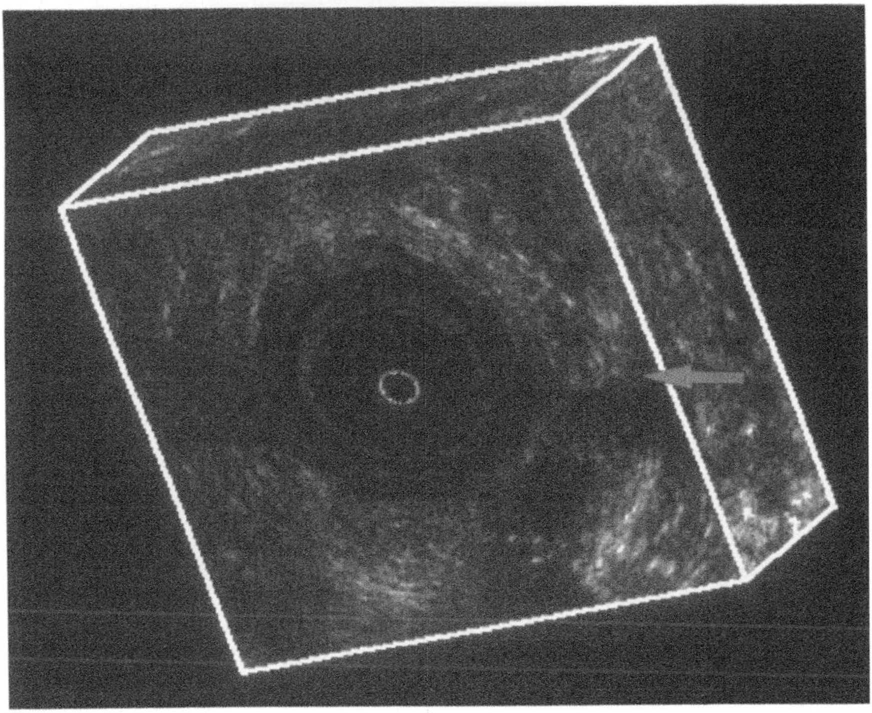

FIGURE 11.21. Three-dimensional imaging of the anal canal.

assessing the sphincters after primary or secondary repair of sphincter defects.

Awareness of the physiological variation in the thickness of the internal anal sphincter and the sexual differences is important in radiological assessment of patients with faecal incontinence. The posterolateral aspect of the external sphincter should be intact at all levels in both sexes, but there is a natural deficiency anteriorly in females at a deep level [53]. Causes of faecal incontinence include obstetrics-related trauma, postsurgical (anal dilatation, lateral anal sphincterotomy, posthaemorrhoidectomy, multiple fistula operations), trauma (accidental and intentional injury, anal rape), and idiopathic.

Childbirth is the most common cause of damage to the anal sphincters. Endo–anal ultrasound has shown a significantly higher incidence of sphincter damage than previously recognised clinically (Figure 11.22, Figure 11.23). Thirty-five percent of women undergoing their first normal vaginal delivery were shown to have endosonographic evidence of sphincter disruption at 6 weeks that persisted at 6 months. One-third had symptoms of

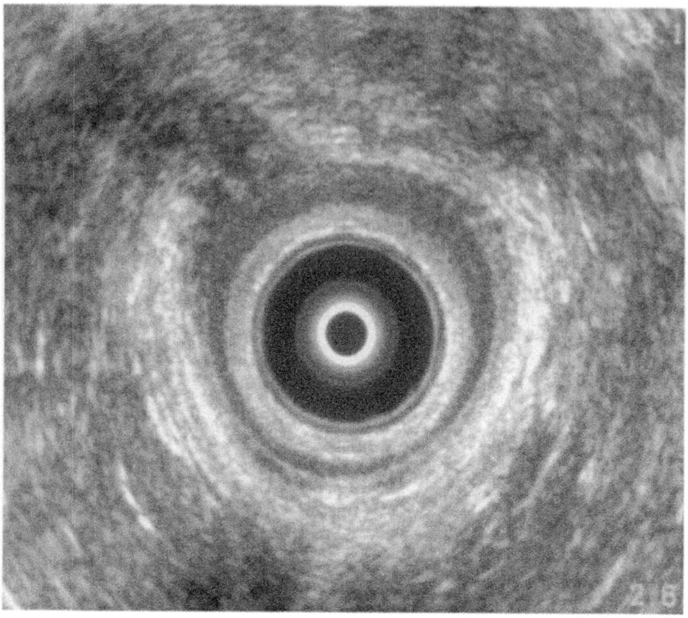

FIGURE 11.22. Endo–anal ultrasound demonstration of external sphincter defect.

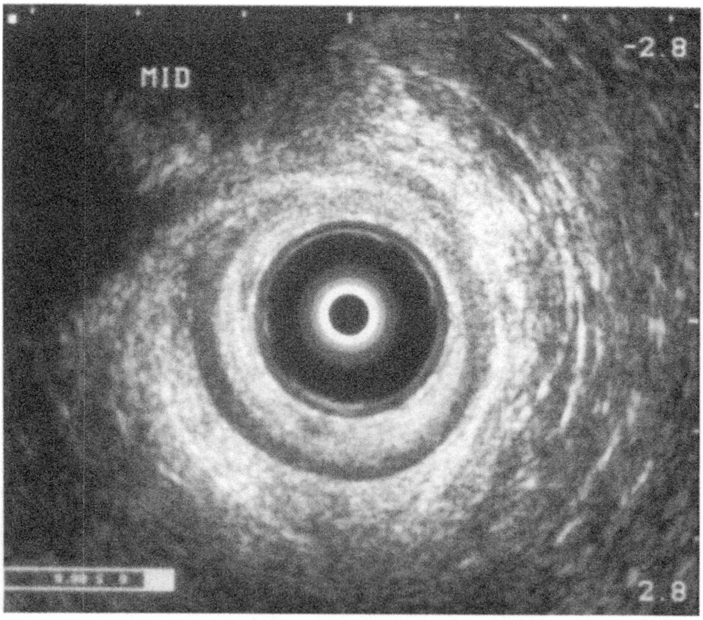

FIGURE 11.23. Endo–anal ultrasound demonstration of combined internal and external sphincter defect.

anal incontinence. Significantly higher incidences of defects were found following forceps delivery (8 out of 10) and those undergoing vacuum extraction were spared [59]. Gold et al. assessed the 3-dimensional EAUS and emphasised the role of EAUS in showing longitudinal and radial extent of the tear, which may have a role in determining the success of surgical repair of sphincter defects [54].

Overzealous manual dilatation of the anus produces varying degrees of tear at multiple points compared with the precise defect of an internal sphincterotomy and both can be delineated by EAUS. Remnants of the sphincter will appear hyperechoic, suggesting fibrotic replacement after manual dilatation (Figure 11.24), while lateral sphincterotomy produces a clean break in the sphincter with well-defined edges (Figure 11.25) [53]. Surgical damage to the internal sphincter can also be recognised after fistula surgery and formation of ileo–anal pouch.

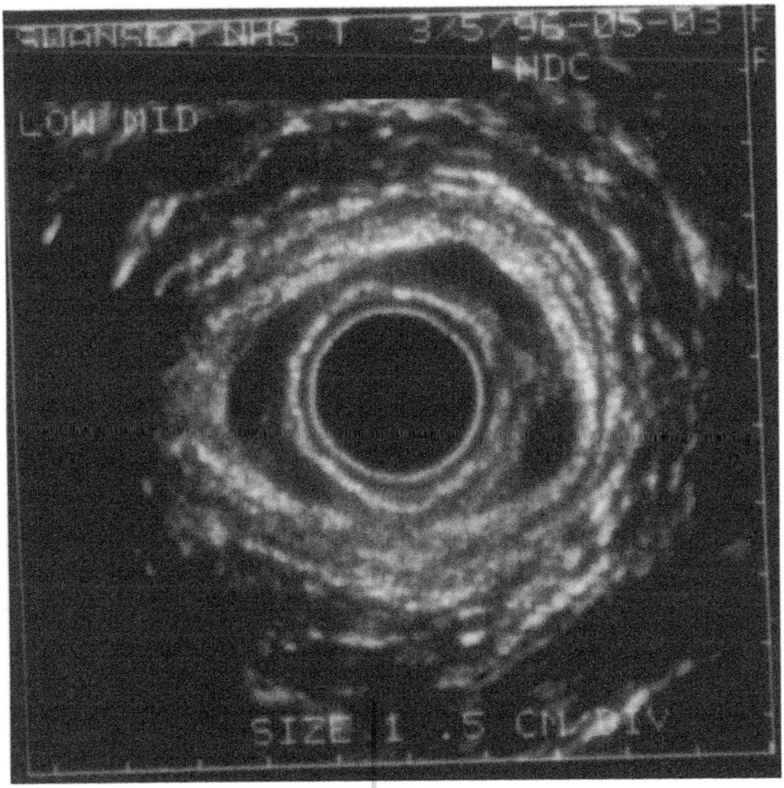

FIGURE 11.24. Internal sphincter disruption following manual anal dilatation.

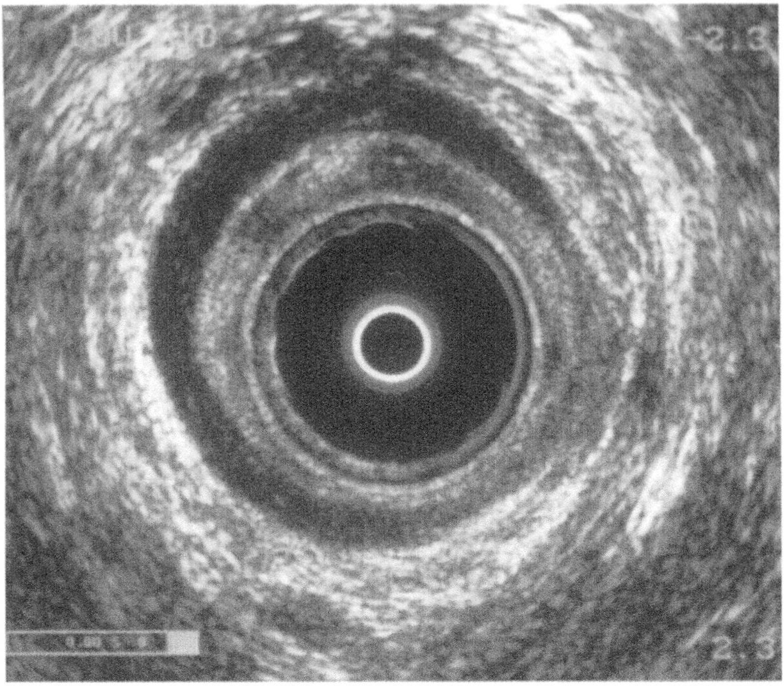

FIGURE 11.25. Internal anal sphincterotomy demonstrated on an anal scan.

Speakman et al. studied 12 patients with faecal incontinence who had manual dilatation for anal fissure and EAUS showed extensive disruption of internal anal sphincter in 10 of these patients [55]. Sixty-five percent of patients undergoing anal dilatation had sphincter defects in a study by Nielsen et al., with 12.5 % of these patients having some degree of faecal incontinence [56]. Bartram et al. have emphasised that EAUS has an important role in making surgeons aware of procedures associated with sphincter injuries [57].

Sultan et al. assessed the effect of internal anal sphincterotomy for anal fissures and showed that women, with their shorter anal canal, are more susceptible to inadvertent extensive sphincterotomy with 9 out of 10 women in his study having the entire length of the internal sphincter divided [58]. Ho et al. showed the usefulness of EAUS in picking up sphincter defects iatrogenically caused by stapling instruments [60]. Other causes of faecal incontinence include trauma (Figure 11.26) and idiopathic faecal incontinence. Idiopathic faecal incontinence is essentially a result of age-related neuropathy, atrophy, fibrosis, and possibly ischemia. Endo–anal ultrasound is required to rule out other cause of faecal incontinence. More recently, MRI using endo–anal coil has proven to be useful in demonstrating these degenerate changes in the sphincters.

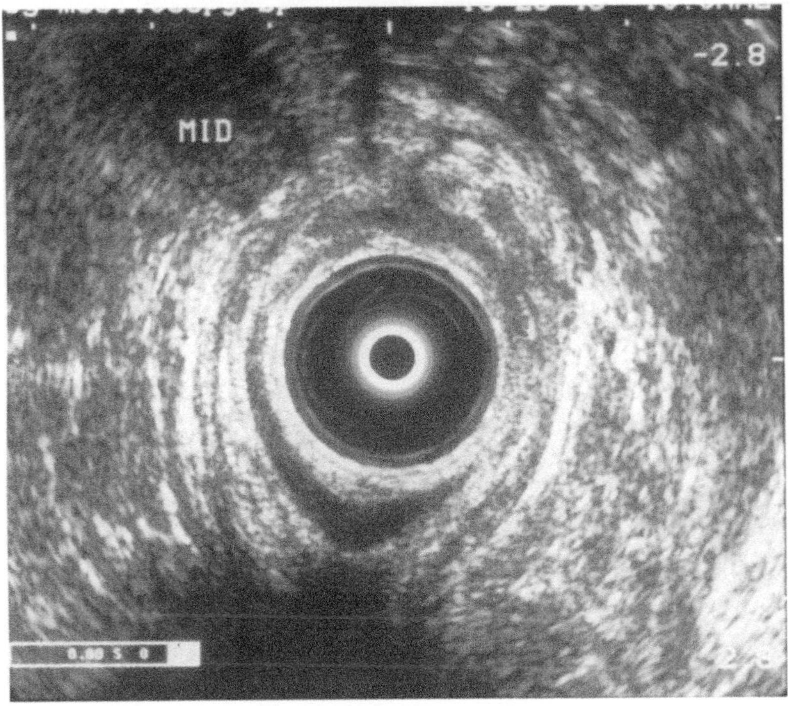

FIGURE 11.26. Sphincter disruption following anal trauma.

5.3. Solitary Rectal Ulcer Syndrome

Halligan et al. showed marked thickness of internal and external anal sphincter in patients with solitary rectal ulcer (SRUS) when compared to asymptomatic controls (Figure 11.27) [61]. The precise aetiology is unknown; however, it has been proposed a combination of mucosal rectal prolapse and increased rectal pressure due to internal anal sphincter thickness could be responsible for SRUS.

Marshall et al., in a further small study, demonstrated the predictive value of internal anal sphincter thickness for diagnosis of rectal intussusception in patients with SRUS [62]. They concluded EAUS has a 91% positive predictive value in detecting internal anal sphincter thickness in SRUS patients having rectal intussusception; however, the negative predictive value was only 57%. It may have a role in patients who failed to evacuate on evacuatory proctography and in pregnant women where radiation exposure is undesirable.

More recently dynamic transperineal ultrasound has been used to demonstrate intussusception, rectocoeles, and enterocoeles, which correlate well with evacuatory proctography [63].

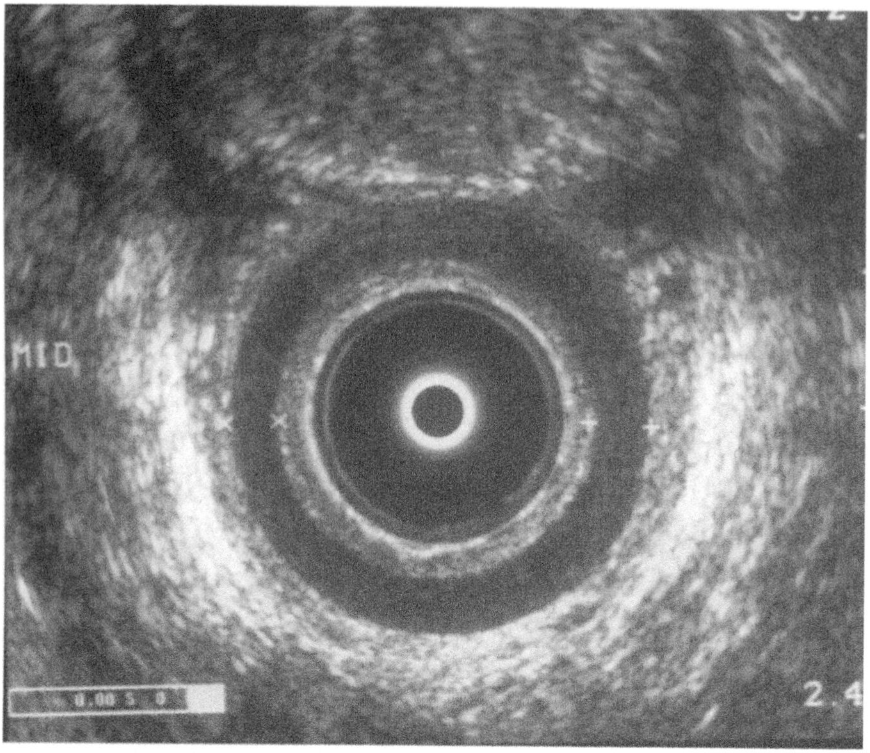

FIGURE 11.27. Increased thickness of internal and external anal sphincter in patient with solitary rectal ulcer (SRUS).

6. Colonic Transit Studies

A colonic transit study is part of the routine assessment in patients with constipation but is also beneficial in assessing obstructed defaecation. It also has a place in assessing patients with evacuatory difficulties following formation of ileo–anal pouch and in assessing drugs altering colonic motility.

Hinton et al. used 20 radioopaque pellets of barium-impregnated polythene and validated his study by comparing the findings with 25 normal subjects [64]. He showed all normal subjects passed the first marker within 66 hours and all except 1 passed 80% of the markers in 5 days. Markers used must not be absorbed, but measurable and must travel at a similar rate to the normal contents and must not alter the activity of the gut. Martelli et al. showed that retention of more than 20% of markers on day 5 is regarded as abnormal, and this is generally accepted as the current criteria for an abnormal study (Figure 11.28, Figure 11.29) [65].

Metcalf et al. used 3 different markers and a single film to assess total and segmental colonic transit time and found age or a modest dietary fiber intake did not affect the transit time [66]. They further showed transit varied in different segments of the bowel. Oral scintigraphic segmental

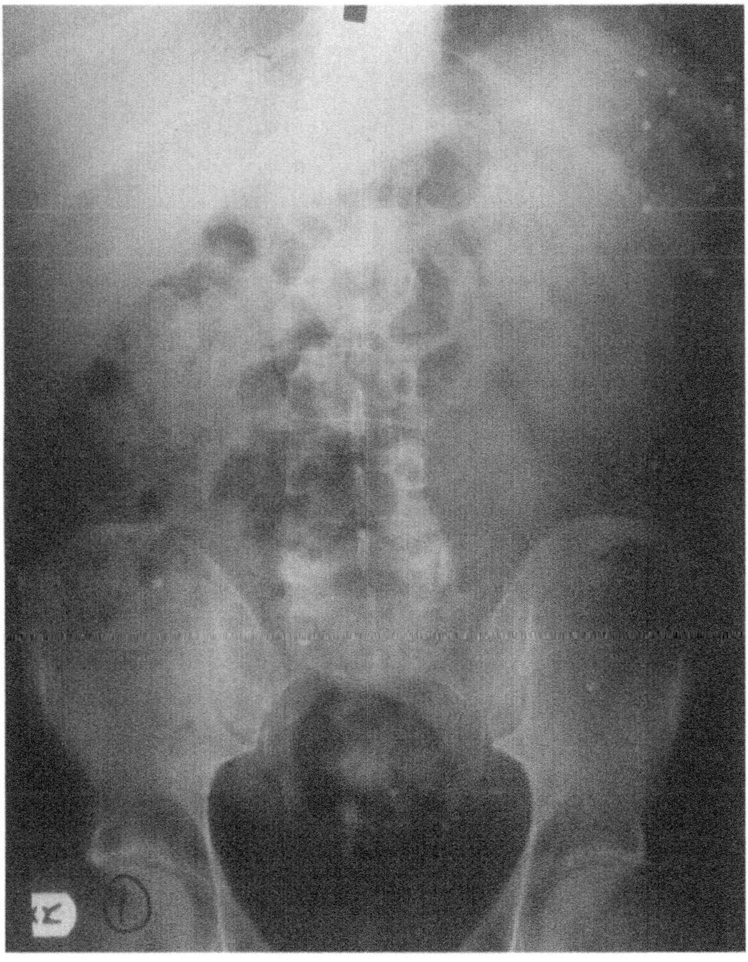

FIGURE 11.28. Shapes colonic transit study.

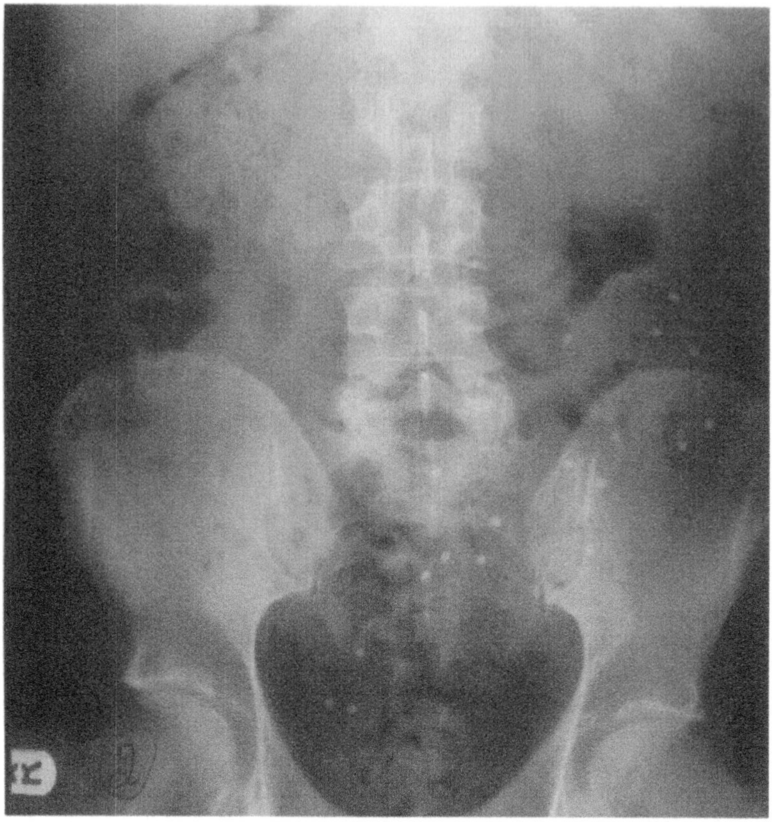

Figure 11.29. Shapes colonis transit study.

transit studies have gained importance with oral In-111–labelled DTPA being used to assess segmental transit (Figure 11.30). Lundin et al., in their study of 28 patients, showed patients undergoing segmental colectomy based on scintigraphy had better results and functional outcome [67].

Recently Technetium 99m tin–colloid has been used to image liquid stools and I-131 microcapsules to image solids in a study to assess pouch function using scintigraphy [68]. The beneficial effects of scintigraphy have also been shown in a technique using In-111–labelled polystyrene particles in assessing incontinent and constipated patients after a retrograde colonic washout [69].

Nam et al. assessed reproducibility in colonic transit and showed a colonic transit study has better correlation coefficient in patients with idiopathic

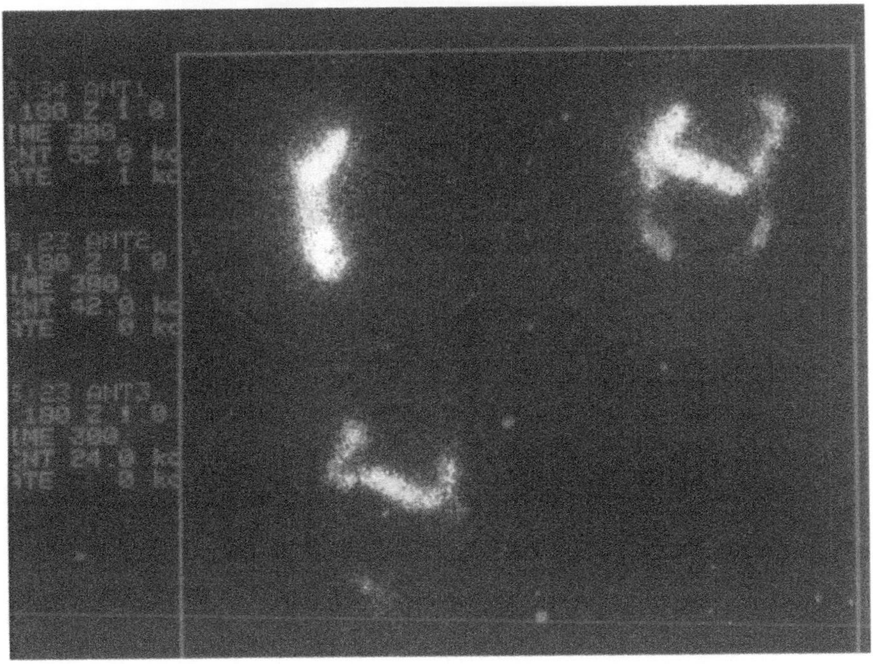

FIGURE 11.30. Oral scintigraphic segmental transit study.

constipation than patients with colonic inertia [70]. They suggested repeating the colonic transit study in patients with colonic inertia.

Colonic transit studies are a part of the investigative algorithm in evaluating functional bowel disorders and play an important role in selecting patients for surgery and in subsequent follow-up care.

7. Summary

The assessment of the patient with a functional bowel disorder is not easy and requires patience and understanding particularly because there may be coexistent problems urologically or gynaecologically. Careful history taking, clinical examination, and use of appropriate investigations are the keys to dealing with these problems. Full assessment should be followed by a careful consideration of the therapeutic options available. Appropriate management of patients with these difficult problems requires a multidisciplinary approach between clinicians with an interest in pelvic floor problems including coloproctologists, urologists, gynaecologists, radiologists, and specialist nurses.

References

1. Bartram C. Radiologic evaluation of anorectal disorders. *Gastroeneterol Clin North Am.* 2001;30:55–75.
2. Stoker J, Halligan S, Bartram CI. Pelvic floor imaging. *Radiology* 2001;218: 621–641.
3. Burhenne HJ. Intestinal evacuation study: a new roentgenologic technique. *Radiol Clin.* 1964;33:79–84.
4. Shorvon PJ, McHugh S, Diamant NE, Somers S. Defaecography in normal volunteers: results and implications. *Gut* 1989;30:1737–1749.
5. Hiltunen KM, Kolehmainen H, Matikainen M. Does defaecography help in diagnosis and clinical decision-making in defaecation disorders? *Abdom Imaging.* 1994;19:355–358.
6. Turnbull GK, Bartram CI, Lennard-Jones JE. Radiologic of rectal evacuation in adults with idiopathic constipation. *Dis Colon Rectum.* 1988;31:190–197.
7. Wald A, Jafri F, Rehder J, Holeva K. Scintigraphic studies of rectal emptying in patients with constipation and defaecatory difficulty. *Dig Dis Sci.* 1993; 38:353–358.
8. Karasick S, Spettell CM. The role of parity and hysterectomy on the development of pelvic floor abnormalities revealed by defaecography. *Am J Roentgenol.* 1997;169:1555–1558.
9. Klauser AG, Ting KH, Mangel E, Eibl-Eibesfeldt B, Muller-Lissner SA. Interobserver agreement in defaecography. *Dis Colon Rectum.* 1994;37:1310–1316.
10. Mahieu P, Pringot J, Bodart P. Defaecography: description of a new procedure and results in normal patients. *Gastrointest Radiol.* 1984:9:247.
11. Bernier P, Stevenson GW, Shorvon P. Defaecography commode. *Radiology* 1988;166:891.
12. Ginai AZ. Technical report: evacuation proctography(defaecography). A new seat and method of examination. *Clin Radiol.* 1990;42:214.
13. Goei R, Kemerink G. Radiation dose in defaecography. *Radiology* 1990;176:137.
14. Roe AM, Bartolo DC, Mortensen NJ. Techniques in evacuation proctography in the diagnosis of intractable constipation and related disorders. *J R Soc Med.* 1986;79:331–333.
15. Bartram CL, Turnbull GK, Lennard-Jones JE. Evacuation proctography: an investigation of rectal expulsion in 20 subjects without defaecatory disturbance. *Gastrointes Radiol.* 1988;13:72–80.
16. Preston DM, Lennard-Jones JE, Thomas BM. The balloon proctogram. *Br J Surg.* 1984;71:29–32.
17. Jorge JM, Habr-Gama A, Wexner SD. Clinical applications and techniques of cinedefaecography. *Am J Surg.* 2001;182:93–101.
18. Halligan S, McGee S, Bartram CI. Quantification of evacuation proctography. *Dis Colon Rectum.* 1994;37:1151–1154.
19. Goei R, et al. Anorectal function: defaecographic measurement in normal subjects. *Radiology* 1989;173:137.
20. Oettle GJ, Roe AM, Bartolo DC, et al. What is the best way of measuring perineal descent? A comparison of radiographic and clinical methods. *Br J Surg.* 1985;72:999–1001.

21. Simkovic D, Smejkal K, Siroky M, et al. Importance of anorectal manometry in chronic anal fissure. *Acta Medica.* 2001;44:105–107.
22. Johnson GP, Pemberton JH, Samson M, Zinsmeister AR. Transducer manometry and the effects of body position on anal canal pressures. *Dis Colon Rectum.* 1990;33:469–475.
23. Azpiroz F, Enck P, Whitehead WE. Anorectal functional testing: review of collective experience. *Am J Gastroenterol.* 2002;97:232–240.
24. Loening-Baucke V, Anwar M. Effects of age on anorectal manometry. *Am J Gastroenterol.* 1985;80:50–53.
25. McHugh SM, Diament NE. Effect of age, gender and parity on anal canal pressures. Contribution of impaired anal sphincter function to faecal incontinence. *Dig Dis Sci.* 1987; 32:726–736.
26. Jorge JM, Wexner SD. Anorectal manometry: techniques and clinical applications. *South Med J.* 1993;86:924–931.
27. Hiltunen KM. Anal manometric findings in patients with anal incontinence. *Dis Colon Rectum.* 1985;28:925–928.
28. Monk DN, Mills P, Jeacock J, Cowie A, Kiff ES. Combining the strength–duration curve of the external anal sphincter with manometry for the assessment of faecal incontinence. *Br J Surg.* 1998;85:1389–1393.
29. Holmberg A, Graf W, Osterberg A, Pahlman L. Anorectal manaovolumetry in the diagnosis of faecal incontinence. *Dis Colon Rectum.* 1995;38:502–508.
30. Hallan RI, Marzouk DEMM, Waldron DJ, Womack NR, Williams NS. Comparison of digital and manometric assessment of anal sphincter function. *Br J Surg.* 1989;76:973–975.
31. Gowers WR. The automatic action of the sphincter ani. *Proc R Soc Lond.* 1877; 26:77–84.
32. Lawson J, Nixon HH. Anal canal pressures in the diagnosis of Hirschprung's disease. *J Paediatr Surg.* 1967;2:544–552.
33. Lewis WG, Williamson MER, Miller AS, Sagar PM, Holdsworth PJ, Johnston D. Preservation of complete anal sphincteric proprioception in restorative proctocolectomy the inhibitory reflex and fine control of continence need not be impaired. *Gut* 1995;36:902–906.
34. Miller R, Bartolo DC, Cervero F, Mortensen NJ. Anorectal sampling: a comparison of normal and incontinent patients. *Br J Surg.* 1988;75:44–47.
35. Saigusa N, Belin BM, Choi HJ, et al. Recovery of the rectoanal inhibitory reflex after restorative proctocolectomy: does it correlate with nocturnal continence? *Dis Colon Rectum.* 2003;46:168–172.
36. Braun JC, Treutner KH, Dreuw B, Klimaszewski M, Schmpelick V. Vectormanometry for differential diagnosis of faecal incontinence. *Dis Colon Rectum.* 1994;37:989–996.
37. Yang YK, Wexner SD. Anal pressure vectography is of no apparent benefit for sphincter evaluation. *Int J Colorectal Dis.* 1994;9:92–95.
38. Kendall GPN, Thompson DG, Day SJ, Lennard-Jones JE. Inter and intraindividual variation in pressure-volume relations of the rectum in normal subjects and patients with irritable bowel syndrome. *Gut* 1990;31:1062–1068.
39. Sun WM, Read NW, Miner PB. Relation between rectal sensation and anal function in normal subjects and patients with faecal incontinence. *Gut* 1990; 31:1056–1061.

40. Ihre T. Studies on anal function in continent and incontinent patients. *Scand J Gastroenterol.* 1974;9:1–64.
41. Voderholzer WA, Neuhaus DA, Klauser AG, et al. Paradoxical sphincter contraction is rarely indicative of anismus. *Gut* 1997;41:258–262.
42. Sorensen M, Nielsen MB, Pedersen JF, Chritiansen J. Electromyography of the internal anal sphincter performed under endosonographic guidance. Description of a new method. *Dis Colon Rectum.* 1994:37:138–143.
43. Sato T, Nagai H. Pudendal nerve complete motor latencies at four different levels in the anal sphincter system in young adults. *Dis Colon Rectum.* 2002; 45:923–927.
44. Vaccaro CA, Cheong DM, Wexner SD, et al. Pudendal neuropathy in evacuatory disorders. *Dis Colon Rectum.* 1995;38:166–171.
45. Gilland R, Altamore DF, Moreira H, et al. Pudendal neuropathy is predictive of failure following anterior overlapping sphincteroplasty. *Dis Colon Rectum.* 1998;41:1516–1522.
46. Thomas C, Lefaucheur JP, Galula G, et al. Respective value of pudendal nerve terminal motor latency and anal sphincter electromyography in neurogenic faecal incontinence. *Neurophysiol Clin.* 2002;32:85–90.
47. Healy JC, Halligan S, Reznek RH, et al. Magnetic resonance imaging of the pelvic floor in patients with obstructed defaecation. *Br J Surg.* 1997;84:1555–1558.
48. Fletcher JG, Busse RF, Riederer SJ, et al. Magnetic resonance imaging of anatomic and dynamic defects of the pelvic floor in defaecatory disorders. *Am J Gastroenterol.* 2003;98:399–411.
49. Matsuoka H, Wexner SD, Desai MB, et al. A comparison between dynamic pelvic magnetic resonance imaging and videoproctography I patients with constipation. *Dis Colon Rectum.* 2001;44:571–576.
50. Lamb GM, de Jod MG, Gould SW, et al. Upright dynamic MR defaecating proctography in an open configuration MR system. *Br J Radiol.* 2000;73:152–155.
51. Sultan AH, Nicholls RJ, Kamm MA, Hudson CN, Beynon J, Bartram CI. Anal endosonography and correlation with in vitro and in vivo anatomy. *Br J Surg.* 1993;80:508–511.
52. Frudinger A, Halligan S, Bartram CI, et al. Female anal sphincter: Age related differences in asymptomatic volunteers with high-frequency endoanal US. *Radiology* 2002;224:417–423.
53. Bartram CI. *Anal Endosonography. Alimentary Tract Radiology.* 5th ed., St. Louis: Freeney and Stevenson, 1994.
54. Gold DM, Bartram CI, Halligan S, et al. Three dimensional endoanal sonography in assessing anal canal injury. *Br J Surg.* 1999;86:365–370.
55. Speakman CTM, Burnett SJD, Kamm MA, Bartram CI. Sphincter injury after anal dilatation demonstrated by anal endosonography. *Br J Surg.* 1991;78: 1429–1430.
56. Nielsen MB, Rasmussen OO, Pederson JF, Chritiansen J. Risk of sphincter damage and anal incontinence after anal dilatation for fissure-in-ano. *Dis Colon Rectum.* 1993;36:677–680.
57. Bartram CI, Sultan AH. Anal endosonography in faecal incontinenece. *Gut* 1995;37:4–6.
58. Sultan AH, Kamm MA, Nicholls RJ, Bartram CI. Prospective study of the extent of lateral anal sphincterotomy division during lateral sphinctertomy. *Dis Colon Rectum.* 1994;37:1031–1033.

59. Sultan AH, Kamm MA, Hudson CN, Thomas J, Bartram CI. Anal-sphincter disruption during vaginal delivery. *N Engl J Med.* 1993;329:1905–1911.
60. Ho Yh, Tsang C, Tang CL, Nyam D, Eu KW, Seow-Choen F. Anal sphincter injuries from stapling instruments introduced transanally. *Dis Colon Rectum.* 2000;43:169–173.
61. Halligan S, Sultan AH, Rottenberg G, Bartram CI. Endosongraphy of the anal sphincters in solitary rectal ulcer syndrome. *Int J Colrect Dis.* 1995;10:79–82.
62. Marshall M, Halligan S, Fotheringham T, Bartram C, Nicholls RJ. Predictive value of internal anal sphincter thickness for diagnosis of rectal intussusception in patients with solitary rectal ulcer syndrome. *Br J Surg.* 2002;89:1281–1285.
63. Gabel MB, Teshler M, Barzilai N, Lurie Y, Malnick S, Bass D, Zbar A. Dynamic transperineal ultrasound in the diagnosis of pelvic floor disorders. *Dis Colon Rectum.* 2002;45:239–248.
64. Hinton JM, Lennard-Jones JE, Young AC. A new method for studying gut transit times using radioopaque markers. *Gut* 1969;10:842–847.
65. Martelli H, Devroede G, Arham P, et al. Some parameters of large bowel motility in normal man. *Gastroenterology* 1978;75:612.
66. Metcalf AM, Philips SF, Zinsmeister AR, et al. S Simplified assessment of segmental colonic transit. *Gastroenterology* 1987;92:40–47.
67. Lundin E, Karlbom U, Pahlman L, Graf W. Outcome of segmental colonic resection for slow transit constipation. *Br J Surg.* 2002;89:1270–1274.
68. Ho YH, Yu S, Ang ES, et al. Small colonic J-pouch improves colonicretention of liquids—randomised, controlled trial with scintigraphy. *Dis Colon Rectum.* 2002;45:76–82.
69. Christiansen P, Olsen N, Krogh K, et al. Scintigraphic assessment of retrograde colonic washout in faecal incontinence and constipation. *Dis Colon Rectum.* 2003;46:68–76.
70. Nam YS, Pikarsky AJ, Wexner SD, et al. Reproducibility of colonic transit study in patients with chronic constipation. *Dis Colon Rectum.* 2001;44:86–92.

12
Innovations in the Treatment of Faecal Incontinence

SUSAN C. PARKER and AMY THORSEN

1. Introduction

The medical condition of faecal incontinence is characterised by two predominant factors: its surprisingly high prevalence and the reluctance of patients to seek treatment or discuss the condition with their physician despite severe limitations in their lifestyle. Community studies using postal or telephone surveys report prevalence rates of 1.4%–4.4% [1–3]. Even higher rates are associated with factors such as age, parity, chronic medical conditions, anorectal surgical procedures, and acute medical problems.

Patients with faecal incontinence are more frequently older and female. A US telephone survey that found an overall prevalence of 2.2% also found that 30% of those who reported symptoms were over 65, and 63% were women. A postal survey focused on older patients (age 65–93) found an overall prevalence of 3.7% [4]. One recent study, which surveyed 10,000 adults over age 40, found a similar prevalence between men and women, but in that same study faecal incontinence was associated with a great impact on the quality of life [2].

The association of faecal incontinence with female gender and, more specifically, with obstetric injuries, has received intense scrutiny since 1993, when Sultan et al. reported a high incidence of sphincter injuries after vaginal delivery [5]. In a subsequent review of 11 studies of obstetric patients, Sultan found that 20%–50% of women with sphincter injuries had symptoms of faecal incontinence within the first year postpartum [6]. Karoui et al. reported that, in a series of 335 incontinent patients, 65% had sphincter defects; this percentage increased to 88% in patients who had a history of childbirth or proctologic surgery. In a series of 115 continent patients, Karoui et al. also found that 43% had sphincter defects, so they caution that sphincter defects alone do not lead to faecal incontinence in all patients [7]. A large number of studies have sought to define delivery risk factors, among them parity, maternal age, birth weight, instrumented delivery, and episiotomy [8–10]. Efforts continue to diminish this significant risk factor for women. The controversy regarding the possible protective effect of Caesarean section has even reached the lay press [11].

The rates of faecal incontinence increase dramatically with increasing numbers of other medical problems. Ambulatory patients reported faecal incontinence at rates of 5.6%–15.9% in Switzerland, and 13.4%–26% in the United States [1,12]. However, higher rates have been reported by patients seeing gastroenterologists, colon and rectal surgeons, and urogynaecologists. Persons with diabetes mellitus, multiple sclerosis, or congenital abnormalities constitute additional high-risk groups. Those with diabetes mellitus have reported frequent upper and lower gastrointestinal symptoms that are possibly related to poor glycemic control; faecal incontinence can occur in up to 20% of such patients.

The influence of duration of an underlying disease on the development of faecal incontinence is debated [13,14]. In a series of 280 patients with multiple sclerosis, 51% experienced faecal incontinence at least once a week. This high frequency was true even of the mildly disabled patients [15].

Despite these alarmingly high rates, even greater numbers of patients are not reporting their symptoms because of embarrassment or low expectations regarding available treatment options. In the United States, only one third of symptomatic patients discuss their incontinence symptoms with their physician. In the United Arab Emirates, 60% of multiparous women with faecal incontinence are similarly reticent to seek medical advice [16]. In a postal survey evaluating defaecation disorders in older US patients, only 23% had seen a physician for their symptoms in the past year [4].

The highest rates of faecal incontinence are found in hospitalised or institutionalised patients. A Canadian study of long-term hospital patients found a prevalence of 46% [17]. Similar results were obtained in a US survey of patients in skilled nursing homes: 47% had faecal incontinence, and the rates rose with lengthening time spent in a nursing home [18,19]. In a survey of 152 patients in acute or critical-care units at a Veterans Affairs Medical Center who were assessed for faecal incontinence, stool frequency, tube feedings, and severity of illness, 50 of them (33%) had faecal incontinence. A greater percentage who had diarrhoea also had faecal incontinence (43% with diarrhoea vs 27% without diarrhoea), but faecal incontinence was not associated with any particular cause of diarrhoea, including *Clostridium difficile* colitis [20].

Thus, it is obvious that faecal incontinence has a high prevalence, that patients are reluctant to seek therapy, and that most physicians—whatever patient population they treat—are likely to encounter untreated patients with faecal incontinence. Patients and physicians alike may be poorly informed regarding the available methods of treatment and the exciting advances in this area of coloproctology. Medical management and biofeedback remain the mainstay of clinical treatment of the incontinent patient, the treatment of this condition now includes new methods of pharmacologic modification, injectable materials, implantable devices, neuromodulation, and muscle transposition. Creation of a stoma—the fear of many incontinent patients—remains appropriate for some patients, but hopefully a decreasing number. For some patients who had a stoma created years ago, bowel continuity can now be restored thanks to a successful innovative procedure.

2. Improvements in Old Techniques

2.1. Medical Management and Pharmacology

Medical management, consisting of dietary changes, bulking agents, and bowel-habit training, is effective for mild faecal incontinence. Antidiarrhoeal medications, such as loperamide, diphenoxylate, and bile acid binders, are widely used for patients with altered bowel consistency and faecal incontinence. Even for surgical patients, research continues into new oral and topical medications. Novel medical approaches include estrogen replacement therapy in postmenopausal women, oral amitriptyline, and topical phenylephrine.

In 1996, Franz et al., using immunohistochemical assessment, found estrogen and progesterone receptors in the smooth muscle fibres and stroma of the anal canal in both men and women [21]. According to a 1997 observational study of 20 postmenopausal women with faecal incontinence, hormone replacement therapy resulted in significant physiologic and clinical changes: After 6 months of treatment, the women's resting pressures, squeeze pressures, and maximum tolerated rectal volume significantly increased, and 5 of them were asymptomatic [22]. The authors of both the 1996 and the 1997 studies concluded that hormone replacement therapy might be of benefit for treating faecal incontinence.

Amitriptyline, a tricyclic antidepressant, has anticholinergic and serotonergic properties. Anticholinergic drugs can alter bowel motility, diminishing symptoms of urgency, evacuation frequency, and nocturnal incontinence in pelvic-pouch patients [23,24]. In an open study of low-dose amitriptyline (20mg daily, as compared with daily antidepressant doses of 75–200mg), anal pressures and incontinence scores improved; the number of bowel movements per day and the frequency and amplitude of rectal motor complexes decreased [25]. Given the above 3 studies, clinicians have already adopted its use, although no randomised, controlled trials of amitriptyline for faecal incontinence have been conducted.

The internal anal sphincter receives stimulatory α adrenergic innervation. This observation has prompted investigators to evaluate topical phenylephrine, an α-adrenergic agonist, for treating idiopathic faecal incontinence. An open study of topical phenylephrine, comparing concentrations of 10%–40%, found that all concentrations increased patients' resting pressures; the effect was sustained for 2 hours [26]. But in one randomised, controlled trial, 10% topical phenylephrine was not effective [27]. In another randomised, controlled trial, involving ileoanal pouch patients with faecal incontinence, topical phenylephrine eliminated nocturnal events in some patients [28].

A topical cream or oral medication that would effectively treat faecal incontinence would have clear advantages. Thus, new formulations are likely to be tested and introduced in the future.

2.2. *Biofeedback*

Biofeedback therapy, a behavioural treatment, is noninvasive and cost-effective, with no morbidity. One large series found that it improved clinical symptoms in 50%–90% of patients—a range comparable to other medical and surgical treatments [29–35]. The goal of biofeedback therapy is to enable the patient to contract the pelvic floor and external sphincter muscles in response to rectal distention. Biofeedback requires a co-operative, motivated patient who can respond to audio or visual cues representing physiologic activity.

Biofeedback protocols may incorporate muscular strength training with anal-canal pressure or EMG (electromyography) feedback, rectal sensory training with balloon-pressure feedback, or a combination of both. A recent meta-analysis comparing the combination technique versus strength training demonstrated no significant advantage to either. The same meta-analysis, however, revealed a significant difference in strength training using EMG feedback (74% mean improvement) versus anal-pressure feedback (64% mean improvement) [36]. Other investigators [37,38] stress the importance of sensory training, despite the high success rates of protocols lacking this component. One of the few randomised trials evaluating biofeedback therapy for faecal incontinence compared EMG strength training versus treatment that added sensory training, a home trainer, or both to the strength program. Although all groups improved substantially, no significant difference between treatment groups was found [39]. Fynes et al. found that pure sensory biofeedback was inferior to augmented biofeedback for treating faecal incontinence after obstetric trauma [40].

Even though diverse patient populations have been treated with biofeedback therapy, no obvious clinical or physiologic predictors of success have been identified. Patient age, cause of incontinence, and duration and severity of symptoms do not appear to affect the likelihood of success [35]. Van Tets et al. found no improvement in faecal control in 12 patients with neurogenic incontinence treated with EMG–strength biofeedback [41], yet some benefit has been observed in patients with mild-to-moderate multiple sclerosis [42]. Pretreatment manometric parameters failed to predict response to biofeedback [34]. The presence of an external sphincter defect or pudendal neuropathy may predict poor manometric results after therapy, but appeared not to affect the clinical results of biofeedback [43]. Biofeedback has also been successful in patients for whom other treatments have failed. Jensen et al. found a significant improvement in 89% of patients who had poor functional outcome after sphincteroplasty for obstetric injury [33].

Some investigators have noted deterioration in the effects of biofeedback over time [44–46]. Such deterioration may be dependent on the treatment protocol, on patient compliance, or on the biofeedback clinician. Gilliand et al. identified the number of treatment sessions—5 or greater—as being the one predictor of success for treating incontinent patients with biofeedback [35]. Paget et al. reported the results of long-term follow up of 120 patients treated with 5 monthly sessions of manometric, ultrasound, or digital-exam–guided biofeedback for faecal incontinence. At a mean follow up of 42 months, 14 patients (17%) had gone on to have surgery for faecal incontinence; 6 of these patients ended up with a stoma (7%). Of the patients in that study who responded to a telephone interview (69% response rate), 75% reported symptomatic improvement and 83% reported improvement in quality of life, as compared with pretreatment. Many patients also experienced further improvement in control after they completed biofeedback. Paget et al. concluded that improvement may be secondary to a strong emphasis on continuing pelvic exercises and that "more treatment was better."

2.3. Sphincter Repair

Described initially by Parks et al. in 1971 [47], overlapping sphincteroplasty has become the preferred surgical treatment of faecal incontinence caused by traumatic sphincter injury. The procedure involves mobilising the sphincter muscles sufficiently to allow them to overlap while the defect is repaired. Scar tissue is not excised, but instead preserved to aid in suture fixation. Modifications of the technique include separate plication of the internal anal sphincter [48] and addition of an anterior levatoroplasty to lengthen the anal canal. Tan et al. noted a decrease, from 44% to 11%, in the incidence of wound infections by using a posterior fourchette incision for sphincter repair [49].

Faecal continence improves in 70%–90% of patients after sphincteroplasty [50–53]. Patients with poor preoperative continence, that is, incontinence to solid stool, may have less satisfactory results [54]. Rasmussen et al. [55] reported poor continence after sphincter repair in patients over age 40. But others found that patient age was not a factor in predicting successful outcome [52,53]. After repeat sphincteroplasty, over 50% of patients may significantly improve [56,57]. The routine use of faecal diversion in sphincter repair adds no benefit in functional outcome or wound healing [53,58,59].

Studies have investigated the ability of anorectal physiology testing to (a) preoperatively predict successful sphincter repair and (b) postoperatively correlate findings with functional outcome. Patients with unilateral or bilateral pudendal neuropathy may be less likely to achieve perfect continence after overlapping sphincteroplasty [60,61]; however, continence may still improve significantly, with minimum morbidity [54,62]. Good functional outcome after sphincter repair may correlate with increases in squeeze pressure [63], anal-canal length [64], or high-pressure–zone length [65]. Residual defects visualised on postoperative anal ultrasound are associated with poor clinical outcome; such patients may benefit from an attempt at repeat repair [66,67].

The use of endo-anal ultrasound to evaluate faecal incontinence has identified a small population of patients with isolated internal anal sphincter defects. Most such injuries are attributed to haemorrhoidectomy, lateral internal sphincterotomy, or fistulotomy. Small series have previously showed poor outcome after isolated internal sphincter repair [68,69]. Recently, however, Abou-Zeid described internal anal sphincter repair by direct apposition in a series of 8 patients. At a median follow up of 15 months, all 8 patients improved and 2 achieved full continence [70]. The long-term results, though, are unknown.

The long-term success of overlapping sphincteroplasty has also been questioned. Functional results appear to deteriorate over time. Success rates decrease to 26%–57% after 3 to 4 years of follow up [71–73]. In a telephone survey, Halverson et al. assessed the long-term functional outcomes in 49 (69%) of 71 patients who underwent overlapping sphincteroplasty at the Cleveland Clinic (1989–1996). At a median follow up of 69 months, 54% of the patients were incontinent to liquid or solid stool, and only 14% were completely continent [74]. Despite these poor long-term results, overlapping sphincteroplasty is probably still the best initial treatment of faecal incontinence secondary to traumatic sphincter injury. As anal continence deteriorates with time, however, other medical and surgical methods may need to be employed.

3. New Techniques

Restoring continence to patients when traditional treatment fails, or when traumatic or neurogenic injuries are extensive, remains a challenge. New techniques for intractable faecal incontinence include the artificial anal sphincter, dynamic graciloplasty, and sacral stimulation. For lesser degrees of incontinence, new options such as the injection of bulking agents or the application of radiofrequency to the proximal anal canal are being tested.

3.1. Encirclement Procedures

The earliest and simplest version of anal encirclement was the use of silver wire, described by Thiersch. The dynamic graciloplasty and the artificial anal sphincter are both advanced variations of anal encirclement. A patient may be a candidate for either procedure. Fundamental surgical differences between the 2 techniques and their complication rates, continence rates, and availability will affect which is chosen for a particular patient.

Dynamic graciloplasty combines transposition of the gracilis muscle with electrical stimulation via an implantable pulse generator. The gracilis muscle is preferred because it has a proximal neurovascular bundle and it can be tunneled under the skin in the proximal thigh and wrapped around the anal canal. Applying electrical stimulation to the gracilis muscle allows conversion of the fast-twitch, fatigable leg muscle to a slow-twitch, fatigue-resistant muscle that more closely resembles an anal sphincter.

Baeten et al. first reported the use of electrical stimulation with a gracilis muscle wrap for faecal incontinence in 1988 and subsequently reported a 72% continence rate [75,76]. In a multicentre trial, the success rate was 63% (defined as a greater than 50% improvement in incontinent events). Adverse events were frequent and often required reoperation. The most common complications were infections, problems with device performance and use, gracilis muscle problems, pain, and thromboembolic events. Only major infectious complications had an adverse effect on function. Experienced surgeons have the lowest complication rates and the highest success rates—the learning curve is steep [77,78]. Despite these limitations, once success is achieved, it can be maintained in most patients (56%) at 24 months [79]. Paediatric patients have also undergone successful dynamic graciloplasty [80]. Use of dynamic graciloplasty is limited to Canada and Europe, because Food and Drug Administration approval was not sought in the United States.

Dynamic graciloplasty can also be adapted for total anorectal reconstruction after abdominal perineal resection. Rullier et al. reported the results of 15 patients who underwent reconstruction with a double graciloplasty wrap. All 15 patients received preoperative radiation and chemotherapy. Reconstruction was done in 3 stages: (1) abdominal perineal resection, coloperineal anastomosis, and graciloplasty; (2) insertion of the pulse generator; and (3) reversal of the ileostomy. The main complication was stenosis of the neosphincter, which Rullier et al. attributed to asymmetrical traction from the double gracilis wrap. After 3–48 months of follow up, no local recurrences had occurred, but 2 patients had distant metastases. Functionally, 7 patients were continent; 2 were incontinent; and 3 had stomas. Rullier et al. recommended a single graciloplasty wrap [81].

Rouanet et al. reported success in 5 patients who were continent to solid and liquid stool after a mean follow up of 32 months, but only 1 patient was able to evacuate spontaneously; the others required enemas to evacuate [82]. Delayed anorectal reconstruction, at a mean of 8 years after abdominal perineal resection, was reported by Rongen et al. but with an even higher morbidity, so they subsequently abandoned the procedure [83].

Thus, while feasible and oncologically safe, total anorectal reconstruction remains problematic. It is probably best done only in select sites by experienced surgeons.

3.2. *Artificial Bowel Sphincter*

In the United States, the limited availability of dynamic graciloplasty contributes to a greater enthusiasm for the artificial anal sphincter (Acticon™ bowel sphincter, American Medical Systems, Minnetonka, MN). The 2 procedures are applicable to many of the same patients, unless perineal soft tissue is inadequate, in which case the artificial anal sphincter is a poor choice. Several features of the artificial bowel sphincter make it a more attractive option than the complex dynamic graciloplasty procedure: it is placed in a single operation, it is operational 6 weeks after placement without the need for muscle conditioning, and it avoids a painful muscle transposition.

The artificial anal sphincter currently in use is a modification of an artificial urinary sphincter (AMS 800). An implantable device, it is composed of a silicone elastomer that maintains continence via a fluid-filled cuff surrounding and compressing the anal canal. The patient controls the device via a pump placed in the scrotum or labia. Squeezing the pump 9–12 times forces the fluid from the cuff into a reservoir balloon, which is implanted in the space of Retzius. Squeezing deflates the cuff and opens the anal canal, allowing the passage of stool. The cuff then automatically and slowly reinflates and occludes the anal canal, providing continence until defaecation is again desired.

Christiansen and Lorentzen first reported implantation of an artificial anal sphincter for faecal incontinence in 1987 [84]. Since then, several groups have reported their experience with the AMS 800 and with later modifications [85–90]. In those reports, infections occurred in 15%–25% of the patients and device explantation was necessary in 20%. The final success rates were often over 70%. Complications could be successfully treated, without major morbidity.

A multicentre clinical trial of the artificial anal sphincter consisting of 19 sites in the United Statea, Canada, and Europe was completed in 2000 [91]. In that trial, 112 patients underwent implantation (86 females). The common protocol consisted of a quality-of-life questionnaire, incontinence scoring, and physiology testing at 6 months and at 1 year. At 1 year after implantation, 75 (67%) patients had a functioning device and 3 were lost to follow up. The infection rate was 25%; 51 patients (46%) had revisional surgery. A total of 41 patients (37%) had their devices explanted; 7 underwent successful reimplantation. Quality of life significantly improved for successfully implanted or reimplanted patients. In the trial, as in other studies, patients with functioning devices had a significant increase in resting anal-canal pressures, as compared with their preoperative status [90,92].

In the trial, a successful clinical result was defined as a decrease in the faecal incontinence score (FISS) of at least 24 points (score range, 0–120), indicating a drop of at least 2 levels. For example, a patient incontinent to liquid and solid stool daily before surgery could report several incontinent events a month, but not weekly, for the procedure to be judged clinically successful. To qualify for the trial, patients needed an FISS of at least 88 or a stoma. After 1 year of follow up, the mean FISS score for trial participants had dropped from 105 (incontinent to liquid and solid stool daily) to 48 (incontinent to seepage). A valid criticism of the trial is the use of a scoring system (instead of diary data) that may not be as accurate, yet patients whose procedure was a success saw a dramatic drop in their scores.

At the University of Minnesota, we recently reported our long-term experience with the artificial anal sphincter [93]. Beginning in 1989, 45 consecutive patients underwent artificial bowel sphincter placement (Group I, 1989–1992, n = 10; Group II, 1997–2001, n = 35). Of the 10 Group I patients, 7 currently have a functioning device (mean follow up, 91 m; range, 29–143 m). Of the 35 Group II patients, 17 (49%) have a functioning artificial bowel sphincter (mean follow up, 39 m; range, 12–60 m). The criterion of at least a 24-point FISS drop (used for the trial to define functional success) was easily met by our patients: their average drop was 54 points at 1 year and 90 points at 24 months or more after implantation. The increase seen after 1 year reflects improvement after successful revisions. Such patients may very well experience unaltered long-term function, as evidenced by Group I patients whose devices have functioned for over 10 years.

Patients who lack sufficient perineal soft tissue pose a particular challenge when insertion of an artificial sphincter is contemplated. We have employed a modified technique for such patients. It consists of initial perineal reconstruction with a gluteal rotational skin advancement flap, followed by delayed insertion of an artificial sphincter. Subsequently, the artificial bowel sphincter is placed with the patient in a prone position, which facilitates creation of the perianal tunnels and placement of the cuff higher than usual within the levator ani muscle. The patient is then repositioned in a lithotomy position, and the implantation of the pump and reservoir balloon completed in the usual manner. Of 3 patients in the above Minnesota series who underwent this modified technique, 2 had a successful outcome.

3.3. Dynamic Graciloplasty Versus Artificial Anal Sphincter

No randomised trials have compared the dynamic graciloplasty versus the artificial anal sphincter. It is unlikely that one could be conducted, given the limited number of surgeons experienced in both procedures. In a 2000 consensus paper on standards for anal-sphincter replacement, leading experts in the treatment of faecal incontinence gave these guidelines for the choice of procedure:

> Implantation of the artificial anal sphincter is indicated in patients with anal incontinence caused by neurologic disease that affects the muscles of the lower extrem-

> ities, or trauma. The gracilis wrap may be preferable to the artificial anal sphincter in patients with very thin or scarred perineums caused by previous obstetric trauma, perianal infections, surgery, or radiation. [94]

This 2000 consensus statement reflected the state of the art in 1998, so it already may be somewhat outdated. As Madoff et al. pointed out, sphincter replacement is still in its infancy. At the time of that statement, promising new techniques, such as sacral stimulation, were untested. The evaluation of such techniques requires objective evidence of improvement in continence and in quality of life. The consensus team preferred daily diary data to continence scores. The suggested quality-of-life instrument was the form introduced by the American Society of Colon and Rectal Surgeons [95].

Patients with intractable faecal incontinence who undergo successful dynamic graciloplasty or artificial anal sphincter placement can expect long-term improvement in continence and in quality of life. But both procedures are associated with high morbidity and high infection rates. Any differences in the degree of continence improvement remain unknown, because different measurement tools (scores vs diaries) have been used for the 2 procedures. Their varied availability (i.e., dynamic graciloplasty and artificial anal sphincter in Europe and Canada, but only artificial anal sphincter in the United States) will influence future studies.

3.4. Sacral Nerve Stimulation

Sacral nerve stimulation, like the artificial anal sphincter, was initially devised for urinary incontinence. In 1995, Matzel et al. introduced the use of sacral stimulation to treat patients with functional, but not anatomic, deficits of the anal sphincter muscle [96]. The procedure entails placing an electrode in a sacral foramen (S2, S3, or S4) to stimulate the nerve roots. The desired effect is maximum contraction of pelvic muscles with minimal stimulation of the fibres to the lower extremity. Once the optimal site is selected, the lead is connected to a temporary external pulse generator for a test period of stimulation, currently 3 weeks. If function improves adequately at the end of the test period, a permanent pulse generator is implanted. Both the initial operation for lead placement and subsequent pulse generator placement are well-tolerated procedures done under light sedation.

Since the initial description by Matzel et al. of neuromodulation for faecal incontinence, other investigators have reported their experience with sacral nerve stimulation. Many have used temporary percutaneous leads or permanent sacral leads, placed via a closed technique or an open laminectomy. Whether used for short-term stimulation (usually under 2 weeks) or for chronic stimulation (for up to 5 years), sacral neuromodulation produces consistently significant results: it decreases incontinent episodes and alters anal and rectal physiologic measurements. But all published reports involve small numbers of patients, and no randomised trials have been done [97–100].

The indications for sacral stimulation are quickly being expanded, given its low morbidity, its promising results in a wide variety of urology patients, and the finding that the stimulation effect is not confined to the striated muscle [101]. Stimulation of the efferent motor nerves does seem to increase anal canal pressures because of contraction of the anal-sphincter muscles. Conversion of muscle fibres may also occur, as with dynamic graciloplasty [96]. Some, but not all, studies have reported an increase in resting anal canal pressures [97–99,101]. Sacral stimulation may modulate sacral reflexes and sacral parasympathetic nerves, thereby altering rectal contractile activity and rectal sensitivity [101]. The initial assumption that a patient needs an intact sphincter and pudendal nerve is already being challenged: sacral stimulation has been successful in patients with sphincter disruption [100]. It has also been successful in patients with constipation, chronic pelvic pain, and complete spinal cord injuries. It modulates bowel and bladder control and decreases care-related costs [97,102–104]. An international multicentre trial evaluating sacral stimulation for faecal incontinence will help define the best patients for this promising treatment.

3.5. Anal-Canal Bulking Agents

Unfortunately, few options remain if standard therapy fails for a patient who is not a candidate for an encirclement procedure or for sacral stimulation (whether because of the degree of incontinence or comorbid conditions). This problematic group also includes patients with minor amounts of stool leakage: the so-called seepers. Adding a bulking agent to the anal canal to augment resting tone has obvious appeal; bulking agents are routinely used for treating urinary incontinence caused by intrinsic urinary sphincter deficiency. Implantable microballoons, autologous fat, and collagen have all been successful in small series, with low morbidity [105–108]. Success may require repeated injections, and migration of the injected material has been reported. Manometric pressures are not significantly altered.

An alternative method under investigation for altering anal-canal resting tone is radiofrequency. A device is inserted into the anal canal with electrodes that, when deployed, pierce the mucosa to apply radiofrequency energy to the muscle. Thermal lesions are created in the muscle to alter collagen contractility and to achieve a tissue-tightening effect, while preserving mucosal integrity [109]. Takahashi et al. reported on a small series of 10 patients whose continence scores decreased by 12 months, but they did not experience a significant change in their quality of life. Bleeding occurred in 4 of the 10 patients. After application of radiofrequency, all 10 patients had a reduction in their initial rectal sensation volume and in their maximum tolerable rectal volume. A multicentre trial is currently underway.

4. Summary

The initial treatment of a patient with faecal incontinence still consists of medical management, biofeedback, or surgical repair. Innovations in standard therapies include the introduction of new pharmacologic options, refinements in surgical and biofeedback techniques, and a better appreciation of the long-term limitations of sphincter reconstruction. Anal sphincter replacement is possible with dynamic graciloplasty or with the artificial anal sphincter; optimal patient selection for each procedure is still being defined. Sacral stimulation does not preclude the later use of either of the 2 anal sphincter replacement techniques; thus, it may eventually be accorded an earlier position in the treatment sequence. Other therapies such as anal-canal bulking agents and radiofrequency have low morbidity, but are largely untested.

Acknowledgments. The authors thank Alexandra A. Broek, BA, for assistance in preparation of the manuscript, and Mary E. Knatterud, PhD, for editorial help.

References

1. Johanson JF, Lafferty J. Epidemiology of fecal incontinence: the silent affliction. *Am J Gastroenterol.* 1996;91:33–36.
2. Perry S, Shaw C, McGrother C, et al. Prevalence of faecal incontinence in adults aged 40 years or more living in the community. *Gut* 2002;50:480–484.
3. Nelson R, Norton N, Cautley E, Furner S. Community-based prevalence of anal incontinence. *JAMA.* 1995;274:559–561.
4. Talley NJ, O'Keefe EA, Zinsmeister AR, Melton LJ 3rd. Prevalence of gastrointestinal symptoms in the elderly: a population-based study. *Gastroenterology* 1992;102:895–901.
5. Sultan AH, Kamm MA, Hudson CN, Thomas JM, Bartram CI. Anal-sphincter disruption during vaginal delivery. *N Engl J Med.* 1993;329:1905–1911.
6. Sultan AH. Anal incontinence after childbirth. *Curr Opin Obstet Gynecol.* 1997;9:320–324.
7. Karoui S, Savoye-Collet C, Koning E, Leroi AM, Denis P. Prevalence of anal sphincter defects revealed by sonography in 335 incontinent patients and 115 continent patients. *Am J Roentgenol.* 1999;173:389–392.
8. Eason E, Labrecque M, Marcoux S, Mondor M. Anal incontinence after childbirth. *CMAJ.* 2002;166:326–330.
9. Zetterstrom J, Lopez A, Anzen B, Norman M, Holmstrom B, Mellgren A. Anal sphincter tears at vaginal delivery: risk factors and clinical outcome of primary repair. *Obstet Gynecol.* 1999;94:21–28.
10. Eason E, Labrecque M, Wells G, Feldman P. Preventing perineal trauma during childbirth: a systematic review. *Obstet Gynecol.* 2000;95:464–471.

11. Springen K. The right to choose. Cesarean sections are on the rise again. Public-health officials want to limit them, but many patients and doctors are resisting. *Newsweek* 2000;136:73–74.
12. Faltin DL, Sangalli MR, Curtin F, Morabia A, Weil A. Prevalence of anal incontinence and other anorectal symptoms in women. *Int Urogynecol J Pelvic Floor Dysfunct.* 2001;12:117–120; discussion 121.
13. Bytzer P, Talley NJ, Leemon M, Young LJ, Jones MP, Horowitz M. Prevalence of gastrointestinal symptoms associated with diabetes mellitus: a popul-ation-based survey of 15 000 adults. *Arch Intern Med.* 2001;161:1989–1996.
14. Epanomeritakis E, Koutsoumbi P, Tsiaoussis I, et al. Impairment of anorectal function in diabetes mellitus parallels duration of disease. *Dis Colon Rectum.* 1999;42:1394–1400.
15. Hinds JP, Eidelman BH, Wald A. Prevalence of bowel dysfunction in multiple sclerosis. A population survey. *Gastroenterology* 1990;98:1538–1542.
16. Rizk DE, Hassan MY, Shaheen H, Cherian JV, Micallef R, Dunn E. The prevalence and determinants of health care-seeking behavior for fecal incontinence in multiparous United Arab Emirates females. *Dis Colon Rectum.* 2001;44: 1850–1856.
17. Borrie MJ, Davidson HA. Incontinence in institutions: costs and contributing factors. *CMAJ.* 1992;147:322–328.
18. Nelson R, Furner S, Jesudason V. Fecal incontinence in Wisconsin nursing homes: prevalence and associations. *Dis Colon Rectum.* 1998;41:1226–1229.
19. Chassagne P, Landrin I, Neveu C, et al. Fecal incontinence in the institutionalized elderly: incidence, risk factors, and prognosis. *Am J Med.* 1999;106: 185–190.
20. Bliss DZ, Johnson S, Savik K, Clabots CR, Gerding DN. Fecal incontinence in hospitalized patients who are acutely ill. *Nurs Res.* 2000;49:101–108.
21. Franz HB, Wendler D, Oettling G. Immunohistochemical assessment of steroid hormone receptors in tissues of the anal canal. Implications for anal incontinence? *Acta Obstet Gynecol Scand.* 1996;75:892–895.
22. Donnelly V, O'Connell PR, O'Herlihy C. The influence of oestrogen replacement on faecal incontinence in postmenopausal women. *Br J Obstet Gynaecol.* 1997;104:311–315.
23. Hallgren T, Fasth S, Delbro D, Nordgren S, Oresland T, Hulten L. The effects of atropine or benzilonium on pelvic pouch and anal sphincter functions. *Scand J Gastroenterol.* 1991;26:563–571.
24. Farrar JT. The effects of drugs on intestinal motility. *Clin Gastroenterol.* 1982; 11:673–681.
25. Santoro GA, Eitan BZ, Pryde A, Bartolo DC. Open study of low-dose amitriptyline in the treatment of patients with idiopathic fecal incontinence. *Dis Colon Rectum.* 2000;43:1676–1681; discussion 1681–1682.
26. Cheetham MJ, Kamm MA, Phillips RK. Topical phenylephrine increases anal canal resting pressure in patients with faecal incontinence. *Gut* 2001;48: 356–359.
27. Carapeti EA, Kamm MA, Phillips RK. Randomized controlled trial of topical phenylephrine in the treatment of faecal incontinence. *Br J Surg.* 2000;87: 38–42.

28. Carapeti EA, Kamm MA, Nicholls RJ, Phillips RK. Randomized, controlled trial of topical phenylephrine for fecal incontinence in patients after ileoanal pouch construction. *Dis Colon Rectum.* 2000;43:1059–1063.
29. Haskell B, Rovner H. Electromyography in the management of the incompetent anal sphincter. *Dis Colon Rectum.* 1967;10:81–84.
30. Cerulli MA, Nikoomanesh P, Schuster MM. Progress in biofeedback conditioning for fecal incontinence. *Gastroenterology* 1979;76:742–746.
31. MacLeod JH. Biofeedback in the management of partial anal incontinence. *Dis Colon Rectum.* 1983;26:244–246.
32. MacLeod JH. Management of anal incontinence by biofeedback. *Gastroenterology* 1987;93:291–294.
33. Jensen LL, Lowry AC. Biofeedback improves functional outcome after sphincteroplasty. *Dis Colon Rectum.* 1997;40:197–200.
34. Sangwan YP, Coller JA, Barrett RC, Roberts PL, Murray JJ, Schoetz DJ Jr. Can manometric parameters predict response to biofeedback therapy in fecal incontinence? *Dis Colon Rectum.* 1995;38:1021–1025.
35. Gilliland R, Heymen S, Altomare DF, Park UC, Vickers D, Wexner SD. Outcome and predictors of success of biofeedback for constipation. *Br J Surg.* 1997;84:1123–1126.
36. Heymen S, Jones KR, Ringel Y, Scarlett Y, Whitehead WE. Biofeedback treatment of fecal incontinence: a critical review. *Dis Colon Rectum.* 2001;44:728–736.
37. Miner PB, Donnelly TC, Read NW. Investigation of mode of action of biofeedback in treatment of fecal incontinence. *Dig Dis Sci.* 1990;35:1291–1298.
38. Chiarioni G, Bassotti G, Stanganini S, Vantini I, Whitehead WE, Stegagnini S. Sensory retraining is key to biofeedback therapy for formed stool fecal incontinence. *Am J Gastroenterol.* 2002;97:109–117.
39. Heymen S, Pikarsky AJ, Weiss EG, Vickers D, Nogueras JJ, Wexner SD. A prospective randomized trial comparing four biofeedback techniques for fecal incontinence. *Colorectal Dis.* 2000;2:88–92.
40. Fynes MM, Marshall K, Cassidy M, et al. A prospective, randomized study comparing the effect of augmented biofeedback with sensory biofeedback alone on fecal incontinence after obstetric trauma. *Dis Colon Rectum.* 1999;42:753–758; discussion 758–761.
41. van Tets WF, Kuijpers JH, Bleijenberg G. Biofeedback treatment is ineffective in neurogenic fecal incontinence. *Dis Colon Rectum.* 1996;39:992–994.
42. Wiesel PH, Norton C, Roy AJ, Storrie JB, Bowers J, Kamm MA. Gut focused behavioural treatment (biofeedback) for constipation and faecal incontinence in multiple sclerosis. *J Neurol Neurosurg Psychiatry.* 2000;69:240–243.
43. Leroi AM, Dorival MP, Lecouturier MF, et al. Pudendal neuropathy and severity of incontinence but not presence of an anal sphincter defect may determine the response to biofeedback therapy in fecal incontinence. *Dis Colon Rectum.* 1999;42:762–769.
44. Guillemot F, Bouche B, Gower-Rousseau C, et al. Biofeedback for the treatment of fecal incontinence. Long-term clinical results. *Dis Colon Rectum.* 1995;38:393–397.
45. Rieger NA, Wattchow DA, Sarre RG, et al. Prospective trial of pelvic floor retraining in patients with fecal incontinence. *Dis Colon Rectum.* 1997;40:821–826.

46. Whitehead WE, Burgio KL, Engel BT. Biofeedback treatment of fecal incontinence in geriatric patients. *J Am Geriatr Soc.* 1985;33:320–324.
47. Parks AG, McPartlin JF. Late repair of injuries of the anal sphincter. *Proc R Soc Med.* 1971;64:1187–1189.
48. Wexner SD, Marchetti F, Jagelman DG. The role of sphincteroplasty for fecal incontinence reevaluated: a prospective physiologic and functional review. *Dis Colon Rectum.* 1991;34:22–30.
49. Tan M, O'Hanlon DM, Cassidy M, O'Connell PR. Advantages of a posterior fourchette incision in anal sphincter repair. *Dis Colon Rectum.* 2001;44: 1624–1629.
50. Fleshman JW, Peters WR, Shemesh EI, Fry RD, Kodner IJ. Anal sphincter reconstruction: anterior overlapping muscle repair. *Dis Colon Rectum.* 1991;34: 739–743.
51. Engel AF, Kamm MA, Sultan AH, Bartram CI, Nicholls RJ. Anterior anal sphincter repair in patients with obstetric trauma. *Br J Surg.* 1994;84: 1231–1234.
52. Simmang C, Birnbaum EH, Kodner IJ, Fry RD, Fleshman JW. Anal sphincter reconstruction in the elderly: does advancing age affect outcome? *Dis Colon Rectum.* 1994;37:1065–1069.
53. Young CJ, Mathur MN, Eyers AA, Solomon MJ. Successful overlapping anal sphincter repair: relationship to patient age, neuropathy, and colostomy formation. *Dis Colon Rectum.* 1998;41:344–349.
54. Buie WD, Lowry AC, Rothenberger DA, Madoff RD. Clinical rather than laboratory assessment predicts continence after anterior sphincteroplasty. *Dis Colon Rectum.* 2001;44:1255–1260.
55. Rasmussen OO, Puggaard L, Christiansen J. Anal sphincter repair in patients with obstetric trauma: age affects outcome. *Dis Colon Rectum.* 1999;42: 193–195.
56. Giordano P, Renzi A, Efron J, et al. Previous sphincter repair does not affect the outcome of repeat repair. *Dis Colon Rectum.* 2002;45:635–640.
57. Pinedo G, Vaizey CJ, Nicholls RJ, Roach R, Halligan S, Kamm MA. Results of repeat anal sphincter repair. *Br J Surg.* 1999;86:66–69.
58. Slade MS, Goldberg SM, Schottler JL, Balcos EG, Christenson CE. Sphincteroplasty for acquired anal incontinence. *Dis Colon Rectum.* 1977;20:33–35.
59. Hasegawa H, Yoshioka K, Keighley MR. Randomized trial of fecal diversion for sphincter repair. *Dis Colon Rectum.* 2000;43:961–964; discussion 964–965.
60. Sangwan YP, Coller JA, Barrett RC, et al. Unilateral pudendal neuropathy. Impact on outcome of anal sphincter repair. *Dis Colon Rectum.* 1996;39: 686–689.
61. Gilliland R, Altomare DF, Moreira H Jr., Oliveira L, Gilliland JE, Wexner SD. Pudendal neuropathy is predictive of failure following anterior overlapping sphincteroplasty. *Dis Colon Rectum.* 1998;41:1516–1522.
62. Chen AS, Luchtefeld MA, Senagore AJ, Mackeigan JM, Hoyt C. Pudendal nerve latency. Does it predict outcome of anal sphincter repair? *Dis Colon Rectum.* 1998;41:1005–1009.
63. Ha HT, Fleshman JW, Smith M, Read TE, Kodner IJ, Birnbaum EH. Manometric squeeze pressure difference parallels functional outcome after overlapping sphincter reconstruction. *Dis Colon Rectum.* 2001;44: 655–660.

64. Hool GR, Lieber ML, Church JM. Postoperative anal canal length predicts outcome in patients having sphincter repair for fecal incontinence. *Dis Colon Rectum.* 1999;42:313–318.
65. Oliveira L, Pfeifer J, Wexner SD. Physiological and clinical outcome of anterior sphincteroplasty. *Br J Surg.* 1996;83:502–505.
66. Ternent CA, Shashidharan M, Blatchford GJ, Christensen MA, Thorson AG, Sentovich SM. Transanal ultrasound and anorectal physiology findings affecting continence after sphincteroplasty. *Dis Colon Rectum.* 1997;40:462–467.
67. Felt-Bersma RJ, Cuesta MA, Koorevaar M. Anal sphincter repair improves anorectal function and endosonographic image. A prospective clinical study. *Dis Colon Rectum.* 1996;39:878–885.
68. Morgan R, Patel B, Beynon J, Carr ND. Surgical management of anorectal incontinence due to internal anal sphincter deficiency. *Br J Surg.* 1997;84:226–230.
69. Leroi AM, Kamm MA, Weber J, Denis P, Hawley PR. Internal anal sphincter repair. *Int J Colorectal Dis.* 1997;12:243–245.
70. Abou-Zeid AA. Preliminary experience in management of fecal incontinence caused by internal anal sphincter injury. *Dis Colon Rectum.* 2000;43:198–202; discussion 204.
71. Yoshioka K, Keighley MR. Sphincter repair for fecal incontinence. *Dis Colon Rectum.* 1989;32:39–42.
72. Ctercteko GC, Fazio VW, Jagelman DG, Lavery IC, Weakley FL, Melia M. Anal sphincter repair: a report of 60 cases and review of the literature. *Aust N Z J Surg.* 1988;58:703–710.
73. Engel AF, van Baal SJ, Brummelkamp WH. Late results of anterior sphincter plication for traumatic faecal incontinence. *Eur J Surg.* 1994;160:633–636.
74. Halverson AL, Hull TL. Long-term outcome of overlapping anal sphincter repair. *Dis Colon Rectum.* 2002;45:345–348.
75. Baeten C, Spaans F, Fluks A. An implanted neuromuscular stimulator for fecal continence following previously implanted gracilis muscle. Report of a case. *Dis Colon Rectum.* 1988;31:134–137.
76. Baeten GMI, Geerdes BP, Adang EMM, et al. Anal dynamic graciloplasty in the treatment of intractable fecal incontinence. *N Engl J Med.* 1995;332:1600–1605.
77. Baeten CG, Bailey HR, Bakka A, et al. Safety and efficacy of dynamic graciloplasty for fecal incontinence: report of a prospective, multicenter trial. Dynamic Graciloplasty Therapy Study Group. *Dis Colon Rectum.* 2000;43:743–751.
78. Matzel KE, Madoff RD, LaFontaine LJ, et al. Complications of dynamic graciloplasty: incidence, management, and impact on outcome. *Dis Colon Rectum.* 2001;44:1427–1435.
79. Wexner SD, Baeten C, Bailey R, et al. Long-term efficacy of dynamic graciloplasty for fecal incontinence. *Dis Colon Rectum.* 2002;45:809–818.
80. Ruckauer KD. Dynamic graciloplasty in children with fecal incontinence: a preliminary report. *J Pediatr Surg.* 2001;36:1036–1039.
81. Rullier E, Zerbib F, Laurent C, Caudry M, Saric J. Morbidity and functional outcome after double dynamic graciloplasty for anorectal reconstruction. *Br J Surg.* 2000;87:909–913.

82. Rouanet P, Senesse P, Bouamrirene D, et al. Anal sphincter reconstruction by dynamic graciloplasty after abdominoperineal resection for cancer. *Dis Colon Rectum.* 1999;42:451–456.
83. Rongen MJ, Dekker FA, Geerdes BP, Heineman E, Baeten CG. Secondary coloperineal pull-through and double dynamic graciloplasty after Miles resection–feasible, but with a high morbidity. *Dis Colon Rectum.* 1999;42:776–780; discussion 781.
84. Christiansen J, Lorentzen M. Implantation of artificial sphincter for anal incontinence. *Lancet* 1987:244–245.
85. Altomare DF, Dodi G, La Torre F, Romano G, Melega E, Rinaldi M. Multicentre retrospective analysis of the outcome of artificial anal sphincter implantation for severe faecal incontinence. *Br J Surg.* 2001;88:1481–1486.
86. O'Brien PE, Skinner S. Restoring control: the Acticon Neosphincter artificial bowel sphincter in the treatment of anal incontinence. *Dis Colon Rectum.* 2000; 43:1213–1216.
87. Christiansen J, Rasmussen OO, Lindorff-Larsen K. Long-term results of artificial anal sphincter implantation for severe anal incontinence. *Ann Surg.* 1999;230:45–48.
88. Lehur PA, Glemain P, Bruley des Varannes S, Buzelin JM, Leborgne J. Outcome of patients with an implanted artificial anal sphincter for severe faecal incontinence. A single institution report. *Int J Colorectal Dis.* 1998; 13:88–92.
89. Wong WD, Jensen LL, Bartolo DC, Rothenberger DA. Artificial anal sphincter. *Dis Colon Rectum.* 1996;39:1345–1351.
90. Lehur PA, Roig JV, Duinslaeger M. Artificial anal sphincter: prospective clinical and manometric evaluation. *Dis Colon Rectum.* 2000;43:1100–1106.
91. Wong WD, Group ACT. The artificial bowel sphincter-results of a multicenter clinical trial. *Dis Colon Rectum.* 2001;44:A5–A26.
92. Ortiz H, Armendariz P, DeMiguel M, Ruiz MD, Alos R, Roig JV. Complications and functional outcome following artificial anal sphincter implantation. *Br J Surg.* 2002;89:877–881.
93. Congilosi S, Spencer M, Madoff R, Jensen L, Wong W, Rothenberger D. The artificial bowel sphincter: long-term experience at a single institution [abstract]. *Dis Colon Rectum.* 2002;45:A26.
94. Madoff RD, Baeten CG, Christiansen J, et al. Standards for anal sphincter replacement. *Dis Colon Rectum.* 2000;43:135–141.
95. Rockwood TH, Church JM, Fleshman JW, et al. Fecal Incontinence Quality of Life Scale: quality of life instrument for patients with fecal incontinence. *Dis Colon Rectum.* 2000;43:9–16; discussion 17.
96. Matzel KE, Stadelmaier U, Hohenfellner M, Gall FP. Electrical stimulation of sacral spinal nerves for treatment of faecal incontinence. *Lancet* 1995; 346:1124–1127.
97. Ganio E, Masin A, Ratto C, et al. Short-term sacral nerve stimulation for functional anorectal and urinary disturbances: results in 40 patients: evaluation of a new option for anorectal functional disorders. *Dis Colon Rectum.* 2001; 44:1261–1267.
98. Rosen HR, Urbarz C, Holzer B, Novi G, Schiessel R. Sacral nerve stimulation as a treatment for fecal incontinence. *Gastroenterology* 2001;121:536–541.

99. Matzel KE, Stadelmaier U, Hohenfellner M, Hohenberger W. Chronic sacral spinal nerve stimulation for fecal incontinence: long- term results with foramen and cuff electrodes. *Dis Colon Rectum.* 2001;44:59–66.
100. Malouf AJ, Vaizey CJ, Nicholls RJ, Kamm MA. Permanent sacral nerve stimulation for fecal incontinence. *Ann Surg.* 2000;232:143–148.
101. Vaizey CJ, Kamm MA, Turner IC, Nicholls RJ, Woloszko J. Effects of short term sacral nerve stimulation on anal and rectal function in patients with anal incontinence. *Gut* 1999;44:407–412.
102. Creasey GH, Grill JH, Korsten M, et al. An implantable neuroprosthesis for restoring bladder and bowel control to patients with spinal cord injuries: a multicenter trial. *Arch Phys Med Rehabil.* 2001;82:1512–1519.
103. Siegel S, Paszkiewicz E, Kirkpatrick C, Hinkel B, Oleson K. Sacral nerve stimulation in patients with chronic intractable pelvic pain. *J Urol.* 2001; 166:1742–1745.
104. Creasey GH, Dahlberg JE. Economic consequences of an implanted neuroprosthesis for bladder and bowel management. *Arch Phys Med Rehabil.* 2001; 82:1520–1525.
105. Feretis C, Benakis P, Dailianas A, et al. Implantation of microballoons in the management of fecal incontinence. *Dis Colon Rectum.* 2001;44:1605–1609.
106. Bernardi C, Favetta U, Pescatori M. Autologous fat injection for treatment of fecal incontinence: manometric and echographic assessment. *Plast Reconstr Surg.* 1998;102:1626–1628.
107. Kumar D, Benson MJ, Bland JE. Glutaraldehyde cross-linked collagen in the treatment of faecal incontinence. *Br J Surg.* 1998;85:978–979.
108. Shafik A. Perianal injection of autologous fat for treatment of sphincteric incontinence. *Dis Colon Rectum.* 1995;38:583–587.
109. Takahashi T, Garcia-Osogobio S, Valdovinos MA, et al. Radio-frequency energy delivery to the anal canal for the treatment of fecal incontinence. *Dis Colon Rectum.* 2002;45:915–922.

13
Surgical Management of Constipation

Ian G. Finlay and Andrew A. Renwick

1. Introduction

Many patients complain of constipation but few require surgery. While symptoms may be improved when surgery is performed, injudicious intervention may make symptoms worse, causing patient discontentment and, all too frequently, litigation. Consequently, a carefully planned strategy is required for the identification of those patients who will benefit from surgery and for the selection of an appropriate operation. In this chapter the authors describe the protocol used in the Department of Coloproctology, Glasgow Royal Infirmary, for the investigation and management of patients with severe constipation referred for a surgical opinion.

Constipation is a generic term that may imply a number of different symptoms [1] and at the outset the clinician requires to elicit which of these symptoms is predominant. In the first instance, it is important to determine the duration of symptoms. Are they life-long, dating to childhood (as in idiopathic slow-transit constipation, Hirchsprung's disease, or megarectum) or do they have a clear precipitating factor (postchildbirth, postpelvic surgery, or after severe gastroenteritis)? What does the patient mean by constipation? Is it the complete absence of the call to stool with bloating and nausea (as in slow transit) or is it a sensation of weight and fullness in the perineum with a sensation of incomplete evacuation (as in perineal descent syndrome and rectal intussusception/prolapse)? Does the patient digitally aid defaecation by supporting the posterior vaginal wall, the classic symptom of rectocoele, or do they attempt to provide support behind the anus, a feature of generalised weakness of the pelvic floor with perineal descent? Finally, it is important to identify whether the most troublesome symptom is pain. Patients who benefit most from surgery for constipation do not report pain as a prominent symptom. The presence of severe abdominal pain should raise the suspicion of underlying irritable bowel syndrome, an absolute contraindication to surgical intervention.

When patients are referred for a surgical opinion for constipation they have usually already had a full range of laxatives and basic investigations.

It is important, however, to be aware of any medications that may constipate such as analgesics, psychotropics, or the use/over use of over-the-counter medicines. All patients should have thyroid function tests and a radiological examination of the large bowel. Every year we identify 2 or 3 patients with previously undiagnosed myxoedema in whom symptoms resolve when thyroxine is prescribed. It should also be noted that myxoedema is associated with rectal prolapse/intussusception. A contrast study is preferred to colonoscopy because in addition to excluding a carcinoma, contrast study gives an indication of the diameter of the hindgut and allows a major distinction to be made between patients. Individuals can be classified as having constipation with a normal caliber colon/rectum or constipation with a megabowel.

A contrast study also gives an impression of the redundancy of the bowel and may identify the presence of colonic volvulus.

2. Severe Constipation and Normal Caliber Colon/Rectum

2.1. Investigations

Having identified that the patient has a normal diameter colon and rectum, the two most useful and easily performed investigations are evacuation proctography and a colonic transit study [2]. The colonic transit study crucially confirms that the patient has objective evidence of severe constipation. The test does not need to be complicated and can be performed in any hospital with X-ray facilities. Patients are given 20 inert markers (Sims Portex®) to swallow and advised to avoid using laxatives or enemata. The presence of 5 markers at 5 days after ingestion on a straight abdominal X-ray indicates constipation, more than 5 markers indicates severe constipation. This is an important initial test because many patients referred with constipation, who consider their symptoms to be severe, will have a normal transit study. Although more complicated scintigraphic and differential transit studies have been described and can be useful, it is not the authors' practice to use these at this screening stage. The value and role of proctography is more controversial and less well defined because it is less objective. It will, however, identify gross anatomical abnormalities and those patients with obstructed defaecation or anismus who are unable to empty even liquid from the rectum due to pelvic-floor spasm. On the basis of these investigations there are 4 possible combinations of results (Figure 13.1) that are used to determine the need for further investigations and the development of a treatment plan. These are: (a) delayed transit and a normal proctogram, (b) normal transit and an abnormal proctogram, (c) delayed transit and an abnormal proctogram, and (d) normal transit and a normal proctogram.

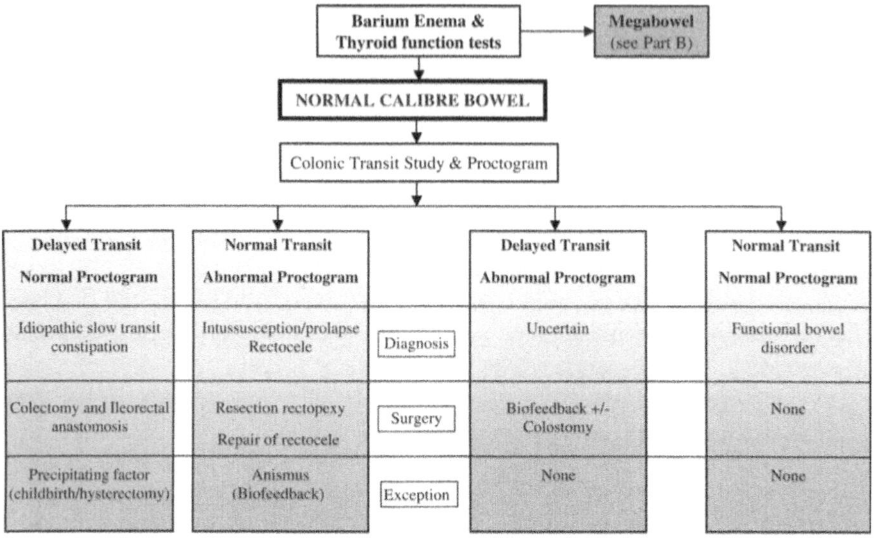

FIGURE 13.1. Flow chart demonstrating the investigative pathway in constipated patients.

2.1.1. Delayed Colonic Transit and a Normal Proctogram (Slow-transit Constipation)

The combination of delayed colonic transit and a normal proctogram typically identifies those patients who have slow-transit constipation, that is, patients who have objective evidence of delayed transit and normal evacuation. The symptoms may be either idiopathic or attributed to a specific event such as childbirth, hysterectomy, or, occasionally, severe gastroenteritis. These 2 distinct clinical patterns probably have a different pathophysiology although they are frequently reported together as a single entity. Classical idiopathic slow-transit constipation (ISTC) is a disorder of young females, in whom the symptoms are life-long, dating to childhood. Patients with ISTC have an absence of the call to stool with symptoms of nausea and abdominal distension. Bowel movements may be as infrequent as once every 2–3 weeks and then only with the use of laxatives. Although these patients may complain of abdominal discomfort (especially prior to evacuation), pain is not a prominent symptom and if present should raise the suspicion that the underlying diagnosis is one of irritable bowel syndrome. Surgery should be avoided in patients in whom pain is the predominant symptom because it is rarely successful [3].

The exact aetiology of idiopathic slow-transit constipation is unknown but it may have a genetic basis because there is frequently a positive family history [4]. Several studies have shown an abnormality of colonic motility characterised by a reduction in the frequency, amplitude, and duration of propulsive contractions in the large bowel [5]. There is a similar abnormality in the small bowel where spontaneous mechanical activity arises from electrical activity of lower intensity and of shorter duration [6] than in controls. It has been suggested that these features may be related to a colonic smooth-muscle myopathy that in turn leads to the inability of the surface membrane to initiate and maintain periods of high-frequency spike activity [5,7].

At the biochemical level, abnormalities have been identified in both nitric oxide synthetase and vasoactive intestinal peptide-containing neurons [8,9], which may explain the observation that there is a myenteric nerve abnormality with a functional cholinergic deficit in response to electrical stimulation [10,11]. Quantitative tests suggest the presence of a small-fibre neuropathy [4]. In addition, it has recently been reported that the interstitial cells of Cajal that are required for normal intestinal motility are reduced throughout the colon and rectum [12,13], suggesting that this is an abnormality of the entire lower gastrointestinal tract. It may also extend to the upper gastrointestinal tract because it has been shown that patients who fulfil the clinical criteria given above for ISTC have evidence of delayed gastric [14,15] and gallbladder [16] (Figure 13.2) emptying with prolonged

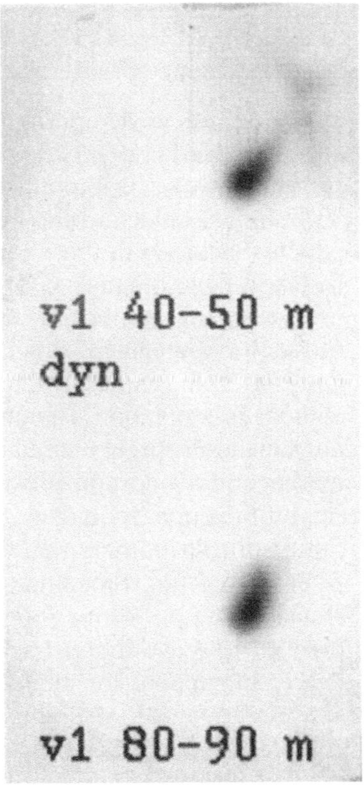

FIGURE 13.2. Cholecystokinin provacation test demonstrating delayed gallbladder emptying.

small-bowel transit [17,18]. It is unknown, however, whether this a manifestation of a pan-gastrointestinal disorder or whether upper gastrointestinal delay is secondary to colonic inertia because it has been shown that inflation of a balloon in the rectum of humans and animals inhibits the entire gastrointestinal tract [19,20]. In an attempt to answer this question, gastric emptying has been measured before and at 1 year after total colectomy and ileorectal anastomosis for ISTC [21]. Although gastric emptying improved in the majority of patients, it returned to normal in only one half of those studied, suggesting that the extent of the abnormality is variable [10]. Unfortunately, the severity of the gastric-emptying abnormality prior to surgery did not predict the functional outcome afterwards.

It should be noted that idiopathic slow-transit constipation as described above is an uncommon condition occurring in <5% of patients referred to Glasgow Royal Infirmary for consideration of surgery for constipation. In reports from the Cleveland Clinic and Sweden the corresponding figures for patients fulfilling the criteria of delayed colonic markers and normal evacuation as assessed by cinedefaecography or electromyography [22] were 13% and 7%, respectively. The authors have not found anorectal manometry, electrophysiology, or balloon evacuation studies helpful in this group of patients when making a decision as to whether these patients should have surgery.

2.1.1.1. Surgery

The most effective operation for idiopathic slow-transit constipation is colectomy and ileo–rectal or ileo–sigmoid anastomosis. The outcome after surgery, however, is unpredictable with reported success rates varying from 30%–100%, reflecting the clinical and physiological heterogeneity of the patients included in these reports. Despite this, some firm conclusions can be made. Fewer than 50% of patients who have a colectomy performed on the basis of clinical criteria alone, without the use of investigations, have a satisfactory outcome [3,23]. Further, failure after surgery often results in an ileostomy. Consequently, patients should never be subjected to surgery without investigation. In contrast, there have been several reports of the outcome after surgery based upon the selection criteria of a delay in colonic markers and a normal proctogram. These show consistently high success rates for the operation of over 90% [22,24–26]. Patients must be clearly consented prior to surgery that there is a risk of either continuing constipation or intractable diarrhoea that may in turn lead to the need for a permanent stoma. When performing the colectomy in these patients it is the authors' practice to leave a short segment of sigmoid colon, preferring to risk a degree of residual constipation rather than incapacitating diarrhoea.

In an attempt to overcome the risk of intractable diarrhoea, segmental colonic resection has been advocated [27,28] and when it is based on scintigraphic transit studies then the outcome may be comparable to total colectomy [29]. Crucially, scintigraphic transit studies have suggested that there may be different patterns of segmental slow-transit constipation with the abnormality restricted to either the right colon or the distal large bowel [30] (Figure 13.3). This later abnormality has been especially identified in those patients who clearly attribute the onset of symptoms to childbirth or hysterectomy. Patients complaining of posthysterectomy constipation have been shown to have abnormal colonic motility with mass inaction extending from the splenic flexure to the rectum [31], leading to the suggestion that this abnormality is related to an iatrogenic autonomic-nerve injury during pelvic dissection. A similar abnormality has been shown in patients with postchildbirth constipation [14,32,33] both on colonic manometry and bisacodyl-stimulated intraluminal scintigraphy [34]. The difference in the pathophysiology between idiopathic slow-transit and postchildbirth/hysterectomy constipation is further emphasized by the observation that gastric emptying is normal in postchildbirth/hysterectomy constipation and abnormal in patients with idiopathic constipation [35]. This raises the possibility that hindgut resection could remove their constipation by removing all colon from splenic flexure to the anal canal. The disadvantage to such a management plan were it to fail is that the patient has lost the option of having an ileal pouch.

In 1990, Malone introduced the alternative surgical approach of antegrade colonic irrigation using an appendicostomy [36]. The Malone antegrade continent enema (MACE) has since proved to be safe and effective in children suffering from constipation secondary to spina bifida or ano–rectal malformations [37]. More recently, it has been used to treat a small number of adult patients with neurogenic colorectal dysfunction and chronic idiopathic constipation [38,39]. Further, using a novel scintigraphic

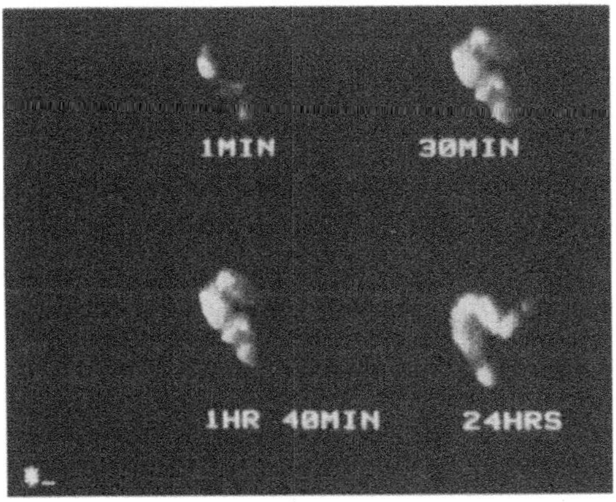

FIGURE 13.3. Radiolabeled scintigraphy scan demonstrating delay at splenic flexure after 24 hours. In normal subjects this would be in the rectum.

technique it has been shown to be effective [40] in clearing the bowel. This technique may have an increasingly important role in the future.

2.1.2. Normal Colonic Transit Study and an Abnormal Proctogram

Videoproctography is the best readily available investigation for identifying abnormalities of evacuation [41]. Newer techniques include dynamic magnetic resonance proctography [42], dynamic anal endosonography [43], and scintigraphic proctography but these have either been studied in only small numbers of patients or remain research tools. Approximately 20%–30% of patients presenting to a specialist clinic with constipation will have the combination of an abnormal proctogram and a normal colonic transit study. Consequently, this is a relatively common clinical problem that requires a clear management strategy. Proctographic abnormalities may be broadly defined as anatomical or functional. The former include evidence of rectocoele, internal prolapse, perineal descent, and atypical herniations including enterocoele and levator ani defects [44]. The principle functional defect is that of anismus or puborectalis paradox.

Anatomical abnormalities of the anorectum are predominantly, although not exclusively, found in female patients in middle and later life. Symptoms include difficulty in evacuation, a sensation of incomplete evacuation, or a sensation of weight in the perineum that initially may be described as pain. Patients may digitally aid defaecation by supporting the posterior wall of the vaginal or by pushing against the buttock behind the anus. Some may digitally evacuate the bowel. Patients also often respond positively to the suggestion that the energy they produce in pushing to achieve evacuation is strangely lost, resulting in a feeling of exhaustion. On occasions patients may be aware of prolapse of either the bowel or the vagina. Frequently patients have already had urological and gynaecological operations including hysterectomy or vaginal-wall and bladder-neck repairs. It is wise to involve these specialists [45] at an early stage and several centres now have joint pelvic-floor clinics involving all 3 disciplines. It is of note that in some countries there is emerging the entity of the pelvic-floor specialist.

In broad terms, these anatomical abnormalities are due to wear and tear and are predominantly secondary to childbirth. It has been shown that even an apparently normal vaginal delivery results in neuropathy of the pudendal nerve with reduced tone in both the external anal sphincter and puborectalis muscles [46,47]. Multiple pregnancies and complicated deliveries involving the use of forceps or other interventions produce an even greater degree of injury. The levator ani muscle may be similarly damaged by either a traction or ischaemic injury to the nerves arising from S2,S3 which course over the ventral surface of the posterior aspect of the muscle, although it should be noted that the exact nerve supply to the levator muscle remains uncertain. It is widely accepted that this is the mechanism that leads to the development of the appearances of perineal descent syndrome

(Figure 13.4) and eventually those of idiopathic faecal incontinence. Many of these features are also present in patients with rectal prolapse although the sequence of events that leads to the development of a prolapse is uncertain. Neuropathy can certainly rapidly lead to a rectal prolapse as evidenced by reports of a rectal prolapse developing within days of spinal surgery that involved transection of the cord. With regard to the present discussion, it is unknown whether a rectal prolapse always begins as an intussusception and

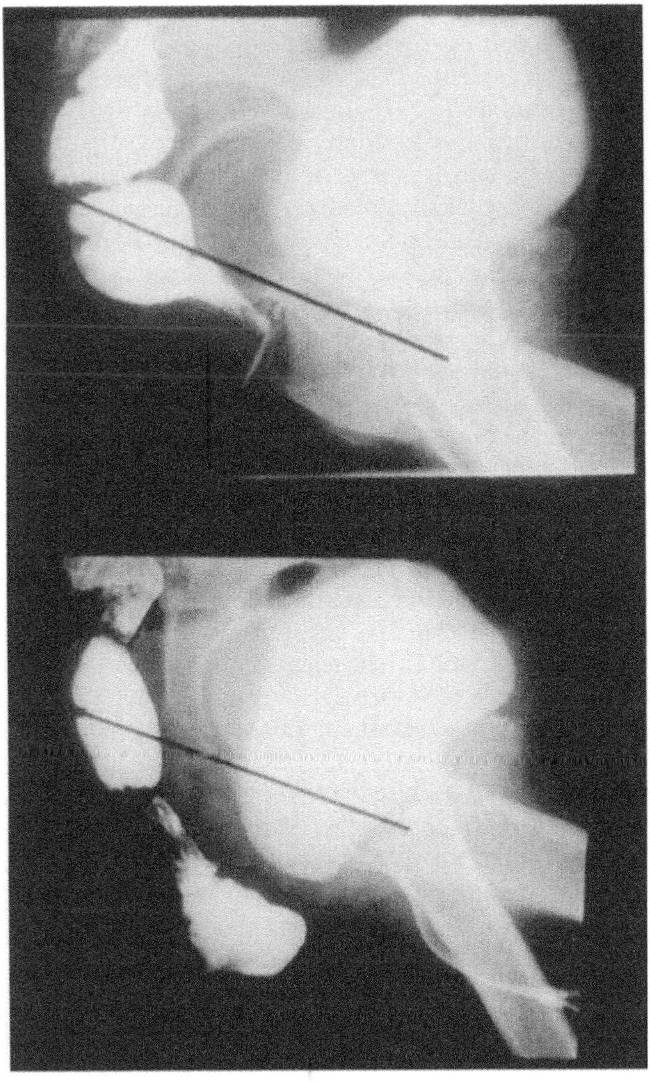

FIGURE 13.4. Combined proctogram and cystogram that demonstrates perineal descent, rectocele, and posterior rotation of the urinary bladder.

if it does, then over what time scale. This has important implications with regard to the selection of patients for surgery who have intussusception on proctography. The management of the common abnormalities found on proctography are discussed below.

2.1.2.1. Intussusception/Internal Prolapse

Patients with symptoms of obstructed defaecation frequently have evidence of infolding of the rectum on videoproctography [48,49] (Figure 13.5). This appearance is known as internal prolapse or midrectal intussusception. Over quarter of a century ago it was recognised that some patients with this feature respond to surgery while others are either unhelped or made worse [50]. For example, in 1975, Ihre and Seligson observed that patients with symptoms of prolapse and incontinence had a good result after rectopexy but the outcome was poor if patients complained of obstructed symptoms or had a solitary rectal ulcer. Several surgical groups have since reported similar results leading to a reappraisal of the indications for surgery in this condition [51–53]. Indeed, in a recent comparative study it has been suggested that biofeedback should be used as the initial treatment for most patients with a rectal intussusception [54]. The reason for this change in opinion with regard to management is directly related to a better understanding of the range of normal appearances on videoproctograms. When infolding of the rectum was initially identified it was assumed to be the principal cause of symptoms in patients with obstructed defaecation. It is now recognized that a small degree of rectal infolding may be present in normal subjects. Further, when it occurs in patients with symptoms of obstructed defaecation it is probably secondary to recurrent straining rather than the primary abnormality. The situation is further complicated by the fact that the infolding may involve only mucosa or include the full thickness of the bowel wall. In either case, the size of the intussusception may vary from <1 cm to a prolapse protruding at the anus. It is also now recognised that very small intussusceptions rarely proceed to overt prolapses, at least over a 10-year observation period [54]. Despite this, an overt rectal prolapse must have a stage when it is a midrectal prolapse/intussusception which does not reach the anal verge. The clinical picture is further complicated by the fact that even overt prolapses may be evident only when the patient strains and can be difficult to diagnose. In conclusion, there are probably 2 distinct entities: mucosal infolding and small full-thickness intussusceptions that are secondary to obssesive straining, and large intussusceptions, which are early prolapses secondary to a pelvic-floor neuropathy.

In order to distinguish these 2 entities, the authors use the following strategy: all patients in whom the proctogram suggests an intussusception proceed to examination under anaesthesia (EUA). An eissenhammer retractor is inserted into the anal canal and the midrectum is drawn downwards using a sponge-holding forcep. When the full thickness of rectum is easily drawn to the anal margin without tension, the patient is considered

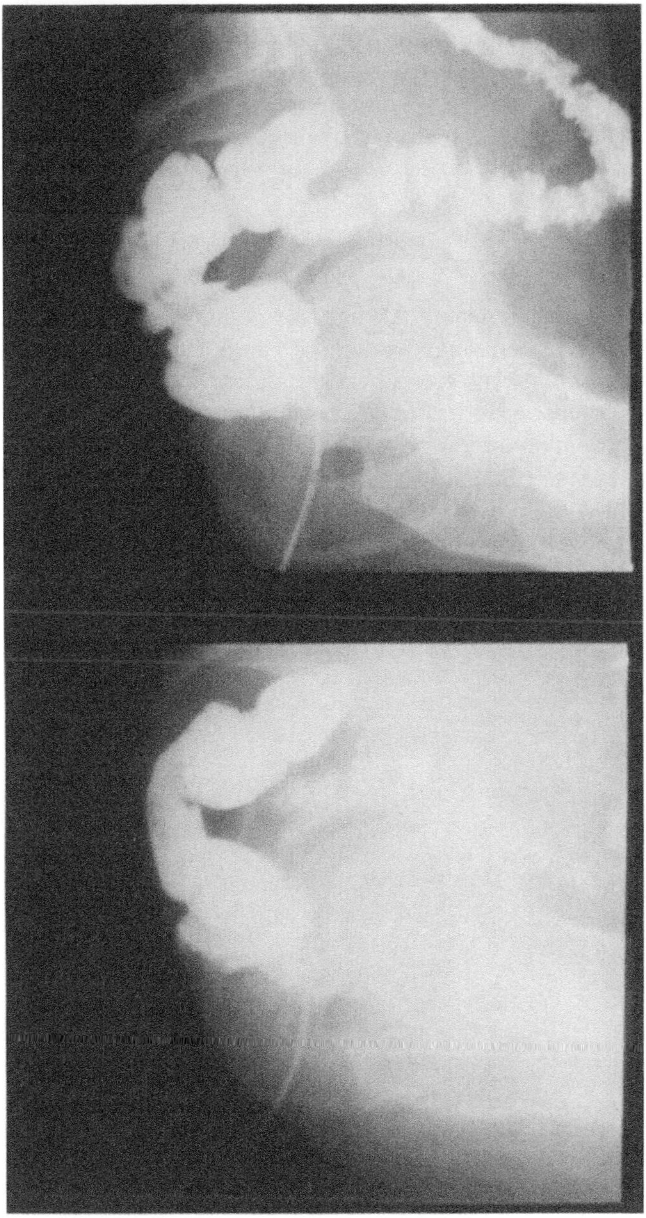

FIGURE 13.5. Defaecating proctogram identifying a midrectal intusussecption.

to have a true intussusception/prolapse. If the patients symptoms correlate with this finding (i.e., sensation of weight, feeling of prolapse) then they are offered a resection rectopexy. Examination under anaesthesia is also performed in those patients who have classical symptoms of prolapse but in whom an intussusception has not been identified on proctography. This excludes or confirms the presence of a midrectal intussusception. Patients selected in this way have a similar outcome to those who have rectopexy for overt rectal prolapse, further confirming that the 2 conditions are interrelated [55]. Those patients who have lesser degrees of intussusception or only mucosal prolapse are treated by biofeedback. This later group includes most patients with solitary a rectal ulcer unless there is evidence of a gross prolapse at EUA.

2.1.2.3. Rectocoele

Rectocoele arises from laxity of the rectovaginal septum. It should be noted that all female patients have a small physiological rectocoele on proctography. Consequently, the rectocoele should have a diameter of at least 5 cm before it is considered to be of clinical significance. In determining whether to offer a patient an operation for rectocoele, the single most important predictive factor is to obtain from the history that the patient is able to achieve evacuation by digitally supporting the posterior vaginal wall. This symptom has been shown to correlates with both the size of the defect on X-ray [56] and outcome after surgery. Proctography alone, however, has no prognostic significance regarding the outcome of surgery [57] (Figure 13.6).

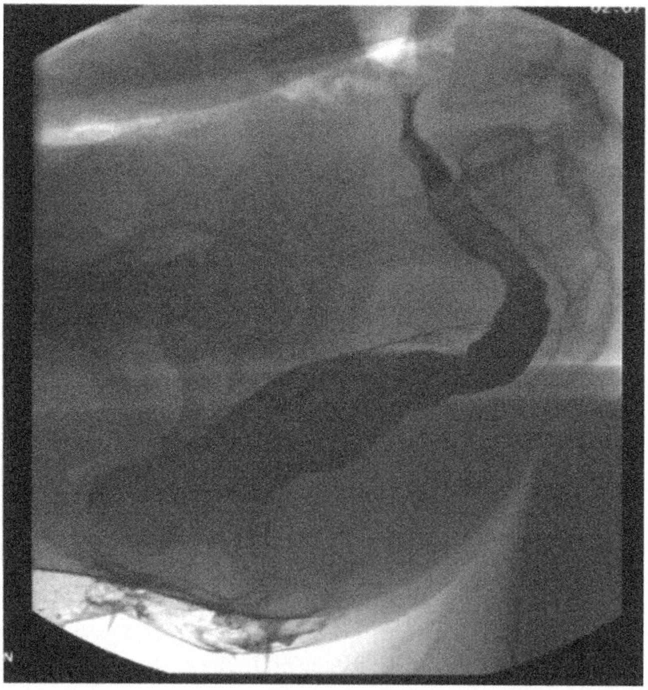

FIGURE 13.6. Defaecating protogram demonstrating a large rectocele.

Rectoceles may be repaired by the transanal, transperineal [58], or transvaginal routes. They can also be repaired using both a transanal and transvaginal approach [64] or by the using circular stapling devices [60]. There are advocates for each technique. The authors favor a modified transanal repair first described in 1968 by Sullivan et al. [61]. The patient is placed in the prone position and using an anal speculum a transverse incision is made in the rectal mucosa. The rectal-wall muscle is then plicated obliterating the rectocele. Although there are few reports of functional assessment after this type of surgery, the operation is considered to be successful in over 80% of cases [62,58]. Ho et al., however, have suggested repair be avoided in those with weak anal sphincters [63]. There are relatively few complications but care must be taken to avoid damage to the vagina, which may lead to a rectovaginal fistula. Similar results have been reported using other techniques including mesh repairs by the perineal route. Prospective randomised trials are notably lacking. Irrespective of the technique used, infrequent stool frequency has been shown to lead a poor outcome [59]. There is variable evidence regarding outcome if the patient also has anismus but this should not be considered a contraindication to surgery [64].

Rectocoele has been observed in men who have had radical prostatectomy [65], but is unknown whether transanal repair helps these patients.

2.1.2.4. Anismus

Anismus is a functional abnormality of the anorectum in which anal-canal pressure rises during attempted evacuation with closure of the sphincter mechanism and failure of evacuation. The condition is variously referred to as obstructed defaecation or pubrectalis paradox. It may be difficult to be certain of the diagnosis because voluntary contraction of the pelvic floor with closure of the anorectum is the normal response to avert the call to stool. It is not surprising for normal subjects to show evidence of puborectalis contraction during straining in the artificial and embarrassing environment of the anorectal physiology laboratory. As a result, anorectal manometry, electromyography, and balloon expulsion tests are of minimal diagnostic value due to the high false-positive rate, but these tests may be useful in monitoring treatment after the diagnosis has been made. The most reliable method for diagnosing anismus is proctography [66]. Although a delay in evacuation of 30 seconds is considered to be important [18], in the authors' experience proctography also has a high risk of producing false-positive results, especially in anxious patients who will voluntarily contract the pelvic floor and sphincter due to embarrassment. Fortunately, in these patients the true diagnosis can be easily confirmed. Those patients with voluntary anismus will empty without difficulty if given the opportunity to do so in privacy. In comparison, patients with anismus will not empty contrast material for at least 24 hours and in severe cases for several days (Figure 13.7).

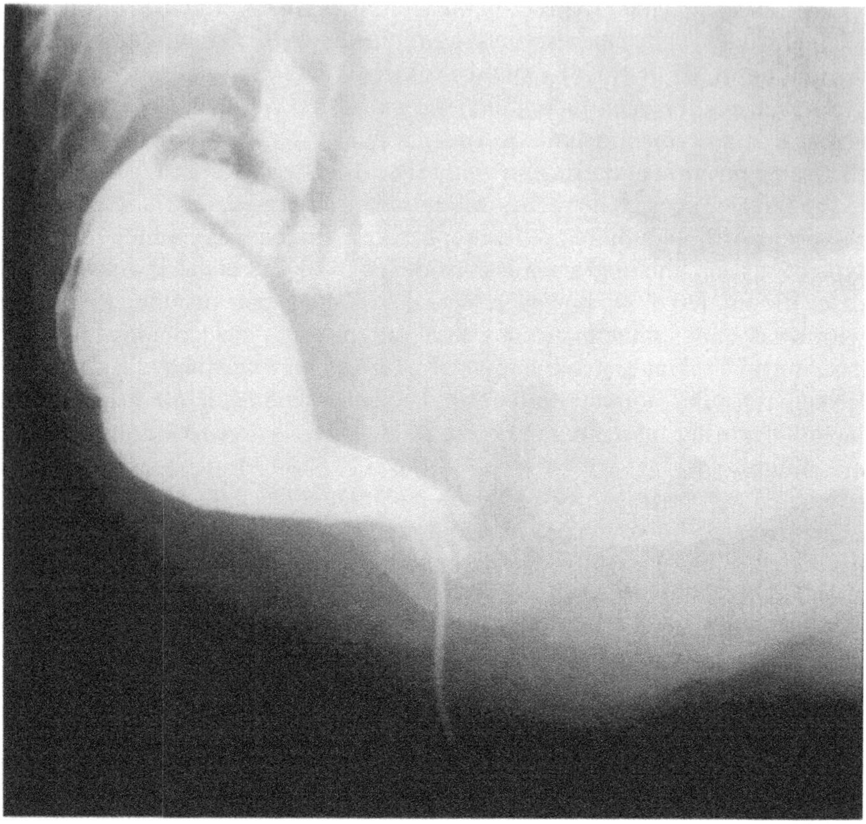

FIGURE 13.7. Defaecating proctogram that demonstrates anismus or obstructed defaecation.

The aetiology of anismus is unknown but it is usually attributed to inappropriate contraction of the puborectalis muscle despite the fact that there is relatively little evidence to support this as the primary abnormality [67]. Further, the mechanism whereby this could occur is unknown although it has been suggested that it may result from a failure of coordination between the hindgut and the anorectum [68,69]. Alternatively, it may simply be a learned event as a component of an obsessive neurotic behavioral disorder. Evidence to support a psychological aetiology may be found in the observation that anismus diagnosed by manometry was found in 97% of individuals who had been subjected to sexual abuse and in only 30% of controls subjects [70].

Surgical treatments for anismus (e.g., puborectalis muscle division) have been abandoned because they are ineffective and have a of risk incontinence. For the past decade it has been widely accepted that biofeedback is the treatment of choice for anismus [71,72] although the mode of action is uncertain. It has been suggested that biofeedback may actually modify higher centre control of defaecation [73]. Several studies have shown that the patients who gain most benefit are those who have no abnormality of the anorectum on physiology studies [74,75]. This suggests that biofeedback is probably simply a form of behavioural or relaxation therapy. Although manometry and balloon expulsion tests are of limited value in making the diagnosis, they are frequently used to monitor treatment and form the basis of biofeedback.

Recently there have been reports of attempts to produce pharmacological puborectalis paralysis using botulinin toxin [76], but the results are variable and often temporary. Prospective randomised trials are required to determine the efficacy of the technique.

2.1.2.5. Solitary Rectal Ulcer Syndrome

Solitary rectal ulcer is an uncommon condition predominantly affecting young adults who complain of tenesmus and recurrent straining. Many also digitally aid defaecation. Fiberoptic examination reveals a spectrum of macroscopic changes, usually of the anterior rectal wall, that range from reddening to ulceration. Microscopic examination from the ulcer reveals collagenous replacement of the lamina propria and thickened circular muscle. Evacuation proctography shows an obvious internal intussusception in 75%–94% of these patients [77,78]. Over one half of the patients will also have incoordination of the pelvic floor with evidence of anismus [66]. Recently, it has been shown that there is a close correlation between high-grade rectal intussusception and a thickened internal anal sphincter on anal endosonography in patients with solitary rectal ulcer syndrome [79]. It is unclear whether this thickening is a primary abnormality or secondary to the mechanical strain of the prolapsing rectum. The aetiology of solitary rectal intussusception remains uncertain; consequently the management is difficult. Patients with evidence of anismus should be treated with biofeedback in the first instance. Rectopexy may be offered to patients with gross intussusception but the results are variable [80], this may also be performed laparoscopically [81].

2.1.3. Delayed Colonic Transit Study and Abnormal Proctogram

The combination of delayed colonic transit with an abnormal proctogram is fortunately uncommon because these patients are especially difficult to assess. It is necessary to determine whether the delay in transit or the outlet obstruction is the predominant cause of the patients symptoms because it has been shown that outlet obstruction may produce secondary transit delay [82]. In animal studies the entire gastrointestinal tract was inhibited when a balloon was inflated in the rectum. It is important not to proceed directly to colectomy in these patients without first correcting the outlet abnormality. Although there are reports of a successful outcome after colectomy in the presence of anismus, the results are unpredictable perhaps because the anismus was diagnosed by balloon expulsion, which is notoriously inaccurate. It is the authors' practice to treat all these patients with biofeedback. In the event that this is successful then the transit study is repeated and if delay persists then a colectomy would be considered. The few patients who fail to respond to biofeedback and continue to have severe symptoms are offered a diagnostic temporary defunctioning colostomy.

2.1.4. Normal Colonic Transit Study and Normal Proctogram (Functional Bowel Disorder)

A surprisingly large number of patients referred for a surgical opinion have no objective evidence of constipation on colonic transit studies and have normal emptying on proctography. These patients should not be offered surgery despite the fact that they often complain of severe symptoms and may be reluctant to accept the objective evidence that gastrointestinal transit is normal. In the authors' experience, it is sometimes necessary to repeat the transit study to convince the patient that the transit is within normal limits. Patients identified in this way typically have symptoms of severe abdominal pain, urgency, and a compelling sensation of incomplete evacuation. Anorectal physiology studies show normal sphincter pressures but there is intolerance of intrarectal balloon distension with a hypersensitive rectum. In brief, these patients have a functional gastrointestinal disorder [83].

Patients with such symptoms are difficult to treat predominantly because there is a poorly understood psychological component to their illness. Antidepressants have been shown to be moderately effective [84]. In a meta-analysis of 12 randomised controlled trials of the use of antidepressants, it has been shown that it necessary to treat on average 3.2 patients to obtain symptomatic improvement in 1 [85]. Psychological treatments including cognitive and behavioural therapies and hypnosis [86] may also be helpful but they are rarely available. Although most trials suggest a positive outcome for psychological treatments, they are often methodologically flawed and as yet firm conclusions regarding efficacy cannot be made.

There is increasing interest in the complex interaction between the brain and the gastrointestinal tract in patients with irritable bowel syndrome. In experimental studies using positron emission tomography, it has been shown that cerebral blood flow is increased in response to inflation of a balloon in the rectum [87]. Of more interest however, the site of this increase within the brain differs in patients with irritable syndrome when compared with controls. Whether this difference arises from an abnormality of the sensory pathways from the gut or a primary abnormality of the brain remains unknown, but it is modified by 5-hydroxytryptamine receptor antagonists [88,89], which may in the future have therapeutic value.

3. Constipation and Megabowel

Megabowel (Figure 13.8) is an uncommon clinical condition that predominantly presents as intractable constipation in childhood or adolescence [90,91]. It may involve only the rectum or include the sigmoid and more proximal colon [92]. Occassionally the condition may be caused by ultra-short–segment Hirchsprung's disease, although this is unusual in the West, where most cases are identified in infancy. Nevertheless routine work up should include anorectal physiology studies with measurement of the anorectal inhibitory reflex which is absent in Hirchsprung's disease. Unfortunately, the reflex is also often absent in patients with idiopathic megarectum due to the failure of the rectal balloon to stimulate the receptors in the dilated rectum. Consequently, it is the authors' practice to perform a full-thickness biopsy (myotomy of the anorectal junction) in all patients presenting for consideration of surgery for megarectum/colon. Although megabowel may also be caused by Chagas disease and chronic intestinal pseudo-obstruction, more than 50% of cases are idiopathic with an intact anorectal inhibitory reflex and evidence of ganglia on full-thickness biopsy. Because the pathophysiology of these idiopathic cases is poorly understood, surgery should only be offered to the most refractory cases and then only after careful consideration.

All cases should be treated conservatively using laxatives and enemata for at least 6 months. Approximately 50% of patients will respond to this regimen, although the degree of improvement is dependent upon the extent of the disease [93]. Patients with megarectum alone do better than those with megacolon. Anorectal physiology studies in isolation have not been shown to be helpful in either selecting those patients who require surgery or the type of surgery to be performed Anal-canal resting pressures are invariably low and the anorectal inhibitory reflex is often absent even when subsequent histological examination reveals ganglia. In addition, few patients with megarectum are able to expel a balloon but known of these findings correlates with surgical outcome.

Many surgical procedures have been used to treat megarectum and megacolon including colectomy and ileorectal/ileosigmoid anastomosis [94,95], proctectomy and coloanal anastomosis [96], pull-through procedures, Duhamel operation [97], anal myomectomy, and, more recently, restorative proctectomy. The outcome after these operations is variable, with poor function leading to a high reoperation rates because of continuing severe constipation. This array of operations reflects the lack of under-

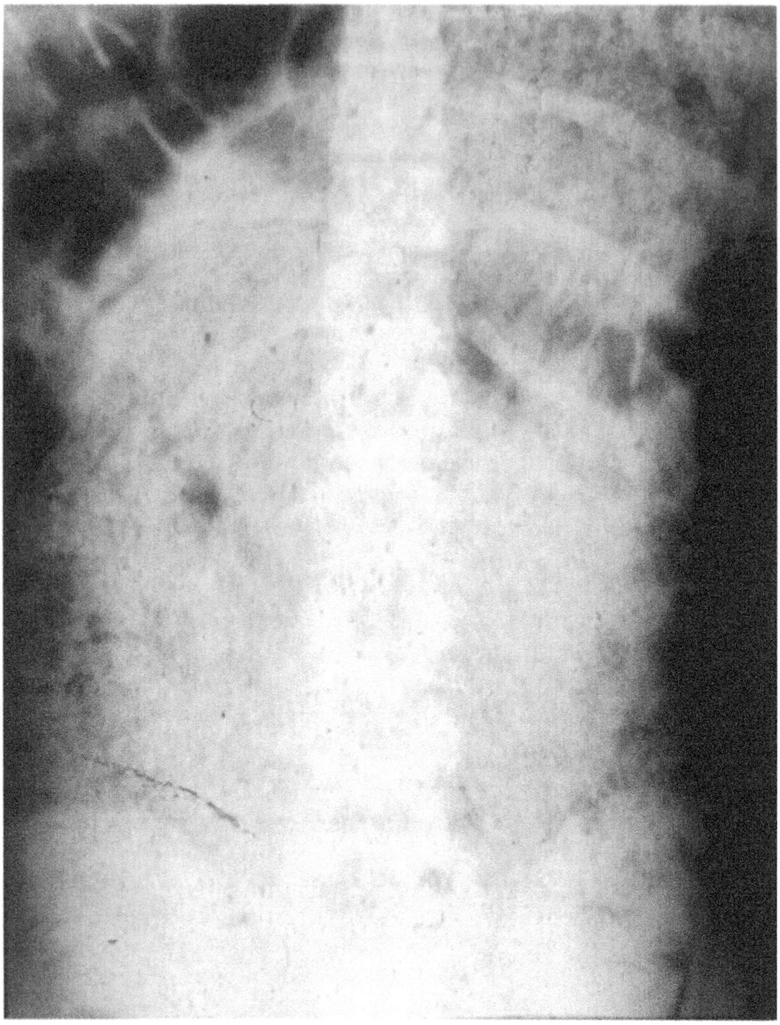

FIGURE 13.8. Faecal loading within a megacolon/megarectum.

standing of the pathophysiology of this condition. For example, it is unknown whether the abnormality is limited to the dilated segment of bowel or extends to involve the nondilated segment. In this respect clinical experience has produced contradictory results. While it has been shown that a stoma fashioned above the dilated segment of bowel works well and a stoma fashioned from dilated bowel usually fails, it is also recognised that megacolon may reoccur despite resection of the entire macroscopically dilated bowel. Despite this caveat, and in the absence of more sophisticated research tests, the author has found the formation of a stoma above the dilated segment to be a most useful way of identifying proximal bowel that has normal function (Figure 13.9).

There is increasing interest in the use of restorative proctectomy for both patients with megarectum and megacolon. The success rate has been reported to be as high as 85% although the largest series has only 14 patients. Surprisingly, despite the fact that these patients all have low anal-canal pressures prior to surgery, there are no reports of postoperative failure due to incontinence. This suggests that any sphincter weakness is a secondary rather than a primary abnormality and recovers rapidly. A review of surgical outcomes suggests that unlike patients with slow-transit constipation and a normal caliber colorectum who respond to colectomy and ileorectal anastomosis, patients with idiopathic megabowel require at least removal of the rectum. An alternative to restorative proctectomy is resection of the dilated bowel with formation of a coloanal anastomosis. Although success rates of 75% have been reported reoperation, for subsequent dilation of the proximal bowel was required in many patients suggesting that the extent of the colonic abnormality is variable. To date there is no foolproof method for identifying those patients who will respond to proctectomy and coloanal anastomosis and therefore avoid a restorative proctocolectomy. Colonic physiology studies have been used as a research tools in an attempt to identify the extent of the colonic motility abnormality, thereby identifying those patients who require restorative proctocolectomy but the number of patients studied are too small to draw firm conclusions.

An algorithm is given for those patients who require surgery for megabowel in Figure 13.9. The principal surgical options are restorative proctocolectmy or proctectomy and coloanal anastomosis. In the absence of sophisticated research tests, it is the authors' practice to offer a pouch procedure to patients with any degree of megacolon. Those patients with only megarectum are offered proctectomy and coloanal anastomosis if a preliminary defunctioning colostomy above the dilated segment works well. Other groups have advocated the use of vertical reduction rectoplasty and sigmoid colectomy with a resultant improvements in clinical and physiological function of patients, but the numbers are small and the work remains to be fully evaluated [98].

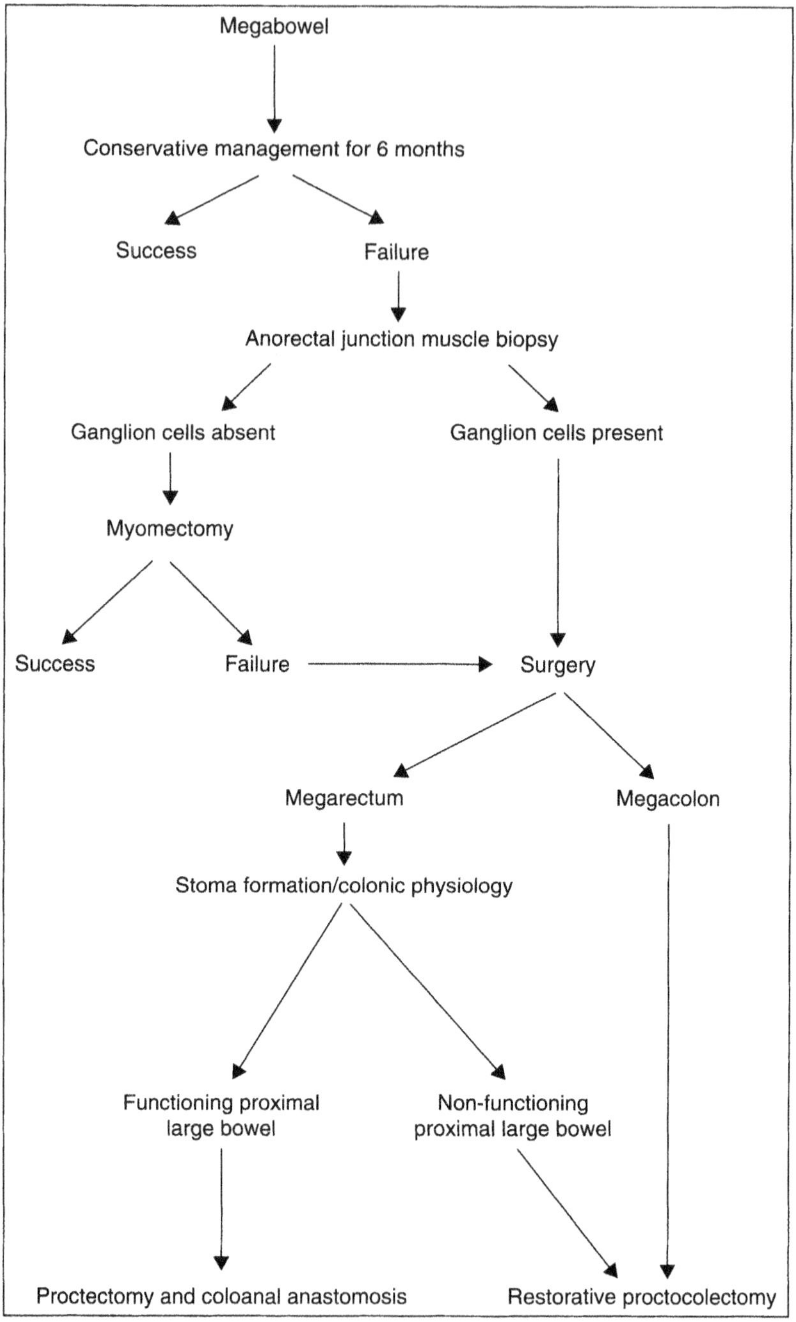

FIGURE 13.9. Strategy for the management of the megarectum and megacolon. (Suilleabhain CB, Anderson JH, McKee RF, Finlay IG. Strategy for the surgical management of patients with idiopathic megarectum and megacolon. *Br J Surg.* 2001;88:1392–1396. ©British Journal of Surgery Society Ltd. Reproduced with permission.)

References

1. Knowles CH, Eccersley AJ, Scott SM, et al. Linear discriminant analysis of symptoms in patients with chronic constipation. *Dis Colon Rectum.* 2001;43: 141–1426.
2. Roe AM, Bartolo DC, Mortensen NJ. Diagnosis and surgical management of intractable constipation. *Br J Surg.* 1986;73:854–861.
3. Platell C, Scache D, Mumme G, Stitz R. A long-term follow up of patients undergoing colectomy for chronic slow transit constipation. *Aust N Z J Surg.* 1996;66: 529.
4. Knowles CH, Scott SM, Wellmer A, et al. Sensory and autonomic neuropathy in patients with idiopathic slow transit constipation. *Br J Surg.* 1999;86:54–60.
5. Slater BJ, Varma JS, Gillespie JI. Abnormality in the contractile properties of colonic smooth muscle in idiopathic slow transit constipation. *Br J Surg.* 1997; 84:181–184.
6. McCourtney JS, Hemingway DM, Muir TC, Finlay IG. Altered small bowel pacemaker activity in idiopathic slow transit constipation. Presented at: Association of Coloproctology, 1998.
7. Hoyle CHV, Kamm MA, Leonnard-Jones JE, Burnstock G. An in vitro electrophysiological study of the colon from patients with idiopathic chronic constipation. *Clin Auton Res.* 1992;2:327–333.
8. Dolk A, Broden G, Holmstrom B, et al. Slow transit constipation. An immunohistochemical study of neuropeptide-containing nerves. *Int J Colorectal Dis.* 1990;5:181–187.
9. Faussone-Pelligrini MS, Infantimo A, Matini P, et al. Neural anomalies and normal muscle morphology at the hypomotile ileo-caecal valve. *Histol Histopathol.* 1999;14:1119–1134.
10. Krishnamurthy S, Schuffler MD, Rohrmann CA, Pope CE. Severe idiopathic constipation is associated with a dinstinctive abnormality of the colonic myenteric plexus. *Gastroenterology* 1985;88:26–34.
11. Burleigh DE. Evidence for a functional cholinergic defect in human colonic tissue resected for constipation. *J Pharm Pharmacol.* 1998;40:55–57.
12. He CL, Burgart L, Wang L, et al. Decreased interstitial cells of Cajal volume in patients with slow transit constipation. *Gastroenterology* 2000;118:14–21.
13. Lyford GL, He C-L, Soffer E, et al. Pan colonic disease in interstitial cells of Cajal in patients with slow transit constipation. *Gut* 2002;51:496–501.
14. MacDonald A, Baxter JN, Bessant RG, Gray HW, Finlay IG. Gastric emptying in patients with constipation following childbirth and due to idiopathic slow transit. *Br J Surg.* 1997;84:1141–1143.
15. Watier A, Devroede G, Duranceau A, et al. Constipation with colonic inertia. A manifestation of systemic disease? *Dig Dis Sci.* 1983;28:1025–1033.
16. Hemingway D, Neilly JB, Finlay IG. Biliary dyskinesia in idiopathic slow transit constipation. *Dis Colon Rectum.* 1996;39:1303–1307.
17. Van der Sijp JR, Kamm MA, Nightingale JMD, et al. Disturbed gastric and small bowel transit in severe idiopathic constipation. *Dig Dis Sci.* 1993;38:837–844.
18. Altomare DF, Portincasa P, Rinaldi M, et al. Slow-transit constipation: solitary symptom of a systemic gastrointestinal disease. *Dis Colon Rectum.* 1999;42: 231–240.

19. Youle MS, Read NW. Effects of painless rectal distension on gastrointestinal transit of a solid meal. *Dig Dis Sci.* 1984;29:902–906.
20. Warren SJ, Lord MG, Rogers J, Williams NS. Neral mediation of the human rectocolonic inhibitory reflex [abstract]. *Gut* 1994;35(suppl 5):S31.
21. Hemingway DM, Finlay IG. Effect of colectomy on gastric emptying in idiopathic slow transit constipation. *Br J Surg.* 2000;87:1193–1196.
22. Piccirillo MF, Reissman P, Wexner SD. Colectomy as treatment for constipation in selected patients. *Br J Surg.* 1995;82:898–901.
23. Walsh PV, Peebles-Brown DA, Watkinson G. Colectomy for slow transit constipation. *Ann Roy Coll Surg Engl.* 1987;69:71–75.
24. Pemberton JH, Rath DM, Ilstrup DM. Evaluation and surgical treatment of severe chronic constipation. *Ann Surg.* 1991;214:403–411.
25. Nyam DC, Pemberton JH, Ilstrup DM, Rath DM. Long term results of surgery for chronic constipation. *Dis Colon Rectum.* 1997;40:279.
26. Sunderland GT, Poon FW, Lauder J, Fnlay IG. Videoproctography in selecting patients with constipation for colectomy. *Dis Colon Rectum.* 1992;35:235–237.
27. De Graaf EJR, Gilberts EC, Schouten WR. Role of segmental colonic transit time studies to select patients with slow transit constipation for partial left sided or sub total colectomy. *Br J Surg.* 1996;83:648–651.
28. You YT, Wang JY, Changchien CR, et al. Segmental colectomy in the management of colonic inertia. *Am Surg.* 1998;64:775–777.
29. Lundin E, Karlbom L, Pahlman L, Graf W. Outcome of segmental colonic resection for slow transit constipation. *Br J Surg.* 2002;89:1270–1274.
30. Roberts JP, Newell MS, Deeks JJ, et al. DTPA scintigraphy assessment of colonic transit in constipated patients. *Dig Dis Sci.* 1993;38:1032–1039.
31. Smith AN, Varma JS, Binnie NR, Papachrysostomou M. Disordered colorectal motility in intractable constipation following hysterectomy. *Br J Surg.* 1990; 77:1361–1365.
32. MacDonald A, Carter K, Baxter JN, Wright R, Finlay IG. Mass inaction: the hallmark of constipation after childbirth. *Br J Surg.* 1994;81:750.
33. MacDonald A. *Constipation after Childbirth and Hysterectomy* [MD thesis]. Glascow: University of Glasgow; 1998.
34. Bassotti G, Chiaroni G, Germani U, et al. Endoluminal instillation of bisocodyl in patients with severe constipation. *Digestion* 1999;60:69–73.
35. MacDonald A, Baxter JN, Bessent RG, Gray HW, Finlay IG. Gastric emptying in patients with constipation following childbirth and due to idiopathic slow transit. *Br J Surg.* 1997;84:1141–1143.
36. Malone PS, Ransley PG, Kiely EM. Preliminary report: the antegrade continence enema. *Lancet* 1990;336:1217–1218.
37. Curry JI, Osborne A, Malone PS. The MACE procedure: experience in the United Kingdom. *J Pediatr Surg.* 1999;34:338–340.
38. Christensen P, Kvitzau B, Krogh K, Buntzen S, Laurberg S. Neurogenic colorectal dysfunction. *Spinal Cord.* 2000;38:255–261.
39. Krogh K, Laurberg S. Malone antegrade continence enema for faecal incontinence and constipation in adults. 1998;85:974–977.
40. Christensen P, Olsen N, Krogh K, Laurberg S. Scintigraphic assessment of antegrade colonic irrigation through an appendicostomy or a neoappendicostomy. *Br J Surg.* 2002;89:1275–1280.

41. Bartram C. Radiological evaluation of anorectal disorders. *Gastroenterol Clin North Am.* 2001;30:55–75.
42. Rentsch M, Paetzel C, Lenhart M, et al. Dynamic magnetic resonance imaging defecography. *Dis Colon Rectum.* 2001;44:999–1007.
43. Barthet M, Portier F, Heyries L, et al. Dynamic anal endosonography may challenge defecography. *Endoscopy* 2000;32:300–305.
44. Kelvin FM, Maglinte DD, Benson JT. Evacuation proctography: an aid to the investigation of pelvic floor disorders. *Obstet Gynaecol.* 1994;83:307–314.
45. Poon FW, Lauder JC, Finlay IG. Perineal herniation. *Clin Radiol.* 1993;47: 49–51.
46. Snooks SJ, Setchell M, Swash M, Henry MM. Injury to innervation of pelvic floor sphincter musculature in childbirth. *Lancet* 1984;2:546–550.
47. Snooks SJ, Swash M, Mathers SE, Henry MM. Effect of vaginal delivery on the pelvic floor: a 5 year follow up. *Br J Surg.* 1990;159:112.
48. Johansson C, Ihre T, Ahlback SO. Disturbances in the defaecation mechanisms with special reference to intussusception. *Dis Colon Rectum.* 1985;28:920–924.
49. Bartolo DC, Roe AM, Virjee J, et al. Evacuation proctography in obstructed defeacation and rectal intussusception. *Br J Surg.* 1985;72:S111–S1116.
50. Ihre T, Seligson U. Intussusception of the rectum-internal procidentia: results and treatment in 90 patients. *Dis Colon Rectum.* 18:391–396.
51. Christiansen J, Hesselfeldt P, Sorensen M. Treatment of internal rectal intussusception in patients with chronic constipation. *Scand J Gastroenterol.* 1995;30: 470–472.
52. McCue JL, Thomson JP. Rectopexy for internal rectal intussusception. *Br J Surg.* 1990;77:632–634.
53. Christiansen J, Zhu BW, Rasmussen OO, et al. Internal intussusception: results of surgical repair. *Dis Colon Rectum.* 1992;35:1026–1028.
54. Choi JS, Hwang YH, Salum M, et al. Outcome and management of patients with large rectoanal intussusceptions. *Am J Gastroenterol.* 2001;96:740–744.
55. Brown AJ, MCKee RF, Anderson JH, Finlay IG. Outcome following surgery for overt and occult rectal prolapse. Submitted.
56. Halligan S, Bartram C. Is digitation associated with proctopraphic abnormality. *Int J Colorectal Dis.* 1996;11:167–171.
57. Van Dam JH, Ginai AZ, Gosselink MJ, et al. Role of defecography in predicting clinical outcome of rectocele repair. *Dis Colon Rectum.* 1997;40:1–7.
58. Lehur PA, Bruley D, Varannes S, et al. Disabling rectocele: rectal plication by perineal approach. *Chirurgie* 1992;118:516–520.
59. Van Dam JH, Hop WC, Schouten WR. Analysis of patients with poor outcome of rectocele repair. *Dis Colon Rectum.* 2000;43:1556–1560.
60. Altomare DF, Rinaldi M, Veglia A, Petrolino M, De Fazio M, Sallustio P. Combined perineal and endorectal repair of rectocele by circular stapler: a novel surgical technique. *Dis Colon Rectum.* 2002;45:1549–1552.
61. Sullivan ES, Leaverton GH, Hardwick CE. Transrectal perineal repair: an adjunct to improved function after anorectal surgery. *Dis Colon Rectum.* 1968; 11:106–114.
62. Tjanda JJ, Ooi BS, Tang CL, et al. Trans anal repair of rectocele corrects obstructed defecation if it is not associated with anismus. *Dis Colon Rectum.* 1999;42:1544–1550.

63. Ho YH, Ang M, Nyam D, Tan M, Seow-Choen F. Trans anal approach to rectocele repair may compromise anal sphincter pressures. *Dis Colon Rectum.* 1998; 41:354–358.
64. Van Dam JH, Schouten WR, Ginai AZ, et al. Impact of anismus on the clinical outcome of rectocele repair. *Int J Colorectal Dis.* 1996;11:238–242.
65. Chen HH, Iroatulam A, Alabaz O, et al. Association of defecography and physiologic findings in male patients with rectocoele. *Tech Coloproctol.* 2001;5: 157–161.
66. Halligan S, Malouf A, Bartram C, et al. Predictive value of impaired evacuation at proctography in diagnosing anismus. *Am J Roentgenol.* 2001;177:633–636.
67. Lubowski DZ, King DW, Finlay IG. Electromyography of the pubococcygeus muscles in patients with obstructed defaecation. *Int J Colorectal Dis.* 1992;7: 184–187.
68. Lubowski DZ, King DW. Obstructed defecation:current status of pathophysiology and management. *Aust N Z J Surg.* 1995;65:87–92.
69. Jones PN, Lubowski DZ, Swash M, Henry MM. Is paradoxical contraction of puborectalis muscle of functional importance. *Dis Colon Rectum.* 1987;30: 667–670.
70. Leroi AM, Berkelmans I, Denis P, et al. Anismus as a marker of sexual abuse. *Dig Dis Sci.* 1995;40:1411–1416.
71. Duthie GS, Bartolo DC. Anismus: the cause of constipation. *World J Surg.* 1992; 16:831–835.
72. Lestar B, Penninck F, Kerremans R. Biofeedback defaecation training for anismus. *Int J Colorectal Dis.* 1991;6:202–207.
73. Papachrysostomsu M, Smith AN. Effects of biofeedback on obstructive defaecation. *Gut* 1994;35:252–256.
74. Mckee RF, Finlay IG. Biofeedback in outlet obstruction constipation. *Br J Surg.* 1999;86.
75. Siproudhis L, Dautrene S, Ropert A, et al. Anismus and biofeedback: Who benefits? *Eur J Gastroenterol Hepatol.* 1995;7:547–552.
76. Ron Y, Avni Y, Lukovetski A, et al. Botulinism toxin in therapy for anismus. *Dis Colon Rectum.* 44:1821–1826.
77. Halligan S, Nicholls RJ, Bartram CI. Evacuation proctography in patients with solitary rectal ulcer syndrome: anatomic abnormalities and frequency of impaired emptying and prolapse. *Am J Roentgenol.* 1995;164:91–95.
78. Womack NR, Williams NS, Holmfield JH, Morrison JF. Pressure and prolapse-the cause of solitary rectal ulceration. *Gut* 1987;28:1228–1233.
79. Marshall M, Halligan S, Fotheringham T, Bartram C, Nicholls RJ. Predictive value of internal anal sphincter thickness for diagnosis of rectal intussusception in patients with solitary rectal ulcer syndrome. *Br J Surg.* 2002;89:1281–1285.
80. Halligan S, Nicholls RJ, Bartram CI. Proctographic changes after rectopexy for solitary rectal ulcer syndrome and preoperative predictive factors for a successful outcome. *Br J Surg.* 1995;82:314–317.
81. Stephenson A, Lumley J, Stitz R. Lap-rectopexy for solitary rectal ulcer syndrome [abstract]. *Tripartite* 2002.
82. Karlbom U, Pahlman L, Nilsson S, Graf W. Relationship between defecographic findings, rectal emptying and colonic transit time in constipated patients. *Gut* 1995;36:907–912.
83. Guthrie E, Thompson D. Abdominal pain and functional gastrointestinal disorders. *BMJ.* 2002;325:701–703.

84. Jailwala J, Imperiale TF, Kroenke K. Pharmacological treatment of irritable bowel syndrome: a systematic review of randomised controlled trials. *Ann Intern Med.* 2000;133:135–147.
85. Jackson J, O'Malley PG, Tomkins G, et al. Treatment of functional gastrointestinal disorders with antidepressent medications: a meta-analysis. *Am J Med.* 2000;108:65–72.
86. Talley NJ, Owen BKO, Boyce P, Paterson K. Psychological treatments for irritable bowel syndrome: a critique of controlled treatments trials. *Am J Gastroenterol.* 1996;91:277–286.
87. Silverman DHS, Munakata JA, Ennes H, et al. Regional cerebral activity in normal and pathological perception of visceral pain. *Gastroenterology* 1997; 112:64–72.
88. Mayer EA, Berman S, Derbyshire SWG, et al. The effect of the 5-HT receptor antagonist alosetron on brain responses to visceral stimulation in irritable bowel syndrome patients. *Aliment Pharmacol Ther.* 2002;16:1357–1366.
89. Berman SM, Chang L, Suyenobu B, et al. Condition specific deactivation of brain regions by 5-HT receptor antagonist alosetron. *Gastroenterology* 2002; 123:969–977.
90. Gattuso JM, Kamm MA. Review article: the management of constipation in adults. *Aliment Pharmacol Ther.* 1993;7:487–500.
91. Gattuso JM, Kamm MA, Morris G, Britton KE. Gastrointestinal transit in patients with idiopathic megarectum. *Dis Colon Rectum.* 1996;39:1044–1050.
92. Pfeifer J, Agachan F, Wexner SD. Surgery for constipation: a review. *Dis Colon Rectum.* 1996;39:444–460.
93. Keighley MR. Megacolon and megarectum. In: Keighley MR, Williams NS, eds. *Surgery of the Anus, Rectum and Colon.* London: WB Saunders; 1993:658–673.
94. Lane RH, Todd IP. Idiopathic megacolon: a review of 42 patients. *Br J Surg.* 1997;64:307–310.
95. Belliveau P, Goldberg SM, Rothenberger DA, Nivatvongs S. Idiopathic acquired megacolon: the value of a subtotal colectomy. *Dis Colon Rectum.* 1982;25: 118–121.
96. McCready RA, Beart RW. The surgical treatment of incapacitating constipation associated with idiopathic megacolon. *Mayo Clin Proc.* 1979;54:779–783.
97. Stabile G, Kamm MA, Hawley PR, Lennard-Jones JE. Results of the Duhamel operation in the treatment of idiopathic megarectun and megacolon. *Br J Surg.* 1991:78:661–663.
98. Williams NS, Fajobi OA, Lunniss PJ, Scott SM, Eccersley AJ, Ogunbiyi OA. Vertical reduction rectoplasty: a new treatment for idiopathic megarectum. *Br J Surg.* 2000;8787:1203–1208.

Index

GPSR Compliance

The European Union's (EU) General Product Safety Regulation (GPSR) is a set of rules that requires consumer products to be safe and our obligations to ensure this.

If you have any concerns about our products, you can contact us on ProductSafety@springernature.com

In case Publisher is established outside the EU, the EU authorized representative is:

Springer Nature Customer Service Center GmbH
Europaplatz 3
69115 Heidelberg, Germany

Batch number: 10755090

Printed by Printforce, the Netherlands